The Last Four Books Of Moses...

- Reveals wisdom that's been lost for

- Unveils the new messages of Moses given to us for our present time.

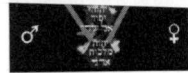

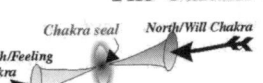

- Uncovers secrets of the Bible not meant to be exposed until now.

- Explains how and why we must move beyond the Law of Moses to the next phase in service of God's Will.

- Teaches you to become one with the Will of God as Moses was.

- Shows how to overcome anything that torments and limits you from being who you were created to be.

- Discusses how the auric field and the chakras function in our present reality of duality compared with how they function in The Garden of Eden.

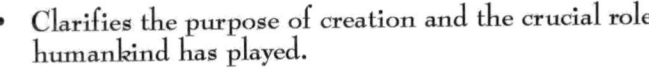

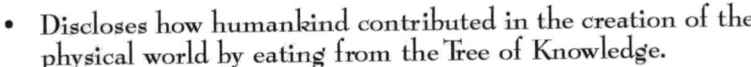

- Clarifies the purpose of creation and the crucial role humankind has played.

- Discloses how humankind contributed in the creation of the physical world by eating from the Tree of Knowledge.

- Shows that the Garden of Eden is a state of being that we are approaching.

- Demonstrates how to let go of Free Will and how your life is freed from all fear and illness when you do so.

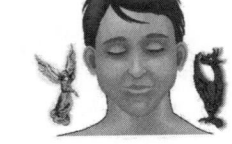

An angel in one ear. A devil in the other.

- Divulges how to cross the threshold between duality and oneness that stands between you and everlasting joy and peace.

- Illuminates the truth about Creation, Noah's Ark, Atlantis, and the Garden of Eden.

You can . . .

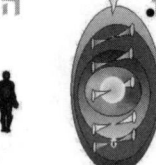

ה

- Dispel the fears associated with letting go of ALL control.

- Understand how you can bring about the Return to Eden and the Messianic Age.

The Four Worlds of the Kabbalah

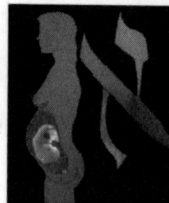

- Harness the power of female energy, bring balance between the male and female within you, and come to peace with yourself and your love relationships.

The Oneness of the Child within the Wom...

- Learn many neologisms depicting new concepts such as allowishing, Ganallisone, Frmee Will, Nabulous, and many Hebrew terms.

- Understand how the human brain creates a reality that is a reverse/mirror image illusion of the way things truly are.

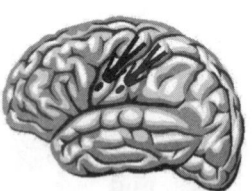

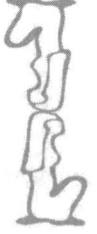

. . . And it's filled with colorful pictures to provide you with a fuller understanding of the concepts of the book.

is nothing less than miraculous. Within only a few days of working with the circles, THE LIVES OF PEOPLE WILL BE VASTLY CHANGED FOR THE BETTER."

—Mathias B. Freese, author, *i*

"Something wonderful has happened! The book that we've all been waiting 4,000 years for. THOSE THAT ARE READY WILL FIND WONDER AND AWE."

— Walter E. Williams, author,
Love Without Limit, A Personal Journey to the Heart of God

"EARTH SHAKING! He has made this total skeptic into a believer. Moshe Daniel explains how to be faithful and true to God without resorting to dogma and without compromising one's own sense of personal freedom. I have finally found what I have been looking for."

— Billie Marie Zal, author, *The Fabric of our Lives*

"IMPRESSIVE. INSPIRED. INSIGHTFUL. Truly life-changing."

— Rev. Basil Sharp, author, *The Adventure of Being Human*

"The book and Web site are among the most beautiful things I have ever discovered."

—Gary Anderson, Syndicated Columnist

"A GROUND-BREAKING APPROACH to dealing with the social ills that we have had little success in healing. THE BOOK IS EXCEL-LENT—a cornerstone for the religious, a buttress for the unchurched, and a map to the Promised Land for those living without direction or purpose."

—Walter Williams, author, *Love Without Limits*

"A prescription for life which addresses the real problems facing humanity, not only the symptoms. A GORGEOUS MESSAGE FOR OUR MODERN CIVILIZATION."

— Dr. Glenda Gnade, author,
Return to Paradise in New Heights of Glory

THE LAST FOUR BOOKS OF MOSES©

Healing the Five—Completing the Nine

Book I

The Letting Go of Free Will

Moshe Daniel Block, N.D.

משה דניאל

Collective Co-op Publishing
5122 Cote des Neiges
P.O. Box 49573
Montreal, Quebec
Canada H3T 2A5
http://www.collectivecoop.com
publishing@collectivecoop.com

Copyright © 2004 by Moshe Daniel Block, ND
moshedaniel@thelastfourbooks.com
http://www.thelastfourbooks.com

ISBN 0-9731406-3-1 (Softcover)

Table of Contents

Meditations/Exercises of Book I

This book is dedicated to
my mother, whose golden nature
of giving, caring, and making people
feel good about themselves has taught
me all the greatest lessons of Kabbalah.

PREFACE

Many years ago, when I was visiting Israel, I became aware of the great potential of the Jewish people, the essence of Judaism and the reason why it was created. I also saw the imbalance that existed in the country, which was divided between extremes of religious dogma and the rejection of spirituality. In my heart, I knew that the Jewish people had to realign themselves with their highest calling, the essence of Judaism and the reason why it was created many thousands of years ago-to heal the World. I felt in my soul a great wish to help the Jewish people understand and achieve their highest calling, so that we could begin the phase of healing the World in a movement as a people. I experienced the most intense and wonderful surging of joy when I discovered this aspect of my soul and understood my life's purpose. It was then that I began to receive new tools and messages, and understand the plan that would help lead to the liberation of the world and the release of all people into abundance and the collective consciousness of love.

In bringing these new insights (which are really the old insights—revealed), it is necessary to challenge some ancient beliefs, both Jewish and global—to make room for all aspects of Freedom. Through the process of receiving the information for this book, I learned and grew so much. All the knowledge that is shared can be just as beneficial for you as it is for me.

The fact that these messages are now available is a sign that we are entering a new era; one yearned for throughout millennia. This is Kabbalah for this day and age and we are now ready to move on to the next phase of our relationship with God, carrying out our service to the planet, bringing peace to all people and the experience of the divine force that unites all of creation.

The essence of Judaism is the same as the essence of other Religions and shared amongst many people, especially those who are healers and

"Light workers," so this book is not only for Jewish people, but for all people interested in healing themselves and others, making the world a better place, and creating Heaven on Earth. Therefore, regardless of what faith you follow, you will find that this book contains universal truths to help you heal yourself, understand reality and the purpose behind creation, and inspire you to be yourself. You will also see that all people are welcome to help carry out the plan of healing the world.

This book is for the secular and religious. It is for secular people who have shied away from their spirituality because of the rigidity of religion today. Discussions in these pages can help you reform a meaningful relationship with the divine by dispelling myths and lofty ideas about God that have made the relationship seem unattainable, so outside of yourself. This book also has messages directed toward religious Jews. Since the Torah acts as the foundation of Christianity and Islam, religious Christians and Muslims can also benefit from reading this book.

These new messages do not try to change *the essence* behind religion. That is, and always will be, the essence of who we are and what we strive for. There is such beauty and honor in the way religious Jews have followed the Torah and the Law of Moses. That dedication and commitment that Jews have had to the Torah, for over three thousand years, is truly exceptional. Yet the service to the Torah and the Law of Moses is not the highest calling of the Jew. The highest calling of the Jew, and any person, is the caretaking of the planet. Therefore, this book calls into question certain Jewish belief systems and traditions that stem not from the Will of the Creator but from human-made conceptions that became incorporated into the tradition of religion and mistakenly believed to be part of the Will of God. The discussions in these pages can help religious people see the freedom to experience God more directly through simplicity and humility of the heart.

These new messages of Moses, which are the old ones revealed, might be what you have longed to hear your entire life. They might also challenge you to look beyond the reality you have adopted as true. I ask that you keep an open mind and really take into consideration what is being said.

Although Book I deals mostly with understanding the importance of, and how to let go of Free Will, one of the purposes of the series of *The Last Four Books of Moses* is to heal the situation in the Middle East. Everyone has their eyes on Israel, the Arabs, and the Jews. Many people are being affected by the situation and a large amount of anti-Semitism is rising up towards Arabs and Jews alike. This hatred is obviously not good for either of the two brother-nations (Ishmael and Isaac, the sons of Abraham), and it is also not good for the planet, as it affects everyone. *The Last Four Books of Moses* are designed to help the Jewish people let go of the past, to find a trust and peace with their neighbors, and to fulfill their purpose toward serving the goodness of the entire planet. I hope this will then be able to help the Palestinians, who are in great need of help right now, having forgotten one of the most important things—the value of human life.

Let us all pray for the resolution of this conflict and all other conflicts in which people, all of whom are really all of the same blood, have forgotten how to love each other. Let us all walk through our lives interacting kindly with people and with a love that shows them they are accepted and special in who they are. When the Nations of Israel and Ishmael are able to embrace each other with love and acceptance, it will be an enormous marker for the return to Eden. Let us pray for peace.

INTRODUCTION

We have all been waiting for a sign in anxious anticipation, with excitement building, that this is the time to fully activate ourselves and be who we really are in service of the world for the good of all people. Signs are appearing now everywhere. They are rising out of the seas and crashing down amidst our cities. They are being written in our crops and portrayed in our films. They shimmer in the heavens and return as fulfilled prophecies. But most important, the call within our souls to go forth and be lights unto all people is louder than ever. This is the most important sign, because in carrying out what our souls urge us to do we fully activate the glow of all levels of Heaven within us, and fulfill the purpose of creation.

If you have forgotten what the incredible glow of your true nature feels like, this book will help you find your way back into the well of your heart and your body where you have always known the way. The path is not always easy. You have chosen (or will choose) a very challenging and special task. As you go about it, with dedication and perseverance, it will simply become an effortless part of who you are.

All can experience the Creator. Now is the time. Many of us feel capable of great deeds, of magnificent healing and creative energies, and of miracles. Because of this knowledge of our true core, we feel unable to rest or feel totally at peace until we have fulfilled our complete true nature. When you have an authentic wish to help others, you know it is a part of you—you cannot give up or turn your back on it. You might think you want to abandon it and postpone it, but your dedication makes you push forward toward being yourself in total and complete freedom. This can lead to a constant and infinite sense of striving. This book will help you understand how to tune into this calling to the greatest degree. It will also explain that there is a way, a point, and a moment in which you become totally and completely what you have longed to be. The Hebrew tradition calls this being *"Or L'Goyim,"* meaning "a Light unto the Nations," or a "whole light being" from another perspective. (This book contains many Hebrew terms like these, new words, and words used in a special way shown in **bold italics**. Definitions are in the Glossary.)

This Light, which is the source that conceived all the religions of the planet, is not limited to anyone and is to be shared equally among all people. Your dreams are not just for you. If you wish just for yourself, or for your people alone, and you don't know how to share the joy of the return to **Oneness** with *all*, then you need some healing. Good. That is what this book is for.

This book is not to be committed to memory in a way that disempowers your ability to know Truth. It is a tool to uncover the well of Knowledge inside you. It is not filled with confining rules or laws you must obey. It is suffused with rubies to spark your true sense of freedom, so that you can see that it is time to let go and trust yourself in being who you are.

This book will address the many belief systems and judgments planted within that limit us and cause the free-flowing nature of our energy to ebb. Such resistance blocks our systems and leads to disease. When you are sick, or exist in any way other than your free-flowing nature, whether or not there is physical pathology, peace and *joie de vivre* are absent. When there is no joy and no peace, there is no **Love**. When there is no Love, the lives and the relationships we create are destructive. Therefore, the path of healing is the process of releasing ourselves from cages that entrap our being. And so the path of healing is really the path of enlightenment and the return to the Garden of Eden. That is why the service that healers and Light Workers offer the planet today is of utmost importance. God bless you all. Your role in bringing us back to the Garden is paramount.

This book draws upon Kabbalah, alchemy, homeopathy, traditional Chinese medicine, the understanding of the chakras, as well as knowledge from other traditions to facilitate our healing. The lost identity of the Tree of Knowledge for Good and Bad is revealed and the immense effects it had on humankind are examined from many perspectives, including how it created our two opposing wills and the reversal of the way we perceive the world. This book explains how the lost Tree of Knowledge can be used homeopathically to release ourselves from duality, so that we may once again eat fruit from the Tree of Life.

The book will help you see why you need not wait any longer—that you are capable and also responsible for creating Heaven on Earth. This involves letting go of what we have called "Free Will," to begin knowing and being totally and completely okay with who you are and who you are created to be, without any resistance or doubt.

Your calling within to save the planet, or in other terms, to help be a part of raising this planet into the state of being as it was originally created to be, is the call to return to the Garden of Eden. This book discusses how we were first created in God's imagination, and that we "threw" ourselves out of Eden and were responsible for beginning duality. Also discussed is *how* to return to the Garden of Eden, and in doing so, how we will be bringing in the Messianic Age and uncovering a lost civilization.

The Garden of Eden is also known as Nirvana or Heaven, a place of divine experience encompassed by many traditions. To be in Eden is to be exactly as we love to be, within our bodies here on Earth. Eden is a state of AllGood, a state of consciousness revealing to you in every moment the unconditional perfection of who you are, where you are, when you are. The energy of Eden is so divine that ecstasy becomes your permanent reality as you surrender to it. No longer will there be the sense of rising into ecstasy and falling into dullness, of the Heavenly and the Hellish, the manic and the depressive, nor ease and joy alternating with the heavy burden of responsibility. To be in Eden is to be totally free of *all* resistance, negativity, and duality.

How many of us truly wish we could be is as a Messiah, not in the sense of being one who will come on a donkey and vanquish enemies, but rather in the sense that the Messiah is a collective movement of many people embodying their true natures of unconditional Love. This Messiah is like the good air we all breath. It awakens first in a few, then in many, then in all. It colors our eyes with pastel-like lights so that we see that there are no enemies, only beliefs we needed to defend. It enlightens us to remember that everything we wish for and seek is peace. Being a Messiah is expressed individually as a person's return to *their* Eden—the place where you see that all you truly are is everything you have wished to be. It reclaims you from all you try to do to avoid being who you really are. Having given yourself totally and completely to who you really are with no more internal resistance, you are capable of great feats and miraculous deeds. Having remembered who you are, you are able to transcend the barriers of earthly reality.

Who are you really? You are Soul. A Worldly Caretaker. A Rabbinical Buddha. A Messianic Merlin. A Christic Priestess. A Many and a One. Truly.

And to become so, totally and completely, you must understand the importance of, and how to go about, letting go of Free Will.

Book I

The Letting Go of Free Will

CHAPTER ONE

THE LETTING GO

OF "FRMEE WILL"

This book is about releasing Free Will and returning to the state of Oneness that is beyond Free Will.

Many of us have come to believe that we are fully free because we have Free Will. What is Free Will?

It is actually a second will that is not part of our true nature. Our first will is the will with which we were created that is One with God's Will, seamlessly aligned and of the very same nature. Free Will is an additional adopted will that goes against the Will of God. With it, we become resistant and believe we must be in control. This causes a duality in a soul that possesses these two wills because they are not harmonious.

It is true that we have the ability to choose, yet we are not fully free to be who we really want to be because we are constantly dueling internally. We are often enslaved by our fears and judgments, which are rooted in our Free Will.

Don't be mistaken, however, in believing that this extra will we were granted is all bad. It is a gift that we were given, because it enables us to experience something impossible had we always remained One with God, in the spiritual and angelic realms. So it is part of God's Will even when it is not. Even though Free Will can be subject to opposition within, it is a necessary tool and a gift.

It is a tool like no other for, like a double-edged sword, it has served a great purpose, and yet we cut ourselves with it. In letting go of Free Will its purpose is fully served.

The paradox of Free Will is, therefore, that we are not completely 'free' when we hold onto the hilt of this double-edged sword. Thus, for the purpose of these books, I have renamed Free Will as a reminder that we are not completely free, when we have it, and so that we keep in mind that having choice is not always what it appears to be.

I have called it *"Frmee Will,"* pronounced For-Me-Will, slurred altogether.

This is the Will of the *self within the self*—the part that became doubled and is trapped within. It is the selfish part—For Me Me Me—that forgets the connection with all things. It is also the will that resides within self-conscience that we experience as guilt. When we are so wrapped up in our own selves, in the conscience of our self, we experience guilt as a result of having lost the connection with all of creation. Frmee Will began right after Adam and Eve ate from the Tree of Knowledge for Good and Bad.

Before eating from the Tree, there was no shame in being naked. "They were both naked, the man and his wife, and they were not ashamed" **Gen 2:25**. This is symbolic; they were completely comfortable with who they were. Nakedness is who you are in the raw, with no mask, nothing hidden—being yourself freely as you were created to be.

Covering up the self is an act of shame. Shame and guilt come from the feeling that something is wrong with you. If we look closely at this, we see that before Adam and Eve ate from the Tree of Knowledge, there was no thought of anything bad. There was nothing to be afraid of, nor was there anything to judge as bad because Adam and Eve were still living within God's kingdom and perceiving all as it was created to be—

good ("And God saw all that He had made, and behold it was very good." **Gen 1:31**). Therefore, Frmee Will is involved in Adam and Eve's changed perception of God's creation from "AllGood" to good and bad. And therefore we can also say that Frmee Will gives a person the ability to think about something and perceive something that really isn't there. Adam and Eve were naked and it was okay, and then they were naked and it wasn't. Which is true? The truth is that being naked is okay. The false perception is that it is wrong and shameful. Since Adam and Eve's "little decision," we have always had the choice to see things either way: true or false, which is the same as good or bad. The bad is the false way of seeing things because our world is really AllGood. We have simply forgotten.

One way we can choose to see is as passive witnesses, grateful for the way things truly are and as they were created to be. This is to perceive the unconditional perfection of Allthatis. It is a way of goodness, of peace and joy. The other choice is not truthful. It is an active way of perceiving by projecting what we believe. It is attempting to be like God controlling reality by deciding what is good and what is bad. Such judgment is the way of perception of Frmee Will. It is not real, nor does it bring us good. This is why we must let go of Frmee Will. Not only does it give us the ability to see things that are not there, it also leads us into trouble and suffering, when we need suffer no longer.

"There is nothing either good or bad but thinking makes it so." Shakespeare — *Hamlet*, Act 2, Scene 2

When we see things in terms of good and bad, things become good and bad. When we release the part of ourselves that sees this duality, we see reality as it truly is, which is AllGood, and what is called "***The Balanced Positive.***"

Frmee Will is an illusion in and of itself and has led us to the experience of forgetting who we are, for we are One with God and have always been. In Eden, there is no Frmee Will, and that's a good thing. So returning to Eden is a surrender, because all the choices that *we* have adopted, all the judgments *we* have divided with, all the control that *we* have enforced has caused our own separation from Eden. God did not cause this.

God is in an eternal state of welcoming of Love and acceptance. We beg God to take us home and yet we clutch and hold on to where we have been. God hasn't asked us to be this way. God did not say, "Here, you have Frmee Will, now you must suffer with it!" God said, "Here, you have Frmee Will" and we chose to suffer and to create suffering with it. Since the dawning of Frmee Will, whether to suffer or not, and whether to be joyous or not, has always been our option.

Yet we have wanted choice. We have wanted "Free Will" or "Frmee Will," as I am calling it. It made possible a Game in which we have been choosing between Love and fear for the purpose of empowering our true nature. Perhaps we didn't fully understand the entirety of what we were getting into as we reached out to take the Tree's fruit that made us begin forgetting our connection with God. Perhaps we didn't see how difficult it was going to be when we adopted the mindset of good and bad. But ultimately there was a sense of trust about the whole process, a sense of faith about it. Otherwise, do you think we, or us as Eve and Adam, would really have embarked upon this incredibly challenging journey—the enterprise that we know as life? Do you think God would have allowed it?

This Game does have a finish line. We are nearing it. The goal is to give up any choices based in fear, or Frmee Will. This will end the journey that has taken us into the realm of Good and Bad, where we have been giving up our true nature of unconditional Love.

Please understand that Love is a realm. It is a state and a way of being. It is strength, kindness and courage. It can say no and be firm in order to establish change. It is much more than our limited romantic or Hollywood association with the word. Love is your true nature. Waking up to that and bringing in the Messiah is remembering what Love really feels like. Therefore, another aspect of Frmee Will is that it gives us the ability to resist knowing, feeling and being Love. In releasing Frmee Will, we become Messianic Beings of unconditional Love whose one and only Will is aligned with the Will of God.

Your heart is your guide, the path the Creator sent you to follow. The marriage of your will with God's Will becomes fully manifest, fully conjoined when you step through **the threshold** in letting go of all control that derives from your Frmee Will.

Frmee Will is a gift that God will not take from us by imposing His/Her Will upon us. If the Messiah and the Return to Eden are coming at all, it is because we are waking up to the **Truth** today and so many are now following the guidance of Truth in their heart. We are steps away from completing a journey that began entirely *for the purpose of making* human beings able to experience the state of God, collectively, in every moment on Earth. Our joy of joys comes pouring in when we serve and share a collective Will that is AllGoodLove and see that as the only reality that exists.

Although we often chose suffering when we could have celebrated, although we have made errors of judgment and held onto them when we could have allowed the Truth to be revealed and constantly renewed, we will find acceptance in the wonder of the planet. We will appreciate this beautiful physical world and give thanks to Allthatis, all that was, and all that ever will be.

For a soul to let go of Frmee Will and achieve the highest potential on earth might seem a little out of reach. Reading this book will enable you to slowly understand that you too are capable of such an enormous feat. The knowledge shared in this book was written to help you heal, and is designed to help even skeptics heal and come to peace with who they are. If you cannot grasp some concepts now, perhaps you will in a future reading.

This book will not try to tell you what the Truth is *all* about, for that is not possible. No book can ever accomplish that because the essence of the Truth cannot be conveyed in words. This book will point to the Truth as it exists in you, to awaken and inspire you onto the path of your true self. It will do so by painting a picture using an ancient model that simply describes what the struggles and joys, growth and suffering of life on earth have been all about.

We will look at the story of Adam and Eve and the progression from paradise, the Garden of Eden, into the furthest reaches away from it— duality. Many have neither adopted the story of Adam and Eve nor the Torah/Bible as their story, nor held it in Truth. No one is obligated to believe it, as if it were the sole Truth. We should never come to see the

Truth as if there is only one way and other expressions are incorrect. There is room for all faiths. We can see the other ways of the world, there are many divine lessons and ways of being. Thus, please accept the model of Adam and Eve as a metaphor that attempts to describe and explain who we are, how we were created to be, and the birth of Frmee Will. We might even look at it as a model that explains much of our existence here on Earth. It is a very simple model that explains much, and is aligned with the Truth, which is also so simple. However, because it is a model, it is not Truth itself, but a tool for understanding Truth. If it evokes and awakens wisdom in the individual as to his or her true nature, then it has accomplished its task. Further, it reveals why we have come to study it and scrutinize it for millennia.

Throughout the book, you will see **CaN**s. They are defined as "**C**hoices that are **N**o Choice." The CaNs are the ways of Love, equality, and harmony with which a person can align him or herself *for the purpose of healing*. The CaNs are arranged into different levels of healing called "circles." The collection of CaNs in all the circles is known as "**The Circle of Nine**" (see **Appendix D** for the entire *Circle of Nine*. The Circle of Nine is a system of healing that I have developed based on the knowledge in *The Last Four Books of Moses* that a person can use to let go of Frmee Will and approach his or her true nature. You are not required to give up any other system of healing, meditation, or prayer to enter into The Circle of Nine. It is not elitist or exclusive. It's only purpose is to heal. You can go to http://www.thelastfourbooks.com to find out more about The Circle of Nine. If you wish, you can enter The Circle of Nine by adding your name to the list of a certain circle, along with others dedicating themselves to manifesting their highest state of Love and most profound wishes. Familiarizing yourself with the Circles and beginning to live by the ways of being within the Circles even now, before you have finished reading this book, will make the CaNs very meaningful.

May every person come to a complete healing of all their ills and limitations of their being.

May the boundaries and borders that separate the different peoples of the earth be dissolved and allow the emergence of the new (and old) order in which we see that we are all of the same nature.

May the defined, controlling energies within us yield to the true might of that which is infinite and undefined so that we might all close the book on Frmee Will and adorn our "Robes with The Golden Glow" (to be explained later).

HEALING
RESISTANCE

IN THE MIND
AND BODY

Healing is the realm that we must all visit, once again allowing ourselves access to our wells of infinite strength and joy. Although we have come to think of health as the absence of disease, health is much more of a continuum between very poor health, in which the body manifests dis-ease, and excellent health, with lots of vibrant energy and well-being. Many people do not have any physical symptoms of dis-ease yet they are very far from being well or feeling good. Others might have something "wrong" with their bodies, yet having found peace with that diseased state they have a great sense of well-being.

The adoption of Frmee Will was actually the very beginning of dis-ease, in which the ease and peace we had with God got dis-embodied. Let's take a close look at what this dis-ease is, how it develops within all levels of being and how it goes beyond the physical definition of disease.

Healing is necessary in order to experience the divine. So let us look closely at what is involved in healing. This will clarify why we chose to adopt a state stuck in the physical with two opposing wills. We can go about bringing ourselves back to a state of absolute well-being which I call absolute "**Beingness.**" Without doing this, we are unable to experience the joy and ecstasy of being that results from letting go of the suppression of feeling.

Below are scenarios that may apply to you. Read the words slowly and allow yourself to imagine how each scenario might relate to you. As you do so, a lot can come up. Give yourself the time and space to deal properly with the letting go that is part of your healing. Breathe, relax, and be brave.

How do you become when you're upset or "uptight?" When you are "stressed out", what happens to your breathing? Is it deep and slow, or shallow and rapid? Have you ever forgotten to breathe altogether? When you are in a situation of tension—during an exam, or before a job interview—what happens to you? Do you relax, or does everything tense up? When you have a major deadline that you are worrying about, what happens to your muscles—are they loose or tight? When something very painful has happened to you, do you embrace it and flow with it, or do you lock it out of your consciousness as much as possible?

All of these situations have something in common—resistance. This is what makes you uptight and stressed out. It inhibits your proper, nourishing breathing and causes your muscles to bunch up. The question is, why do we resist certain situations and not others? Is there something common to all situations causing us to feel the need to go into a resistance reaction? There is. It is **the judgment** of the situation deeming it bad (no good) that causes us to resist that situation. From this judgment, resistance, stress, and disease take root.

For example, if you did something that you have judged as wrong, then you might feel guilty and ashamed of it. Most of us, instead of allowing ourselves to feel ashamed for a short period of time to quickly clear that energy and realize, "Hey, it's okay to screw up," will use a resistance reaction to the guilt and shame. We will not allow ourselves to feel. Our whole system will become involved in not allowing ourselves to think, feel, or connect with the feelings of guilt and shame. In fact, the feeling of shame is not due to the initial error, but to the effort we put into avoiding the fact that we made an error and accepting that. We all make mistakes. Isn't that okay?

One way to know which of your parts is affected by resistance is to see which parts are tired when you wake up in the morning. These are the places where resistance blocks your energy. In these places, you will continue to shut down your energy for the rest of the day and there will be a lack of vitality because you don't allow yourself to feel. The places where you feel tired upon waking are the places where you need healing.

Healing is feeling. When there is feeling, there is flowing. We know within the healing world, for example, in Chinese Medicine, that when the flowing of the different body systems or acupuncture meridians stop that disease can begin to manifest in the body. Feeling is also energizing. It is flowing and allowing. When you do not allow yourself to feel in certain situations, you block the flow of your feelings.

Blocking "bad" feelings also blocks your energy and your positive emotions. When we block a feeling or sensation that feels unpleasant (e.g., shame, anger, insecurity, jealousy, sorrow) it is felt in the *same space* where the corresponding positive emotion is felt.

- Where we feel insecure is in the place of self-esteem.
- Jealousy in the place of trust.
- Feeling wronged and victimized is in the place of empowerment.

Negative emotions are exactly that, *they are the negative* of positive emotions. When you shut down self-esteem, block it, resist it, freeze it, then you will feel insecurity in its stead.

Because these negative emotions exist in the same space as the ones that we love to feel, if we resist feeling the negative, if we push it away or try to eradicate it, we will not be able to feel the positive either. The negative is our very own true nature turned around on us. If you are feeling insecure and you continue to resist feeling that, then you are increasing the negative space and the feeling of insecurity. This furthers you from allowing yourself to feel your self-esteem and self-confidence.

"Negative" emotions that arise only become more because we resist them. They then grow in importance in our minds due to our inability to face them and allow them to flow. When they are allowed to flow, they no longer exist as negative, because a negative emotion is *the resistance of being.* That which we judge as bad and do not accept, or allow ourselves to feel, becomes blown out of proportion. It builds in your mind into something much more terrible than it really is. Suppose you fear that a meeting with someone will go terribly. You worry about it constantly until the time comes and you see that it wasn't nearly as bad as you *made it out to be.*

When we have lived too long suppressing our feelings, we become so completely blocked and frozen that we don't even remember the wonderful feeling of the state of flow. We have forgotten. That is why, for our return to a state of joy, ecstasy and well-being, it is of utmost importance to allow ourselves to feel. And to allow ourselves to feel, we must accept ourselves unconditionally. No matter what we have suppressed and tried to control within, the acceptance is the magical ingredient that removes self-judgment, allowing our true nature to return so that we can be well.

Acceptance is of utmost importance. Try it. Try accepting all of who you are and who you have become. It is interesting to note that by accepting yourself, you are not admitting that you would like to remain an anxious or jealous person, for example. You do not carve yourself in stone as you do when judging yourself. Rather, you reverse the process of dis-ease when you accept yourself, because the very process of dis-ease begins by judging who you are as bad. Whenever you say 'Bad' to something, you resist it. Dis-ease can snowball when you begin to judge yourself for being a certain way and then you get worse because you're fighting it so much and struggling so much. It is not that you really want to be jealous, or anxious. But what you're doing by focusing on it so much is just making it bigger and worse than ever. By accepting dis-ease and allowing it to be, it will heal. Try trusting this process and you will be amazed at how great you feel about yourself. You should. You are great.

Blocking ourselves with judgment weakens us. Strength is not only a physical attribute. It is also a principle of Love and a principle of healing, because the path of healing is the way of Love. A person who has more muscle may have less strength than another who has less muscle. We often think of strength as a physical force, as per muscular action, but is not strength also involved during difficult tasks, like child-bearing and birthing, long-distance running and standing up for your rights during an onslaught of opposition from every direction? Strength is energy that comes from within. It is the empowerment of being.

Imagine now: what is energy that animates the body? What gives long-distance runners the guts to push themselves further? Who is commanding the muscles to move? Our Will does. Yet blocking our feelings and emotions also blocks our strength and energy, because stopping feeling stops the source of our strength and energy. We will lack *the Will to live as we Love*.

When we see how we can generate strength with the gentlest of Wills, we will be able to unveil and remove the illusion that strength must be forced. You will need a lot of gentle Will to see outside this "strong" belief. Gentle Will is related to the function of our **hara** which is our *Will to Live*. The hara is an energy center located just beneath the navel that gives us great physical strength when we are connected with it in that gentle fashion. It is the propeller of Forwardness (see Figure 1). It also generates great inner strength.

Inner strength doesn't feel like muscle strength. Inner strength comes from the hara, deep in the guts and the heart. To do something very challenging or to get something stuck to flow again, you connect with the will of the hara, becoming more and more grounded into your body. Then, because of the nature of the hara's energy, you no longer need to muster any effort. You can give up effort, allowing strength to flow *simply because you can feel and allow it to flow*.

To heal stuck energies and beliefs, you get your energy flowing by allowing yourself to feel through acceptance. Once your energy has begun to flow, you don't need to do anything more. Simply allow.

I have developed a simple meditation by which you may demonstrate to yourself this gentle effort connecting to the hara, then effortlessness in the action of the various muscles of the body. (See the Effort-Effortlessness meditation at the end of this chapter.) This meditation also demonstrates the difference Gentle Will makes in the strength of your body. Gentle Will is not a trying will, but a Will of **allowishing**. It is one that you guide, but in an allowing sense, not forcing or trying. Trying is the same as resistance. Trying comes from doubt in your capacity; you believe you must try to make something happen. The belief that says 'The more I try, the more I do,' is only an illusion. Allowishing is the source of all power within. There is a long lost way of moving that we have forgotten. We have become stuck, believing that we must force, rather than just allow our actions to move us. The lost way is in allowishing, where feeling and movement are One. There is no separation. All is Light. It occurs, in part, when we have released the notion that we are trapped in the physical.

The point at which you've gone as deeply as possible within a belief or a stuck feeling is the *limit* of the belief system or blocked energy. Once the connection to this limit is accomplished, you may give up the struggle and just be beyond the belief system, allowing the empowerment of all you do.

The opposite of allowing is resistance, and that is the way we stop our feelings (see Figure 2). This resistance is part of the **Yetzir Hara**— The 'bad' Will, which is the same as Frmee Will. We use our *Will to resist* to stop the feelings or experiences that we have judged as bad. We tend to judge difficult feelings, like shame, guilt, grief, and anger, as bad. Sometimes we also judge feelings when they can be quite good. For example, we might have learned, and subsequently believed, that it is bad to feel proud of ourselves. Perhaps when we were feeling great self-esteem in the past somebody said "Why do you think you're so great?" with a negative intention that we took to heart. Or on another occasion, we were happy and all others were depressed or miserable, so we created the false belief that we shouldn't be so happy. We took on the belief that it's not fair to others if we're so happy and they're not. Self-esteem and happiness thus could have become "bad" to feel.

When we feel disempowered and weak, we have a *need* to use more of our *Trying Will* just to get through the day. You might also say that we need more Will to move because we are "putting on the brakes" within our system. This causes fatigue. My friend Rob asked me why I thought humans needed to sleep. I said I think it is because we resist what we don't want to feel.

Remember how we get when we are afraid or stressed out? situations in which we are afraid, or in situations that we judge as bad for us, we tend to tense up. Tensing up uses a lot of your Will to resist the unpleasant situation that causes you fear, anger, pain, guilt, worry, stress, etc. Any negative reaction to a situation can cause you to tense up in this manner. It will cause you to block the flow of your energy that blocks your strength which, in turn, makes you use your Trying Will more. That tires you out, makes you feel weaker, and makes you use your Trying Will more—a vicious cycle!

Dis-ease results from resistance to the natural flow of the body. We are fluid creatures. As with nature all around us, nothing living remains stagnant. Chinese medicine explains this in the philosophy of "*the Three Treasures*" which states that there is a relationship between mind, Qi (energy), and blood, in which the mind governs the Qi (energy) which governs the blood. If the mind blocks the flow of Qi by a resistance reaction (see Figure 3), then the blood will eventually stagnate as well, leading to lack of nourishment of the tissues and eventual disease. We can translate the Three Treasures of mind, Qi, and Blood as Mind, Emotions, and Body. In Kabbalah, these are the worlds of **Bria** (Mind), **Yetzirah** (Emotions) and **Assiyah** (Body).

The mind oversees all bodily systems. And to be precise, it is in the *rational mind* where control takes place. This doesn't necessarily mean, however, that the rational mind is *supreme*. It's just bossy. The control panel of resistance exists in the rational mind. It says "yes" or "no," depending on what it decides to allow or resist. The rational mind doesn't only resist in a linear direction. *It can resist in a cloud, or resist when it's proud. It can grab like a snare, or a balloon filled with air. It can boss to be King and to freeze up the sting.*

Dis-ease begins in the rational mind. Some ask: "What if you broke your arm or had internal bleeding which then led to disease? That is not rooted in the mind!" This is true to some degree, yet people have a disposition to injuries, accidents and traumatic events. This susceptibility is rooted in the rational mind. A constant fear of injury will dispose some people to injure themselves. Also, when someone does injure him or herself and disease develops, that is because of the suppression of the mind and emotions, not because of the injury itself. The body has an innate ability to heal and repair itself. Your body spontaneously heals unless you resist facing the cause of injury in the first place. In other words, if there is an unwillingness (resistance) to release the initial suppression that caused weakness and allowed the body to be injured, then the body is prevented from healing.

This understanding is also aligned with one of the principals of naturopathic medicine's philosophy: *Vis medicatrix naturae,* the healing power of nature. This principles states that the body has a natural ability to heal itself once the causative factors of disease are removed. It is the same with a river. When a dam is removed, the flow of water resumes naturally. The cause of disease, the dam, is our rational mind's resistance.

Let's look at the way our nervous system carries out resistance. The body conducts information via two major routes: the direction that sensations flow and the direction that actions go. These are **afferent** (sensory) and **efferent** (motor) conduction pathways (see Figure 4). Generally, on the physical plane, afferent flow is from a place of sensation (e.g., skin, toe) to the organ (brain) where we perceive through the senses. The brain sends efferent information out to the rest of the body.

It is possible to use part of the efferent system to counteract the flow of the sensory inputs. For example, the Corticospinal tract, a bundle of nerves, carries the brain's commands to the muscles. This is what happens when we wish to suppress and resist a feeling or sensation we do not like. In the physical dimension, our will is carried through the corticospinal tract fibers into the area where we want to numb or block our senses from feeling. Injured people tense up immensely. You may have witnessed someone break a leg, perhaps their tibia (big bone of the shin). Many muscles in the area and above, in the thigh and the hip joint, will become very rigid. This is due to pain the injured person cannot bear. He or she will use Will to force the feeling of pain away. The pain hurts so much, it will naturally be judged as bad, and so the mind will resist the feeling. This activates mostly the efferent corti-cospinal tract (there are other nerve tracts that are involved as well), tightening the muscles, which limits the amount of movement in the area. This will help to control the pain. With decreased movement, there is less muscle spindle and golgi-tendon organ activation. Together, the muscle spindles and golgi-tendon organs act as an afferent pathway to the brain, telling the brain a part of the body is localized there. When movement ceases due to pain, this is an attempt to shut down all affer-ent, sensory fibers. We thus lose our body's awareness when we are in pain and we resist feeling.

When rigidity and suppression occur long enough in an area, local-ization inputs will cease to inform the brain. In some very traumatic injuries, the pain is so intense that the brain will altogether freeze the feeling. This can lead to paralysis in the affected area, but it will more likely contribute to loss of body awareness. The person will adapt slow-ly to the loss of perception of the different body parts and forget how the true, healed state of the body feels. They have become numb.

The cells store trauma underneath the layers of unfeeling ice. The body is frozen *and* the pain is still there, buried, like a cold fish at the bottom of a frozen lake. The pain will continue to be there as long as it is frozen. This is an important understanding of healing. Even though someone might have long ago forgotten the pain of a traumatic emo-tional or physical event, the pain can still be there *and* be frozen, thus the pain is not perceived. When healing begins, which happens by doing nothing more than allowing the flow to resume in the stagnant area, the pain will initially be felt again. This is equally true for both physical and emotional pain.

With time, the trauma in the body or mind fades into the past and there is no longer any pain. The person can continue to use, for instance, a leg, but will not even realize that the area is frozen because the freez-ing process occurs gradually. If you were to take a pin and poke the per-son in a frozen trauma site, he or she would most likely wince or scream, because they are not completely numb. Their nerves still feel unless there has been nerve damage. So the term frozen doesn't neces-sarily mean to *all* feeling. It means to the true feeling of the body beyond just the physical sensation—the true, vibrant, flowing, strong, poised, balanced, light feeling.

The difference one feels before and after the flow is allowed to resume is astounding. There is a great difference between the life we live in suppression and the life we live free. We just don't know it until we can experience the rebirth.

Very often people get really worried and upset about certain pains and think they are sick or dying, rather than moving toward a space of better healing. I have become so accustomed to feeling long-forgotten wounds and traumas coming to the surface and causing pain that I never think of them as bad. I do not worry. I know that my body and being are coming out of suppressed hibernation. I am healing. This is profound because so many people think something is wrong with them when pain surfaces that they immediately take a pill, which only serves to further suppress the healing process. So many of the ills and pains we feel need no intervention. With the simple understanding of what is truly happening and a simple shift in mindset, those little ills and pains naturally give way to our true strength and health.

Homeopathic medicine recognizes the phenomenon of pain emerging from long-lost traumas and calls it an "*aggravation*"—meaning things get worse before they get better. But truly, they are not getting worse, they are getting better because we are returning to the ability to perceive our body in its true, flowing nature. The very term "aggravation" is misleading because it has negative connotations and there is absolutely nothing negative in resuming the natural flow of the body. Although it may feel painful or sad or lonely, for example, letting it flow and feeling it is part of healing. Imagine the body as coming alive again after you have been outside in the winter and you have frozen toes. It hurts, yes, but if you want to feel your body the way it really is, then some discomfort must be accepted.

The reason for this clarification is that we have become so indoctrinated with quick fixes for our pains that to tell someone that they are going to aggravate, as in getting worse, will cause them to focus on this negatively. The alternative is to help the body heal with positive intention, excitement, and knowing that what they are feeling is their healing process and the awakening of frozen parts. The mind-set that is aligned with judgment will instantly feel something unpleasant and continue to suppress it. But if we all knew and understood how such suppression is really killing us, we would come to love the flow of feelings, no matter how difficult or painful.

And this is really the secret. Let the pain be twice or three times as much. *The secret is allowing yourself to feel it more, thereby reversing the resistance that has caused it to hamper you.* You are clearing it for good! When you feel that twinge of the blocked feelings that scare you, like loss, grief, anger, jealousy, pain in the back, neck or head, do not *try* to feel so that you can get rid of the blocked feelings. That won't do it. Trying to get rid of the blocked feelings by fighting them will just make them stay. You must willingly allow the feeling, not by trying, but by letting it be. This is acceptance.

When we begin to fully understand how pain and discomfort can be stored in the body simply because they haven't been allowed to exist, and that suppression confines us in little boxes of numbness, we will likely see the positive in letting all feelings resume their natural state. There is comfort in coming back alive by *diving into the pain completely,* but gently, and thawing out faster than if we dabble between allowing and resisting. As a result, the health of the world will improve.

The muscles in the area of a frozen site have also lost their full capacity, especially since they are the agents that the mind uses to resist, rather than employ for proper movement. The muscles simply cannot function optimally when they are used to resist pain and trauma. They have one foot on the brake, so to speak. If you want to give them gas, they just will not feel right, as if something is holding them back. If you ever feel this in your muscles, then you can be sure there is some resistance going on.

This is also true for frozen emotional trauma. If you have frozen your heart to numb the pain of loss, you will lose the feeling of Love. *This is how the mind and body become separated and divided.* In our true nature, the mind and body are one. This state of perfect harmony is beyond all judgment and fear. But for most of us, there is a great degree of separation between the mind and body because of how much we judge. We then pull our awareness out of our body up into our mind to avoid feeling anything we have judged as bad.

Some diseases that are becoming more common these days are fibromyalgia and chronic fatigue syndrome, although it is possible that they are the same condition. In these diseases, an immense mental-emotional cause is draining the person's strength to the core, causing the whole body to ache and be weak with fatigue. People with these illnesses are not willing to face something and that is sapping their vitality. They exert immense resistance in order to avoid feeling certain emotions. The mental and emotional suppression is different for each person, thus each individual must be considered uniquely.

One way we will compensate for this loss of feeling, e.g., in a broken leg, is by relying more on the use of another part of the body to balance the frozen zone of the leg. You can imagine how this can lead to more tension and trouble in the other parts of the body that must make more effort to keep the machine running. We use more control in other parts to avoid the original feelings of fear/pain, or whatever we have judged as bad. When a part of the body gets too overworked, then it too will collapse, putting added strain on the rest of the body that is still up and running. The ultimate result of this cascade of resistance is death. Didn't God tell us we would die if we ate from the Tree of Knowledge, a.k.a. The Tree of Allow and Resistance?

The sympathetic nervous system is responsible for getting us geared both in times of stress and for strenuous activities, like sports. When used over a long period of time, it leads to hypertonicity, meaning a higher degree of tension, in the muscles. More tension in the area, more muscle activity and firing, more energy catabolism (energy burning), more sympathetics, more muscular fatigue—a vicious cycle of muscular fatigue *and* tension. Forcing your Will over the Corticospinal tract (efferent) activates it in a greater proportion to the Spinothalamic tract (sensory/afferent) which leads to an even higher degree of muscle spasm. This also means tension—the opposite of relaxation. This causes an increase in activity by the sympathetic system, everywhere, overpowering the parasympathetic nervous system which is responsible for relaxation. This then leads to decreased functioning of our immune, digestive and elimination systems.

When we sleep, the tensest parts of our body get the least nourishing sleep in proportion to the amount of tension stored in the muscles and tissues. Instead of going into a state of rest, they will take a while to relax. Only then comes the rejuvenating energy of sleep, which allows complete relaxation and proper oxygenation of the tissues. One of the purposes of sleep is to release all resistance generated while we were awake.

We are truly a tough species. We have learned to adapt to survive. Rather than trusting in the process of life, life has become about the struggle against pain and weakness, rather than allowing and just being. I am truly astonished at how some people persevere day to day with their burdens. They go on, somewhat laden, somewhat downtrodden, yet they go on all the same. The struggle and hardships bend them over, as they wither under intense strain through the years—yet they persist. "What other choice do we have?" they might ask. We take pride in the fact that we can survive anything. It is truly commendable that we have endured terrible suffering, over oceans of time, as individuals and as a collective. Yet life need not be all about survival, nor should we pride ourselves about our ability to survive. When life becomes about living to survive, it is because we must survive against all the oppression *we have created for ourselves* by not allowing ourselves to just be and by creating enemies of Nature. It is time to say goodbye to the limitations and pain by letting go, even though we have lived with them for thousands of years. We can unlearn them or, rather, we will remember the way of our true nature. Then we will thrive, not merely survive.

The *chakras* are also involved in the way in which we use our will to resist feelings that we judge as bad. A chakra (Sanskrit for 'wheel') is a funnel of spinning energy. There are seven chakras located on the body and nine in the energetic system in total. Each absorbs energy and carries out a different function (see Figure 5). Those seven chakras located on our body are at different locations, on the front and back of the body, one is on the crown of the head, another at the base of our spine. The chakras draw in the universal energy that is the source of all life.

When we examine how our chakras are affected by our Will, we see the similarity to the affect on the nervous system, and the holographic pattern of nature becomes more apparent.

The energetic system of the chakras and the nervous system are intimately connected and constantly influence each other. As Barbara Brennan shows in her book, *Hands of Light* on page 46, the front chakras are the feeling and receptive chakras (afferent) and the posterior chakras are the Will chakras (efferent).

When we wish to avoid pain, our chakras have a response very similar to our nervous system. *We use force with our Will chakras to avoid pain.* This takes energy from our back Will centers right through to the front and influences the receptivity of the front chakras, just as we use the corticospinal tract to slow or stop the signals of the afferent nerve fibers (when we don't want to feel something). The resistance of the Will chakra causes a decrease of the flow of the feeling chakras (see Figure 6). So when we do not want to feel something we have judged as bad, soon enough, we will accomplish this.

Emotional trauma has the same relationship to chakras as physical trauma—we lose the awareness of how we truly feel. All the times we were wounded by hurtful words, neglect, or rudeness, we knew no other way than to resist the feelings. For example: a situation occurred where we felt betrayed by the behavior of a friend. The pain of this could be felt anywhere, but let's say it was felt in the solar plexus. The Will to resist this hurt feeling comes from the rational mind which judges the feeling of hurt and betrayal as bad. The rational mind exerts its efferent control through the rear/Will efferent solar plexus chakra and makes it stop the flow of the front/feeling solar plexus chakra. Blocking the solar plexus will stop the feeling of the solar plexus chakra. This leads to a frozenness of the feeling of self-esteem, because self-esteem is felt in the solar plexus chakra. To take this a little further, the decreased flow of the feeling (afferent) chakra and increased use of the will (efferent) chakra causes an increased sympathetic response in that area of the body. The energetic system of chakras is closely related to the sympathetic (Will) and parasympathetic (feeling/allowing) nervous systems. It is called the autonomic nervous system, because it is believed to be beyond our control. There is, however, a direct link to our Will and how we choose to use our energy, because with the use of the rear/Will chakra, the stomach area will begin to receive more sympathetic response. This can lead to a dysfunction of the stomach's digestion. Malnourishment, nausea, or stomach ulcers are some of the examples of physical conditions that can result from the initial emotional suppression of third chakra feelings.

All our power and energy come from allowing the flow of the feeling chakras. That is the source. If we look at the word "acceptance" again in this light, we see that one of the definitions of acceptance is "the willingness to receive." Isn't that interesting? In accepting ourselves and our situation, we are actually allowing the harmonious flow of the feeling chakras to nourish our body with healing energy, vitality, and gentle strength.

By exerting too much of our Will in trying or resisting, which most of us tend to do, the Will chakras act as the brakes against the natural flow of the feeling chakras. Everything becomes such a struggle that we must constantly maintain by being in control. When we try too hard to be a certain way, or if we resist feelings, we stop the flow of our feeling centers and we stop feeling our sense of well-being in that chakra area.

Just because the front chakras are called feeling chakras does not mean they are related only to emotions. Each feeling chakra has a different function. So when we discuss the feeling of the 6th chakra, or third eye, it is experienced as an intuitive awareness. The feeling experience of the 5th chakra, which is at the throat, is faith, and the 7th crown chakra is direct knowing. Does the experience of direct knowing give the sensation of feeling something? Well, yes, kind of. And also no. It just is.

If the flow of energy is decreased through the feeling chakra, this causes a decrease in the nourishment of the nerve plexus/centers and nearby organs. For example, the front, feeling heart chakra nourishes the thymus gland, the heart, lungs, and surrounding muscles and tissues. The nerve supply will also become undernourished when the flow of the feeling chakra is blocked by the resistance of the rational mind, which is carried out through the rear, will chakra.

When a trauma becomes frozen, it also blocks the acupuncture meridians that flow through the area (see Figure 7). The acupuncture meridians are little channels, or rivers of energy, that flow inside our bodies, nourish us, and bring us life. The energy that flows through the acupuncture meridians is absorbed by the chakras from the Universe. If you break your radius right near your wrist, there is a good chance that you will block the flow of the lung, large intestine, pericardium and triple burner channels in that area, and possibly other channels as well. Because the flow of blood follows the flow of Qi, this leads to long term health difficulties and a continual decrease in the sense of lightness of being in the body.

The acupuncture meridians follow closely along with nerves. A local excess in an acupuncture meridian will ensue if it is blocked by a will chakra. In other words, because the energy of the acupuncture meridians is like the energy of little rivers, if not allowed to flow, it acts as a dam, and a build-up will occur. Such excess also contributes to rigidity, which we know from traditional Chinese medicine, and will lead to rigidity in the muscular system that follows the flow along that meridian. This is in harmony with the explanations of the nervous system, in which resistance leads to more rigidity. Amazing to think that suppressed grief or anger can lead to rigidity. Rigidity is the antithesis of life and healthy living.

To resist the pain is to amplify it. By resisting you give pain, and anything else you resist, power. This contributes to the scariness of letting it go because it will feel like you are taking on the pain of the whole world. Pain only feels huge when it is stagnant. Once it begins to flow, it will feel very manageable. So even though it feels beyond possible to face the feeling of sadness from the loss of a friend, or the scariness of standing up for yourself when you've let yourself be dominated for a long time, or the feeling of insecurity around speaking your Truth and being yourself, know that it only feels that way because it has long been frozen. In the state of stagnation, there is fear. As soon as it starts to flow, even a tiny bit, you will feel that you are okay.

It is thus quite important to feel the pain and accept the sensations stored in our muscles, cells, and energy centers without judgment. You may want to think about what might have caused the suppression, i.e. what judgment you are holding onto that resists the feeling, so you can work on releasing it. This helps let go of the pain so that the whole system can start to feel again.

When the body starts to feel again, the original pain that was frozen within begins to be experienced again for a brief period. This can be a few minutes to a few days, weeks, months, depending on how much you are able to allow it to surface. If you truly allow, healing of the body can occur in a very rapid manner. There is really no rush though. The simple knowledge that you can be healed as you wish and when you wish helps. It is funny when people say they are not ready, because of course you are not ready if you say you are not ready. But there is really nothing about you that isn't ready. You choose not to be ready. It is only your choice not to be ready. You can take the leap at any point because you're really okay. The healing is simply in allowing the flow to resume so that you feel the cosmic 'I am okay.' Of course, don't rush or hurry for the finish line, for it is important to move at the rhythm that is best for your healing. Don't feel bad if it is taking you a long time, for some patterns of suppression can stem from an experience in utero, or even beyond. Simply be aware that an immense amount of healing *can* occur in a short time for those willing completely to accept pain and judgment and allow feeling. Because in our true nature beyond all illusion, we are purely Light beings. Such bodies can heal quite quickly.

This way of allowing yourself to feel is essential for anyone on a healing journey or for anyone seeking spiritual enlightenment. Those who force all negative feelings away are distancing themselves from true enlightenment. It is easy to force away issues and say "I feel no issues in me," "It's all good," but this is what contributes to the **unbalanced positive**. It is not that you have no issues. It is that you have numbed yourself and you are in denial. But when you face your issues and let them flow, what an incredible sense to have your body and soul restored to their natural feeling. They feel warm, strong, full, light and loose. All the things that you fear and worry about fall away. Then you can say "it's all good" and it will be real.

Take time to become aware of the ways you are suppressing and resisting your feelings. To feel, you simply allow. It is hard to describe such a process in words. But once you align your intention to remembering how to go about it, in no time you will be a champ at feeling again. Your hardness will melt. When you are hardened, you cannot feel. You cannot feel goodness, Love, God, nothing can you feel, for you have severed yourself from the well of your divine feelings which swirl about you like the silk scarves of fairies and pixies, magically sparkling with golden dust, caressing you and bringing you the totally clear knowledge that you are good.

Allowing feeling is a process that will naturally and effortlessly return you in time to the point where you first started to control and resist. That deepest point in you where you first began to resist is the time you first adopted Frmee Will. When you are so deep in your lifetime that you are at the point where you first stepped away from Oneness into duality, then you will feel like Adam, or Eve, or both, because you are at the gates to the Garden of Eden.

Most men (and some women), whose entire basis of reality is rational and mental, find allowing feeling especially difficult. For them, feeling can seem foreign and wrong because they feel vulnerable. This may be because of how the emotions have been judged as bad through the ages. A person's defenses are an attempt to control any feeling of vulnerability. Faith and trust are infinitely important in order to make the leap from the controlled, rational world into the feeling world. Once you yield to being vulnerable, you see that there is no vulnerability and that the nature of Universal Truth is witnessed by acceptance and allowing, not holding on.

Embodying our absolute state of joy and healing requires absolute healing. The foundation given in this chapter is very important to understand the very deep concepts of letting go of Frmee Will and the return to Eden. I will elaborate on them in later chapters.

Why do we enter into states of disease and disharmony, pain and suffering, suppression and frozenness? Why does life involve going through difficult times and losing feeling with our true nature? In order to understand this, it is necessary to venture back in time, to where life, as we know it, began. The purpose of our lives here on earth will become understandable and we will free ourselves to experience what we have most longed for since the beginning of Time.

These questions will be answered in the next chapters, but first, a meditation!

Effortless-Effort Meditation

This meditation is quite physically challenging and can be used to strengthen your legs, buttocks and stomach muscles as well as the connection to your hara. The connection to the hara and the ability to use the will of the hara is vitally important in letting go of the past and propelling you forward to meet life head on. Sit with your tailbones flat on a chair. Make sure you are on a non-slippery surface. Tilt the chair forward so that it is at a 45° angle. You may want to put the back two legs of the chair securely against the wall when you achieve the proper angle to make sure the chair doesn't slip. Lean forward so that much of your weight is now supported by your legs and the chair is supporting less weight. You can vary the amount of weight that you put on your legs by varying the angle of the chair. You might want to start with less weight or you can jump right in with more weight. Relax in this position and allow your legs to take up the weight. Soon you will feel your legs begin to burn and grow tired. As soon as you feel this, let go and *allow* your legs to take up the weight *effortlessly*. This is done by letting go of all *effort* to maintain your body in this position, but maintain the intention and the allow—Will to do so. The goal is to give up the effort and just allow your legs to take over. Drop the mental forcing and trying that you do in your head, neck, jaw, and shoulders.

You will be able to tell whether you are doing this properly because when your legs are tired, *further effort will tire them more*, whereas less effort with gentle intention will strengthen them. This shows us that *trying* is like putting on the brakes. Note the difference in this meditation between *try* and *allow*. This exercise also helps you remember what action without effort is like. When you succeed in this meditation, you will feel your legs harden incredibly and your mind will be very calm. If you think too much about what you are doing, or when you say "Wow, look what I am doing!," you will interfere with the effortlessness and your legs will burn and become tired again.

Chapter 2: Summary

To be free of physical symptoms or physical pathology is not necessarily to be well. Wellness is experienced as a great joy and lightness of being. It is to feel peace inside. Throughout our lives, when we have received hurt or experienced trauma, whether physically, mentally or emotionally, we have the tendency to suppress the hurt and pain so that we don't feel it. This freezes the pain inside our cells and inside our system and even though, through time, we no longer feel the pain, it is still there, *and* it affects our health by numbing our sense of peace and well-being and freezing the flow of energy through our bodies. The reason we hold back from feeling this pain is because we judge it as "bad." We also hold back from allowing other feelings we have judged as bad, even if they are part of our true nature, like sexual excitement or feelings of greatness (if we believe such things are bad). With this judgment of bad, an act of the rational mind, we inhibit ourselves from allowing experience to occur. The secret to understanding healing is that once you accept who you are and how you feel without any resistance, and allow yourself to feel whatever you are holding back, it will clear itself and leave you to feel good naturally and well in the space that the pain/negative emotion and suppression occupied. We often try everything under the sun to "heal" ourselves except face and accept the original hurt and see that it is not so bad after all. Once you feel okay within the original hurt, it begins to flow and that is when the healing and sense of well-being return. Ironically, it is when the pain and emotions are stuck and do not flow that they feel bad to us. Allowing them to flow is to be healed. To be healed is to feel good and at peace. To feel good and at peace is to be free to Love, an act true to your nature.

ESSENCE OF THE CHAPTER

Allow yourself to feel. Don't resist anything in your body. Don't resist your feelings. Don't resist any uncomfortable or painful sensations. Don't resist your thoughts. Allow everything to be. Acceptance is your path to healing.

CHAPTER THREE

THE BEINGNESS

OF GOD

Where shall we start? We will start with the Universal Truth. The desire to live within Universal Truth is so powerful that it drives us ever onward throughout our days, whether we realize it or not. The quest upon which we all embark, the journey we all undertake, is for Truth. This drive is really for the reward that the Truth offers. It is the reward of Freedom.

Yet the path of Truth is not easy, nor is it free of conflict. No other subject or topic has gotten us into more trouble than the Truth. Yet speaking about the Truth is not what has caused bloodshed and unhappiness through the centuries. Believing that the Truth must be guarded and enforced is what creates violence and destruction. Believing that the Truth is something *external* has caused the difficulty. *Defining* the Truth and living by it as if it is a rational concept gets us all tangled and twisted.

It is not possible to define the Truth, hold onto it in that definitive manner, and still experience it. Any definition, rational construct or idea about the way things are, and how we should therefore be, simply limits the nature of Truth.

Yet we can *experience* Truth and *be* full of Truth. We all have the capacity to connect with the feeling of Truth on an intuitive level, and experience it directly. Through that experience we come to know and be as we were created. That is what makes all the difference.

To experience Truth requires that we give up what we adopted and which initially caused us to forget it. That is to release Frmee Will. If we look back to our origins in the Garden of Eden, we see that the serpent deceived Adam and Eve into believing that they could be like God in having possession of "Knowledge." The serpent said: "you will be like God, knowing good and bad." **Gen 3:5**

Believing this to be true resulted in Adam and Eve being thrown out of paradise. Living in paradise is living as One with God. God and the Truth are one and the same. Therefore, the point at which we made a choice that got us kicked out of paradise was also when we started to lose touch with the Truth. This is all due to the fact that we adopted Frmee Will and the desire to be like God in knowing the Truth. This was our error because we really had all there was to have of the Truth when we were One with God.

Before the Tree of Knowledge for Good and Bad, there was pure Beingness. There was no separation between the self and the moment, nor was there any separation between the self and Allthatis (God). At this time, there was pure Oneness. The experience of this pure Oneness is something beyond words. It is something so divine and magical that it melts us into pure Light when we touch it. It is the Garden of Eden.

This Garden of Eden is not a garden of finite boundaries, surrounded by an ivy fence with a few benches and a nice bird bath in the center. It is a state of being for humans to exist in. We have already described some of the attributes of this state of being. Partly, it is to exist with no resistance as One with the Will of God. It is the pure ecstacy of the Truth of who you are and all your splendor. It is also beyond "time" as we know it. So what was the Universe like before the beginning of time?

Our language is limited because it doesn't entirely make sense to say *before* the beginning of time, although we can understand what that refers to. Also, when referring to God, the undefined, the Infinite, it is not accurate to say "God was this…" because "was" implies a definition and a time constraint, both of which are not possible. Yet, for the purpose of this book, it is important to write in *some* way so that we can understand what is being said of a time that we perceive, relatively, as the past. As we will soon see, this idea of past is only an illusion. The phrase "return to Eden" is also problematic because there is no such thing as a return to an eternal place. There is just closing and reopening the eyes.

Before the beginning of time, God's existence was perfect and so beautiful that if we were to perceive it it would melt our minds. It is impossible to *mentally* conceive of this existence. With the most imaginative mind, we can only gain a glimpse into this existence. The rest is a mystery that can only fully be experienced once all control is released. This is the **Ain Sof**—the Hebrew אֵין סוֹף "without end." It is the infinite and undefined.

Contrary to popular belief, it is not true that a human cannot experience the state of being of the Ain Sof. You can, but *it can only be felt*, not understood on a mental/rational level. And since this divine Being (think of the word "Being" in both senses of the word—entity and existence) existed in an undefined state, these words must not be committed to memory as *if this state is that way*. In fact, no concept in these pages is ever to be regarded in that manner, or to be held onto as *if it is that way* and that's final. These words are for inspiration and for the awakening of your innermost knowledge, nothing else. To try to speak of the undefined in concrete terms is to pigeon-hole the Truth. We can approximate the state before the beginning. Flowery analogies and metaphors can brush up on the essence of the Truth. But in all actuality, it doesn't matter what is "right" or "correct," especially because the issue is not at all about *knowing* the Truth. It is about *being* the Truth, *feeling* the Truth. What does matter is that these words trigger a memory in you, a searching within for the feeling that can connect you with the Truth. From the connection to that feeling, you have re-plugged yourself into the source of your guidance, and need nothing external to guide you toward your absolute Beingness. So don't just read. Imagine. Wonder. Feel. Even though you read with your rational mind, let this book be a journey to release you from your rational mind.

Rene Descartes' famous statement from his *Meditations,* "I think therefore I am," reveals a philosophy based in the rational mind. Throughout my discussions with people and in examining current and widely-held belief systems, I have found that for these belief systems, the nature of reality is rational-mind based. This means that their arguments on a certain subject—like science, the Universe, or existentialism—are derived from *the actual belief itself* that our true nature is rational. Ultimately, beyond all fear and illusion, we are not rationally-based creatures. The belief that we are rationally-based creatures became possible when we forgot our true nature (upon the dawning of Frmee Will). This simple point is one of the most important Bottom Line Truths (**BLTs**) of this book and the books to come. To understand these words is to see an all unifying Truth that will enable you to achieve the level of freedom you have sought for a very long time.

Descartes' statement places great limitations on us. "I think therefore I am" is only true within *duality* consciousness in which we perceive ourselves to be separate entities from God. In the rational, there is only the empty reflection of Truth. To use the rational mind is to look back to see what you know, or think you know. But past thoughts are held in a finite, limited way. Holding on to the past limits the experience of the undefined to what you believe to be true, which is what we do with our Frmee Will. We are holding onto our thoughts with our own will based in the past. This interferes with and opposes the experience of the Ain Sof, which is not defined, and which dwells and is experienced in the every changing moment of the now.

What you need to be afraid of is not the unknown, because that's where we live all the time. What we need to be afraid of, if anything, is the known! Because the known is the rigid patterns of past conditioning that imprison us in a prison of space, time, and causation—squeeze us into the volume of a body in the span of a lifetime. When that's not the way it really is. *A talk at the Seattle Center on May 18, 1991, given by Dr. Deepak Chopra, M.D.*

We are coming to a point at which all things defined will melt into the Oneness, like sand castles into the sea, as stated in *The Essene Gospel of Peace*, p. 20, "but as for tongues they shall cease, and, as for knowledge, it shall vanish away."

Thus, *there is a very important purpose* in stating that Descartes' dictum would more accurately depict a Universal Truth if it were written in the opposite way: "I think *because* I AM". This is a deeper Truth beyond the rational idea of his statement. There can only be awareness or thought *of* something or *by* something which truly *is*.

How can thought exist without something else existing before the thought? Where would the thought come from if not from an entity that *is* already?

Buddha said, "The thought becomes the word becomes the deed becomes the habit becomes the character." Since there is no thought without an entity, a Being, to think the thought, we may add to Buddha's statement the following: "Being becomes the thought becomes the word..."

—Yes, okay, but where did this Being come from? Who created the Being? ("Who created the Creator?" is a common philosophical stumbling block, and one of Religion's fundamental questions, which Buddhism answers as "There is no Creator, everything just is, was, and always will exist in a 'cause and effect' world." (A somewhat scientific-like theory about the nature of the Universe) The idea that everything is, was, and will always be is similar to the Kabbalistic notion of Ain Sof, except that the Kabbalah acknowledges a Creator. It is my feeling, and also the gist discussed in the book, *Buddha—Life and Work of the Forerunner in India*, that Buddha, when he became enlightened, was strongly stressing the importance of Brahma, the Creator, to the Hindus, who were, at the time, overemphasizing the other gods of Hinduism, particularly Shiva. I don't understand why modern Buddhism has evolved to choose a "no Creator" philosophy.)

There is a Creator. The Being/Creator is eternal. It is Ain Sof. What has no end has no beginning. This is beyond our rational comprehension. Feel this. It is so pure. It extends into the reaches of infinity right in a tiny point.

What existed before the beginning had the *capacity* to think, yet existed even without thought. Because there is thought, there is an entity, a Being, an am, thinking the thought. If we exist *because* we think, then what happens when we stop thinking? The answer some offer is that we cease to exist, but that is not true. We simply exist in a state that ironically is very difficult for us to understand due to our constant state of rational thought. We are so used to existing within a constant state of rational thought—a perpetual flurry of mental activity—that it is very difficult for us to imagine an existence with *no* thought of this nature. Beyond the rational flurry of thoughts holding onto the past, you enter into a state of Beingness, so that you are what you are. You become a human *being*.

So we can say, "I am, therefore I *can* think." The difference is subtle, yet it is actually a complete reversal, a flip, a mirror image. Mirror images can seem quite similar to each other, can they not? This is an example of such a flip: you look closely, you see they are the same image, yet one is real and the other is the opposite reflection. If you believe that you exist *because* you think, then you will be incredibly afraid when you feel the last threads of rational thought slipping away. If your entire being exists *because* you think, you will have a lot of fear at the **zero point** threshold, a state of mind in which we completely stop thinking in a linear fashion. This will feel like entering into non-existence. Here, at this zero point, there is a great hurdle to overcome. It is the belief that says: "I am because I think," or "I think therefore I am." This is a deep-rooted belief and the source of the primordial control of the ego-mind. Translated differently, this belief really states "I create myself because I think" which means "I am the ultimate controller of my reality." In truth, we do form ourselves by what we believe ourselves to be, but we did not create the source of who we are, nor our essence. That came from God, the Creator.

Your ego-mind knows that if you were to completely stop using its rational thought processes *it* would cease to exist. This is true. But your ego-mind is not the real you. It is your true nature turned around on you which you have adopted by choice. It is the part of the mind with the capacity to judge the self as separate from the Oneness of the Universe.

This means that your ego-mind, which is the same as your rational mind, will never want to stop thinking or exerting some control over your consciousness, for if it did, it would die or cease to exist. The rational mind holds onto control of all that we know or think we know as the Truth. Releasing all rational mind control leads us to the undefined, which we may fear. This stems from the ego-self, because the true self does not know any fear.

A common misconception is to assume that without the counterpart or opposite of something, that something does not exist. For example, light is thought not to exist without darkness, which is the absence or opposite of light. This is not true. Light does exist without darkness. It just is. And what is that? Undefined! Undefined does not mean "non existent" although it can seem like that when examined from a perspective within the defined. (See **Appendix A:** Common Misconceptions.)

Many have trouble imagining a state with no rational thought and no judgment. Yet this state does exist, and it is time for all people on the planet to let go of the rational; it will be an experience for all people of the planet to go through, whether they like it or not.

We have received certain clues that can prepare us for this and other planetary changes to come. Gregg Braden, for example, in his work *Awakening to Zero Point* also discusses this. These changes have to do with the dissolution of the Earth's magnetic field. When this occurs, our ego existence will be challenged because without the magnetic field of the earth, the ego cannot exist. Our ego remains in us because of the gravitational pull of the Earth. The pull that we experience from gravity is due to the Earth's influence on our energy polarities. This is explained later on. If the magnetic field were to become zero, then the ego-minds that keep us aware of ourselves in duality, or indivi*duality*, where we experience ourselves *only* as individuals, would be dissolved, not instantly, but quickly. When the gravitational pull is zero, then we lose the feeling of being stuck to the physical. Dr. Hurtak speaks of this in *The Keys of Enoch*, as the foundations of earth dropping out from under us. When gravity is nullified, then you feel exactly as if the foundation of the Earth is dissolving underneath you. (see Figure 8.)

What does gravity give us? It gives us the feeling of standing on something, the perception of up and down, the ability to feel our physical bodies in a location. When nothing holds you to Earth, you will not feel as if you are on anything. This doesn't mean that you will start to drift aimlessly in space. You can still stand on the ground, if you choose, yet you have no feeling of standing *on* anything. Up and down suddenly don't exist as two dimensional directions, for they were only defined when you knew what down was by the direction in which things fell due to the gravitational pull. Other directions also cease to *matter* as your mind lets go of its defining control. *Infinity* in all directions replace the rational definitions of your body's dimensions. You begin to feel all around in all directions stretching out into infinity. This sense of self is far beyond the ego's identification of self, localized in the dimensions of the physical body. You feel One with the undefined.

Once you embrace the feeling and sense of infinity, you become One with what is infinite. Infinity is undefined, for what is infinite? How can you define it? At this point, you become one with the Ain Sof. Where we merge with the Ain Sof into the infinite reaches is what I feel Barbara Brennan has described as the Core star level in *Light Emerging*. This is also the World of **Atzilut**, from the **Four Worlds** of the Kabbalah.

In the state of undefined Oneness, we are not aware of the self solely as an individual. We know ourselves as part of the collective whole, a part of all that is, the **Ibeall** world.

In thinking about becoming One again and in the complete surrender of the self within the self (giving up *all* control), there can be much apprehension, fear of the unknown, and fear of death. It makes sense to think that the mind, which is based entirely in the known, will fear something that is completely foreign. But don't forget that it's AllGood. When you have faith in this, you can let go. If you were standing on the edge of a precipice where you couldn't see the bottom, it would be very difficult for you to let go and leap off the edge. But if you knew, *knew* without doubt because you could feel it, that below the precipice you would be caught by magical winged creatures, you could leap.

Imagine this: a place of AllGood, where all is One within a state of Love. Allow yourself to actually consider and imagine this. Allow yourself to stay within such a space. Can you feel it or do you rush through it?

The work of Harry Palmer, founder of the Avatar Program, offers insight into how the ego-mind goes through a kind of insanity as it loses control over consciousness. Palmer developed an isolation chamber in which he suspended himself in an Epson—salt water solution, in order to float as one would in the Dead Sea. He was, thus, beyond the experience of gravity. He was isolated from any external stimuli, such as noise, temperature, or light and was completely alone with his internal processes, that is, his thoughts and his feelings. Without the distractions of the physical, external messages constantly bombarding us, and without the normal sensation of the physical body due to gravity, Palmer's ego-mind lost control. One might call this "losing your mind." When they start to lose control, many people panic and demand that they be removed from the situation. This is because the ego-self feels that it is dying. Fear of this surrender process can make it a negative experience, but if you have faith and trust in knowing that when you let go completely of your ego-self, that there is still an existence that you slip back into that is who you truly are and where you have come from.

Palmer remained in the chamber long enough to confront his mind's cacophony circus. Others have experienced this as a whirl of cartoons, images, both fantastic and horrific, and varied sounds, gongs, chimes, and drums. It is much like completely losing all grips on "reality," like traveling through an internal cartoon of complete nonsensicalness. Long suppressed images can arise as they free themselves from the past confines of your mind. The mind goes through this in order to be beyond the control of the ego-self. It is as if you lose your grip on what is real and the conversion process brings you to Oneness, to your foundation where you experience what is true, which has nothing to do with what we often think of as real.

How will you ever experience the glory of unity with all things if all of your beliefs, judgments and mental laws remain intact? However, the way to letting go of Frmee Will is not through the isolation of the body and removing all factors of "distraction." This experiment is wonderful to witness, but is not a balanced way to achieve our highest potential because it removes the body and other physical factors from the equation. The modern monk of the world has the responsibility of achieving a state of grace while remaining within all challenges, standing firmly on the ground, for that is the purpose of the game of life. What kind of game is it, if you remove all challenges and obstacles by going to a cave or a mountaintop in order to achieve enlightenment? Doing so is similar to make-believe. It can feel good, yet it is not real. You cannot go through the zero point into total and complete Beingness without the body because, through all the suppression of the pain we feel inside, our mind has separated itself from our bodies. Lasting true peace is achieved by facing all that is in our bodies. As discussed within Chapter 2, when we resist feelings in our bodies and emotions, we become frozen. Without feeling your true nature, you can only have the *mental awareness* of the infinite and undefined (I AM), *not the full experience felt in your entire being* (I AM that I AM).

Marrying your mind to the "I am" consciousness versus actually being One with the "I am" with your body and mind matching in vibrations are very different. When a person sees the Truth or gets insight to the Truth, they can believe that they have arrived at full enlightenment or have fulfilled their absolute destiny, yet their mind is still not connected with their body. Rifts in the mind-body connection are caused by pain, judgment, and suppression. Although the person understands the Truth of the universe, only when their body and mind are in perfect harmony and synchronicity with the consciousness that is One with the Creator, can that person enter the state of **Adam Kadmon**. This is the original state of existence of Eve and Adam before the fall.

In terms of the Four Worlds of Kabbalah, achieving the marriage of mind and body is to bring heaven down to earth, or to bring the Oneness of the spiritual realms down to the world of Assiyah, the world of action in the physical realm. That means that to achieve absolute potential and fully set oneself free, you must go through life's challenges and succeed in being who you would most love to be. By being in the world as a modern monk, instead of just experiencing a mental I am, you experience the marriage of the mind and the body, which is I am that I am. Wow!

> "Moses said to God, 'Behold, when I come to the children of Israel and say to them, 'The God of your forefathers has sent me to you,' and they say to me, 'What is His Name?'—what shall I say to them?'

God answered Moses, 'I Shall Be As I Shall Be.'" **Exo 3:13-14**

The answer God provides in Hebrew is "***Ehye Usher Ehye***," אהיה אשר אהיה meaning "I am that I am" put in the future tense: "I shall be as I shall be." If you were to ask an entity existing in the state of Oneness what they were, the answer could simply be "I shall be as I shall be," for there is no other answer that wouldn't pigeon-hole that entity (see Figure 9). This is the statement of the Oneness Being and it has everything to do with the nature of time that you experience when there is no resistance. This is the answer that God gave to Moses. Any other answer would have required God to give *all* that God *is* and that would have taken many more stone tablets than Moses could have carried down Mount Sinai, or that he could have written in the Torah and kept it reasonably sized for the chagbah aliyah (the honour of holding up the Torah during prayer services). But in saying "Eyhe Usher Eyhe" God has given us an incredible way to gain an insight into the Truth about God's nature.

God's name, Ehye Usher Ehye, I am that I am, uses the verb "To Be," which is another part of this message: God's nature is beheld within Beingness. The Beingness of the Creator existed before *all* other things. In fact, the Being is the force, the energy, the entity, that gave birth to all of Creation, which includes thought. This also gives us a clue as to why, the *purpose* for which we were created. God's name will help us understand *why* we were given Frmee Will and to where we strive to return.

Chapter 3: Summary

Truth is beheld within the experience of being. It is not something perceived within the rational mind. To conclude that we exist because of our ability to think thoughts, as in Descartes' famous dictum "I think therefore I am," assumes that we are rational creatures. Ultimately, beyond the physical, which has become our reality for so long, this is not true. The physical reality on this dense, gravitational planet gives us the misperception of our identity as purely physical bodies. The density caused by the gravity also gives us the capacity to use the rational mind, so that we perceive ourselves only as individuals. The thought of stepping outside such a rational-based existence can be frightening for it is accompanied by the feeling of slipping into non-existence. This fear is the fear of the unknown.

If you understand that the ego's rational way of being is incredibly limiting and stifles the experience of who you really are, then you can experience the freedom of existence beyond the rational—a consciousness without fear and judgment.

ESSENCE OF THE CHAPTER

Beingness is the basis for all of creation, including thought. When we let go of all thought, we still exist. This is the experience of the undefined.

CHAPTER FOUR

THE BOREDOM

OF GOD

W hen something is infinite and occupies all existence, as the Creator did before the beginning of time as we know it, anything else is absent. There is nothing to compare it with. We see this stated in *Conversations with God* by Neale Donald Walsch:

> In the beginning, that which IS is all there was, and there was nothing else. Yet All That Is could not know itself—because All That Is is all there was, and there was nothing else. p. 22

There is also an innocence of being that is associated with being Allthatis when there is nothing else. It creates a kind of a celestial dilemma, an inability to fully experience oneself. We call this "boredom."

In *The Only Planet of Choice*, on page 82, it is asked "If you couldn't challenge your own mind, would you become bored?"

(The answer is, of course, yes).

"Therefore first there was the thought. Then the necessity to challenge the thought, do you understand?"

Page 22 of *Conversations with God* goes on to say:

> Now All That Is knew it was all there was—but this was not enough...
> the experience of itself is that for which it longed, for it wanted to know
> what it felt like to be so magnificent. Still, this was impossible, because the
> very term "magnificent" is a relative term. All That Is could not know what
> it felt like to be magnificent, unless that which is not showed up.

The existence of God, Allthatis, could not *experience* itself, for it was all there was, and there was nothing else. So what is that? What is this that I am, if I am Allthatis and there is nothing else? What does it feel like? It is just as it is! Without something to compare, it cannot be experienced. All souls and all of Creation have longed for this *experience*. Without that, God is bored.

The dilemma of the Creator wishing to experience itself was the motivating factor creating the opposite of Allthatis. Something opposite or *other* than God's nature had to come to be. So when God existed without anything else, God was aware of the potential to be *something more*. The concept that this wonder, this great Being, God, can become more of what God is, may be difficult for some to understand. In his work on the Kabbalah, *Sparks of the Hidden Light*, Rabbi Moshe Shatz explains:

> "*Everything that is* can be more than what it is now. Later, it can develop
> into a greater whole than what it is now."

The return to the Garden of Eden (a place of AllGood), during the Messianic Age (a time of AllGood), is to experience the Garden of Eden as more than what it was. We experience *the same state of Being*, but *with something more*, an added element. As T.S. Eliot wrote in *Little Gidding*:

> We shall not cease from exploration,
> and the end of all our exploring will be

to arrive where we started and to know
the place for the first time.

When something does not grow, it is stagnant. Knowing this, God
sought to create a situation so that Allthatis could expand to something
greater. Something had to come into existence to reflect God. The creation of something *other* or *opposite* to itself was necessary in order for
the Oneness Being, the Ain Sof, and all that exists to experience itself.

What was created to reflect God, to be that which God is not, and
to challenge "the thought," is our Frmee Will. We have been given the
will that opposes, that goes against, or that is not God's Will.

The Tree of Knowledge for Good and Bad splits according to its
name, or more accurately, alters our perception of reality so that we for-
sake AllGood, for Good and Bad. God's true nature is AllGood. All that
God created is Good. Adam and Eve, representations of the image and
likeness of God, were also created AllGood. When Adam and Eve ate
the fruit of the Tree of Knowledge, it split them from the Oneness into
duality; they each went from having one will, to having two.

The *Tree of Life* in the Kabbalah is a model used to describe the different levels of reality and the nature of a human being. On the Tree of
Life, there are 10 branches called the *Esser Sefirot*, which have specific
attributes, just as the different chakras located on our bodies have different attributes (see Figure 29). In fact, many people are using the different branches on the Tree of Life to represent the chakras and consider them the same. The Tree of Life can be represented on a human
being, with, for instance, the crown of the head being the branch called
Keter (Hebrew for crown). The root chakra is represented by the branch
of the Tree of Life called Malchut (Hebrew for kingdom). In a state of
Oneness, a human being *is* The Tree of Life, for the Tree of Life represents Oneness.

Let's look now at two of those branches, which are called **Chochma**
(חכמה) (wisdom) and **Bina** (בינה) (understanding). When combined,
Chochma and *Bina* create another branch that is usually hidden and
called **Da'at** — (דעת) which means *knowledge* (see Figure 10). True
knowledge of something is the *experience* of that something. For how can
you have true knowledge of something unless you experience it? Thus

Da'at is the knowledge that comes from direct experience. It is also the experience that God and all of creation longed for when there was nothing with which to compare.

The Tree of Knowledge created that which is not in Adam and Eve by transforming their Chochma and Bina from their Trees of Life into two opposing things. When Chochma and Bina are One, Bina is the understanding inherent in intuitive wisdom. For instance, you have the direct experience that Love is the most powerful force in the Universe. You touch with this Truth and know it to be absolutely infallible because you experienced it directly. The feeling of this Truth comes from the intuitive wisdom of Chochma. Once you have a feeling, an extension is understanding what you are feeling. You gain the understanding, for example, from the intuitive feeling that Love is the most powerful force in the Universe. The feeling (Chochma) is received as the basis. When combined with the understanding (Bina) of what you're feeling, you experience Da'at, the experience of what you felt/intuited to be true.

When Wisdom (Chochma) and Understanding (Bina) exist separately, they are in a state of duality. When we became split in two, Good and Bad, instead of our parts acting in harmony with each other, they oppose one another. When Bina (Understanding) is separate from Chochma (Wisdom), *Bina turns into the rational mind*. Therefore, divisive action of the Tree of Knowledge created Bina-in-separation-from-Chochma, which I have called **Bina2** (2 for duality). It became the ego-mind which is in opposition to true nature, because our true nature is undefined, infinite, and it is *based* within the intuitive and feeling nature of Chochma. When Bina is separate from Chochma, it is split from its source and attempts to perceive Truth with its own will, on its own, by holding on to and projecting what it believes to be true. This is how the rational mind holds on to the past and can believe an illusion. It attempts to label Truth according to what *it believes* to be True. Instead of receiving the Truth from the Universe, the Bina2 mind has always attempted to control reality by projecting what it holds to be true.

The *experience* of true nature can therefore only occur when the limiting nature of the rational understandings of **Bina2** (belief systems held in the past) is released. This allows the true knowledge-experience, in which Chochma and Bina are one, to be reestablished as the basis of reality. *You cannot have experience of the Truth while you are still within the duality of the Bina2's rational mind.* You can only have what you believe to be true projected and reflected back to you. This kind of experience of reality is control-based and it is an illusion. Bina2 is the reflection of the Truth, an empty shell. It might have the appearance of Truth, but it is only the reflection of Truth.

Let's connect this with what we established in Chapter Two about the feeling and will centers. *What is received* is equivalent to the feeling chakras. So on the Tree of Life, Chochma can be represented by a feeling chakra, since Chochma is receptive in nature. Specifically, Chochma is the front 6th chakra (the third eye). Bina is therefore the will aspect of the 6th chakra. In fact, the entire right column of the Tree of Life is symbolic of the feeling centers. The left column symbolizes the will centers. Will can oppose the flow of feeling. So Bina2 tends to oppose Chochma. The left column of the Kabbalistic Tree of Life got turned around after Adam and Eve ate from the Tree of Knowledge, which we can call the Tree where Will opposes Feeling. If you understand this, then you will see that the left column is the source of duality in us. However, we must not attempt to push away or to cut off the left column, or the rational process of Bina2. That would not help, because Bina2 is Bina, our true nature, turned around on itself. What we can do, instead, is to accept ourselves as deeply as possible. Then the root cause of what made us feel we must oppose our very own nature will turn around, allowing the left column of the Tree to return to its proper position.

If Bina2 opposes the left column and attempts to project what it knows as the basis of reality, no true knowledge is experienced. True knowledge is not a reflection of Truth, but the very direct experience of Truth itself. Truth is not to be found in answering the question "How much do you know?," and "How much have you studied and learned?" If someone believes that Da'at (Knowledge) from the Kabbalistic Tree of Life means something possessed by assembling pieces of learned information, then I simply ask: "What does this give you? How does it feel? What experience do you gain from this kind of knowing?" The answer is simple. It gives you little and it feels like nothing in relation to experiencing our true nature. Compared to the immense kind of knowledge that comes from being, it is nothing. Desire for this kind of knowledge is a trap.

How is the temptation of Adam and Eve in the Garden of Eden written in the Torah? The temptation was to be like God *in knowing Good and Bad* and the Serpent tempted them. "The serpent said to the woman, 'You will not surely die: for God knows that on the day you eat of it your eyes will be opened and you will be like God, knowing good and bad.'" **Gen 3:4-5**

This temptation to know Good and Bad, which is finite knowledge, is the Serpent's trap and the Bina2 mind implements it. It really has no choice but to see things in separation, because it is separated from the source itself. This is not to see things as they truly are, AllGood, but an illusion.

These questions often arise: How can we do anything without the rational? How would we create technology, use it, and fix it? Do we need to use the rational to survive on the planet?

Perhaps what occurred is that Adam and Eve had no rational minds so the rational was created for them so that they could increase their intelligence and advance their civilization? Like where we are today, with all the technology? Is this true? Can we know what a phone is by direct knowing? Know how to use it? Know how to live and function fully and freely? These are very important questions that come up quite often.

In our world, if you wish to use technology, then you must go through the process of learning about that technology, especially if you want to build it or repair it. This process involves learning from a source outside yourself. If you wish to learn how to speak a language or play an instrument, you have to go through a process of learning as well. However, in terms of being who you are, you do not need to learn, nor must you rationalize to yourself about how you should be. The "shoulds" and "should nots" get in your way of just being. They are the antithesis to being. Even for survival, the best way of being does not involve the rational. The whole process of living rationally actually creates the duality that leads to strife and disharmony that you must then survive.

In the World to Come, which is beyond this duality, there *is* great technology, although not necessarily in the way that we might imagine it. This technology involves inherent wisdom; simply direct-knowing of principles of technology. There is no disconnection from the source, so all knowledge is directly accessible from the collective consciousness. You are one with the mind of God, balanced, and, yes, God does know how to operate a VCR.

Only from the perspective of the rational mind does the world beyond seem like complete nonsense. And it would have you think that way in order to maintain its control over existence.

The potential of direct knowing also gives you the ability to communicate directly to someone without the limitation of rational, word language. Soon we will be connected on a level of awareness that enables us to know anything we wish by having a direct line to Allthatis, in the infinity of the moment. So it won't be necessary to sit down to learn things. You will simply place your hand onto something, intuit its function and allow the Will of One to come through you.

Ever play a piano in a dream and you just knew that you were playing it not only correctly but incredibly well, but you've never studied piano? It is like that kind of knowing. It exists. It is simply opening yourself up and feeling the marriage with the act.

Therefore, of course Adam and Eve knew how to communicate with each other without rational language. Set yourself free. Trust once again in your direct knowing. There's nothing you need to prove. *There are no mistakes in Love.* Fear of making a mistake or of appearing stupid holds us back from the sea of the unwritten knowing. Thus, letting go of the fear of making a mistake is also releasing the fear of what it means to seem ignorant of something that you think you should know. This clears the way for bigger and better things. This doesn't mean you should take no part in the knowledge of the world. It means that it shouldn't matter if you do not know something.

[*3rd Circle:* CaN #5—I do not need to know or to be right all the time. I can make mistakes whenever I wish. I let go of the need to be perfect. I let go of making hierarchies according to what a person knows. I value my guidance as something more aligned with my true nature than my rational understanding.]

The rational mind doesn't realize *how* confused it is, how limited in its understanding and perception it is, compared to the experience of the self that is free from the self. For only when there is a choice to adopt a nature that is opposite to true nature, could the rational, fragmented mind exist. Other civilizations in the Universe have far greater intelligence than we currently do. These civilizations do not think with rational thought processes. There is great logic in the Oneness mind, but this clarity and understanding stems from wisdom, not by having seen things and, therefore, knowing from that past experience, or thinking you know, but by simple, direct knowing in the now.

The rational, Bina2 mind must break things down to their parts so that it can understand. Because of this tendency, very rational people often tend to see the negative side of situations. We all have this tendency when we get very rational. It is part of the rational-ego mind's way of picking on things and finding faults where there are none. Our negative part is always looking at what is wrong and is always disapproving. It will find what is wrong, even if there isn't anything wrong. This is because it is based in illusion.

I once heard from a Rabbi that a King (Hebrew—Melech מלך) is a King because he rules with his mind which also begins with the Hebrew letter Mem, מ, from the Hebrew word Moach, מוח, which means brain. This Rabbi then told me that a fool (the Hebrew word for fool is Lemach, למך, also meaning Clown) is a fool because a fool rules with their heart, which begins with the Hebrew letter Lamed, ל, and the Hebrew word for heart, Lev, לב, also begins with Lamed.

I couldn't disagree more with this Rabbi. There is much wisdom in the ways of the fool, is there not? And the fool is a major arcana in the tarot deck represented by a "0," a very nice lesson in and of itself, because it represents the undefined nature of God.

This Rabbi's lesson truly reflects a mistaken perception of the brain or the rational mind's importance and all the emphasis placed within knowledge of a finite nature (Bina2). Yet his lesson hinted at another message of which he was unaware. A king who rules *over* people is not one with them. He sets himself above them. A ruling human is trying to be like God. That is why, in this example, the King uses the rational mind, which rules *over* the body just as the King rules over the people. A good King rules amongst people, in their collective heart. The heart is situated in the center. It resides amongst the people, as one with them, on the same level. Equality is aligned with Love. So is the fool. And a great King not only laughs at his fool, but sees the wisdom in the comic gestures.

The kind of knowledge that comes from the brain, Moach, and Bina2, is a trap when it is embraced as if it is the Truth itself. It is not experience. Any experience is cut quite short when the rational mind jumps in to examine it, like in kissing, meditating, or making love. The passion, the pleasure, and the joy disappear when we step out of the moment of experience to look at things rationally. If you are being and also looking at yourself being, it makes you double. The two are really not separate. Many people, during deep meditations, remember intense feelings of time stopping, or becoming One. These quickly disappear when they make a mental note of the feeling. "Wow, look how deep I am into my meditation!," the feeling disappears. To focus on the fact that you are kissing during a kiss diminishes the experience of the kiss. The very act of focusing on a state of being in your mind is an act of separation. You cannot take rational note of what God *is* like. The nature of such rational knowing limits it because it separates us from the experience. The state of being is beyond definition, yet it still *is* and can be *experienced*.

We are coming full circle, back to simplicity, back to the joy of being. We will come to experience God, have true Da'at, when the infinite Chochma is absolute and the finite Bina2 is released as the foundation of our physical experience. Until we release *all* control from the rational mind (Bina2), we will not be able to experience the true Bina, which is the understanding of Truth, unavailable to us since the Tree of Good, Bad and Ugly.

Frmee Will is the will created by the separation of Bina and Chochma and is something to which we have grown accustomed and ultimately still hold onto. When we release Frmee Will, we may experience the Bina within the Chochma and use it to carry out our will of being rather than be enslaved by it, the norm of most of our days here on Earth.

When you *hold* onto knowledge in your mind, no matter how wonderful that knowledge is, it will only limit you to a lesser reality. We only *hold on* to knowledge if we doubt its true existence. If you knew something was true, absolutely with no doubt, you would not need to hold on to the idea, because you simply know it is, because you experience it right where it is, in nature, in reality all around you, as if it was the sky you were standing beneath or the sea you were swimming in. When you know it is, you let it be. There is no effort on your part. How can you control reality? Like the child who clutches onto toys for fear that they will be taken away, we become limited to the rational state of mind in order to *hold on* to what we believe because we fear we will be nothing if what we believe is removed. When you let go of *that* knowledge, you allow yourself the opportunity to experience what you believed to be true. When you let go of a belief system (stop thinking it), or an ordered, rational idea, you give yourself the opportunity to determine whether or not the belief or idea is true. This is like the expression, "If you love someone, set them free." If the person is free, will he or she return? Can your belief withstand the test of letting go? Then and only then do you actually have true knowledge, for when you release a belief from the fragmented thoughts of your rational mind, you are able to experience first hand whether or not it is true.

While day by day the overzealous student stores up facts for future use, He who has learned to trust nature finds need for ever fewer external directions. He will discard formula after formula, until he reaches the conclusion: Let nature take its course. By letting each thing act in accordance with its own nature, everything that needs to be done gets done. Lao Tzu, *Tao Te Ching*

Those with a deep sensitivity and/or a lot of meditation experience can more easily grasp the concepts discussed in this book. Let not the person who doesn't understand them instantly be easily turned. We all must start somewhere. Feeling and connectedness didn't come easily for me either, yet I knew that what I wanted was to become more and more aware and acutely feel the Truth. I continue with this intention every day, and it helps me grow. Don't be discouraged. Rational processes are everywhere we go, everywhere we turn, in our schools, the way we think, the way we communicate. This means that wherever we go, they are encouraged or enforced. We get the message that in order to learn something, we must do so from the outside—from a teacher, a book, a rabbi, or a priest. This is the way of learning of the fragmented Bina2 mind. Like all lines tapping into the Internet, we all contain Truth via a direct connection. To return to this source and our divine confidence in our own abilities, there is much unraveling to do, and so we will.

> Without opening your door,
> you may know the whole world.
> Without looking through the window,
> you may see the ways of heaven.
>   Lao Tzu, *Tao Te Ching*

Maharishi, the creator of Transcendental Meditation, goes into meditation for long periods of time and returns with immense wisdom from the Universe. He also brings back ways of expressing the awareness of the Universe using the principles of modern physics. Yet amazingly, those working with him on physics cannot always grasp the complexity, or perhaps simplicity, of certain steps in his formulae. His answer to physicists is always "Meditate." They say, "We understand this step, but how did you go from this point in the equation to this?" His answer? "Meditate!" They persist: "Yes, but…" "Meditate!" he says gently, yet persistently.

Meditation helps us reconnect with God. The meditations in this book are designed to help you reconnect with your true nature.

Whatever meditation you do, it is essential to dedicate the time and the place to realign with the source of Truth within and detach yourself from all illusions of your limitations. Take the time to calm your mind which is in constant motion, pulling you away from who you really are. Take the time to reacquaint yourself with the Oneness within. All you need is provided by having a direct relationship with God.

What is God? What is this entity that was everything when there was nothing else? What is this Entity that is Everything-that-is, all-knowing, all wonder encompassing all and, sitting alone in a void with nothing to compare itself with cannot experience its own nature? What is this perfect existence that becomes bored because there is nothing with which to share the experience of itself?

"Are you prepared to know who God is?"
"Love is God", *The Only Planet of Choice*, p. 14

Man can try to name love, showering upon it all the names at his command, and still he will involve himself in endless self-deceptions. If he possesses a grain of wisdom, he will lay down his arms and name the unknown by the more unknown...by the name of God.

C. G. Jung, *Memories, Dreams, Reflections*, p. 354

The nature of the Creator is to take what is and improve it. The Creator is so divine a state that it must share the experience of itself, just like Love. The natural inclination of Love is to share. The purpose of creation is to give rise to something more—more Love, more joy, more creativeness. That is a pretty good definition for any kind of creation: *giving rise to something beyond what existed before.*

Yet the evolution of the Universe has not yet been entirely achieved. In other words, the purpose of all creation has not yet been fully realized. We are still in the process, along the production line, in which we still hold on to rational thought. It will not be possible to experience Love within the totality of the Universe until enough people, a critical mass, allow the absolute Love to completely enter them so that the planet becomes a vessel of Love. When enough people do flow with this infinite Love, *which each will have dedicated themselves toward*, Love will spread like wildfire. It will spread rapidly, for true Love is very difficult to resist. Actually, it is irresistible. There is no resistance to an energy that knows no judgment. When we see others living within the divinity of Love that flows from them, it is impossible to not be triggered at our very core to remember our deepest longing. Love that is true is Love that is experienced. Then and only then do you have true *knowledge*, beyond doubt, that Love is real and the ultimate reality of Allthatis. The *experience* of Love for all of creation is the World to Come, the return to Eden, the *experience* of who we really are, the "something more."

Love is the *experience* of God.

Chapter 4: Summary

Before the beginning of time as we know it, the Creator, the existence that was then, was all there was and there was nothing else. For this reason, Allthatis could not experience this state of self, because there was nothing else with which to compare. This gave rise to a kind of celestial boredom. Therefore, God created the opposite so that something other than God's true nature would then exist and be comparable. The rational mind is the means with which we are able to experience the opposite of our true nature, for the rational mind only understands fragments, which is the opposite of the all-unifying nature of the experience of Oneness and Love.

We have become trapped in the experience of the opposite of our true nature, which, in part, is to have become trapped within the rational mind and to see things in separation and in a judgmental way—Good and Bad. We have lost the essence of who we really are, believing our present existence to be our true existence. When we release ourselves from the opposite way from our true nature we can then come to fully experience and appreciate who we really are, which is Love. Experiencing Love is the purpose of the creation of the physical reality in which we live.

Within the Kabbalah, Chochma (wisdom) is aligned with the source of who we are, and its balance is Bina (understanding), which carries forth and gives meaning to the Chochma. The Tree of Knowledge caused Bina to turn in upon itself and create the opposite, Bina2, which is rational understanding. In order to have the Balanced Positive of Da'at, direct knowledge by experience, you are required to give up holding onto Bina2, in order to experience what we have all longed for since the beginning of time. The ordered, defined nature of the Bina2 process limits the experience of Truth and must be transformed into its original nature, which is Bina or true understanding.

ESSENCE OF THE CHAPTER

To experience Beingness, it must first be challenged. Rationality, the mind of separation — Bina2 — challenges Beingness. Once the challenge has been set into motion, you must release the rational in order to experience Beingness.

CHAPTER FIVE

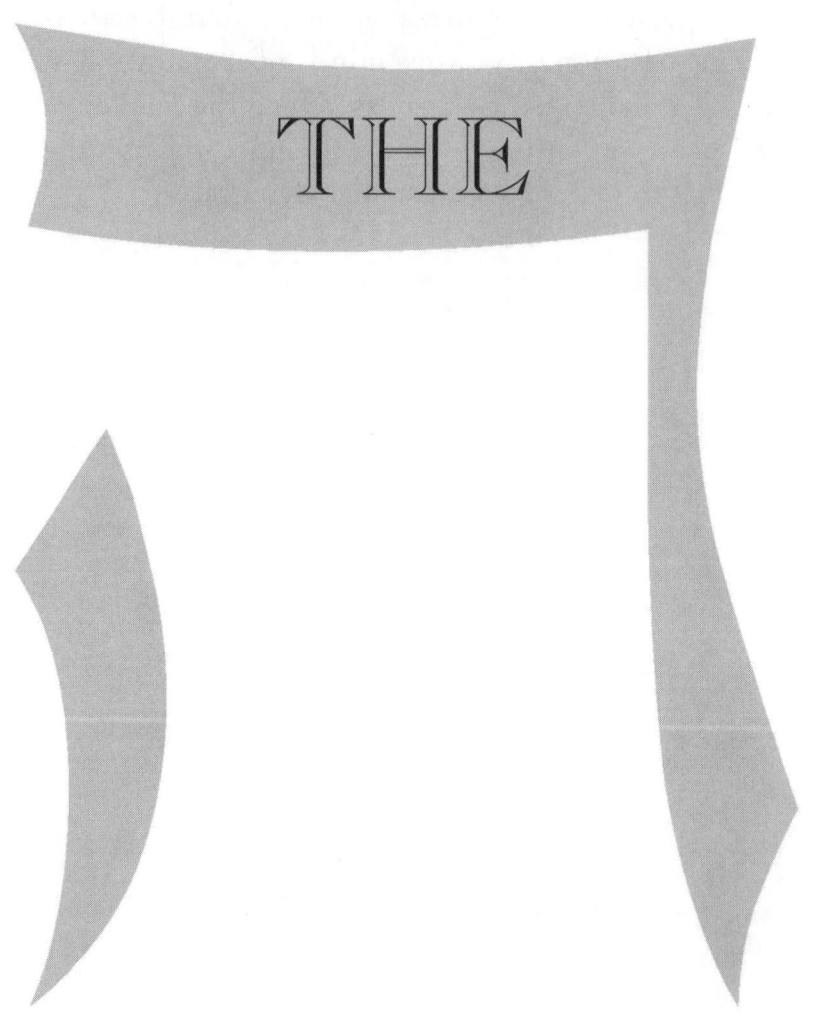

GAME

"Over a period of time—if you play a game with your mind in your head—you reach a point in your mind where you know every game, is that not so? Therefore to create a game in which all parts of you had a choice to do as that part wished, but were connected, it would then create a game in which you did not know the results. Would that not be more joyful?

It was the releasing of the energy of the Creator that created. The intelligence that said; "I know all I do, now I do not know all I do and I know all I do." If you were to tell humankind it is a game, they would not understand." *The Only Planet of Choice*, p. 21

The creation of Frmee Will gave rise to a Game, in which the children of God (us) became divided in two. It is a Game in which we are tested and given the option to choose between Truth and illusion, or in other words, between Love and fear. Because you have the ability to experience fear of your own volition, when you release fear-based

choices, it leads to fully experiencing the nature from which you disconnected and which you forgot.

This is the ultimate purpose of the Game: to makes choices based in
Truth and bring the experience of the Creator to all.

There are many ways of understanding the Game. Throughout the
book, you will see the phrase "This is the Game." Allow your mind to
encompass the different contexts where you see this phrase and see
what understanding you gain about the Game. The better we play The
Game, the more joy it brings and the more Love we can feel for ourselves, others, and all of creation. Can you remember how much fun it
was and how good it felt? Can you recall how it is to be ourselves totally and completely?

The answer does not lie in the question "What is real and what is
not real?" How do you know what is real and what is not? It is difficult to know for sure what is real. What we have *conceived* to be real is
so large. All our interactions are so immense and intricate that it
becomes overwhelming *to try to figure out or solve* what is reality and
what is illusion.

The answer lies in contemplating the question: "What do I *want to
be* real and what do I *not want to be* real?" or "What do I want to be and
what do I want not to be?" That is the question.

A great way to decide what you want to be, is if you feel who you
are and you love it. Another way of saying this simply is *"You choose how
you love to Be!"*

These words can seem so ridiculously simple that you will chuckle
when you understand the intention behind them. But these words convey the way the Creator can have experience of itself. It can do so if it
is given the ability to choose its own nature according to what it would
Love to be. By putting us to the test and separating us from the source,
the very nature of the Creator is being put to the test, for we are one
and the same.

All the souls go through a deep forgetting because they chose outside of their true nature. Forgetting then actually enables us to choose
our true nature which gives power to the experience of who we really
are. If we fully remembered who we were, we would have no choice. It

wouldn't be possible for our fears and judgments to seem real. The experience of the opposite would not be possible. We would have no choice other than to be ourselves. When there was just Being, there was no choice in that and thus no ability to experience that true nature. The ability to choose outside your true nature actually gives great meaning and power when you finally decide to choose *within* your true nature.

Imagine that you have always had a wallet in your pocket. Because you've never been without it, you have no sense of appreciation of that wallet or what it means to you. Well, one day, you lose the wallet. You panic, suddenly realizing how precious that wallet is to you. You search frantically. You plead with the heavens. You call all your friends and curse them for not looking hard enough. In a whirlwind of desperation you think of all your credit cards, your driver's license, money, etc. that you lost. You give up and feel despair. Then you realize that it just slipped underneath a cushion on the sofa. Suddenly, you are *so* happy that you have it. Before, it was just your wallet. No big deal. Now, it is a cherished and prized artifact. And it's the same wallet. (see Figure 11)

The *potential* to forget and choose outside of your true nature empowers your true nature *when* you choose it. This does not mean you continuously choose outside of your true nature. It means that the potential to choose lets you experience your true nature when you choose it. So we see that, *from one perspective*, the original sin of eating from the Tree of Knowledge was not a sin at all. It was a choice. We chose for ourselves, to see for ourselves. It also does not mean that we must experience fear to experience Love. It doesn't mean that Love only exists *because* fear exists, or that Good only exists with Bad. This is a common misconception (Appendix A). It means the *potential* to choose between Love and fear gives power, meaning, and experience to Love *when* you actually choose it. There is power in the choice of Love when there is also the choice of fear. And remember, a great way for you to decide what you want to be is when you feel who you are and you love it.

As soon as Adam and Eve touched the Tree For Better or For Worse, they started to forget their true nature. Their first action to make their previously public parts their private parts showed that they had already forgotten the Truth that there was nothing wrong with their bodies to be ashamed of. In fact, the very judgment of their nakedness as bad has led to a lot of control and suffering.

It is not purposeful to suffer. Suffering isn't fun, nor is it joyful. It doesn't bring Love or happiness. It is not how we want to be. Therefore, *from another perspective*, it *was* an error to disobey the Will of the One by adopting choices outside of the Truth of the One. God said, "Here you have choice between Good and Bad, now do as you will (and please, oh please, just choose your true nature)." As soon as we chose the Bad, we fell. What do you do when you fall down? You pick yourself up. End of story. The purpose of the fall is over once you have fallen. You don't stay there on the ground and say "There was purpose in my fall. I must stay on the ground." No. You dust yourself off and then it is time to rise again.

Inside all the negative choices we have made, we have forgotten who we really are and have become frozen. When we touch the Truth again and have a most powerful release of the pain, guilt, fear, and frozenness, we awaken to the memory of our true selves. This moment, *after* the release of the negative and opposite, manifests the experience for which we have longed.

We are being nudged by all that is around and within to see that the Game that we have embarked upon is ending. The boxing match is over, the bell is ringing, so if we continue to throw punches, we are hurting others and ourselves for no reason. The very fact that there is *anything* separate, divided, apart is only an Illusion. The very fact that even one person suffers shows that we are still forgetting, somehow, somewhere.

This means that when we are living in illusion and choose from Frmee Will as if that is our true Will, we are being controlled. When we live in fear, we are being controlled. To set ourselves free, we must wake up to the fact that we do have total and complete choice in everything. If you do not see that you are choosing to be a certain way, especially if you don't really want to be that way, then you have no choice; you are being controlled by your fear, judgment, and belief. If you choose something that is not good for you that is controlling you, you must realize that you have made the choice. Then you can choose to be empowered.

But if you do not see the choices you are holding onto and believing, you will never have the power to set yourself free. We have choice over everything we believe and everything we do, including our health, professions, and relationships. We have choice over how we feel and what thoughts pop into our minds. We must wake up to the fact that we have choice in everything to be able to let go of the choices. You cannot release what you do not know you have. If you know you hold a rock in your hand, you can drop it. If you do not realize that you, yourself, are sticking a needle into your foot, how can you stop? You cannot. If you believe one of God's commandments is to stick a needle in your foot, then you are being controlled by what you believe. If you understand that you have choice totally and completely, what are you going to do with that choice? Stick a needle in your foot?

You decide how you love to be.

This is the greatest BLT (Bottom Line Truth) of this book. It far surpasses any other truth that I can convey. You are truly free to be as you love to be.

So when you say, "I cannot. I must not. I am unable. I shouldn't. God wants something else of me," (when you would really love to do something else or be another way), you are not seeing that you have choice. When you are not happy and suffering, when you do things that are really not who you are, you are being controlled by your beliefs about yourself and reality. When you see that you can be as you love to be in every aspect of your life (and God wants that for you too), you set yourself free from the challenge, the Game you play with your opposing selves of Good (true nature—Free) and Bad (reflection/opposite of true nature—trapped).

Therefore when we say that you must give up control, that is not saying you must let God swoop down and start doing things for you. It doesn't mean that you do not have the power to do as you wish. It actually means the opposite. Giving up control means giving up trying to control others, situations, and trying to hold power over people. It means ceasing to control how you feel. Giving up control actually means that you have total and complete freedom, power and ability to be as you would love. Allowishing is the will that makes all this happen. It is that simple. Is God involved? Of course, completely, in every breath you take and in your every action. It is God in you that *is* you.

Can you see that there is never a reason to want to be what you do not love? It is also true that you will only want to be who you *are*, for why would you ever want to be who you are *not*? In fact, it is not possible *to be* what you *are not*! You can only pretend. You can only use Frmee Will to try to be what you are not. It is also not possible to *try* to be who you are. You can just be. But we do try, a tendency we have had for a long, long time.

You will only ever *want* to be what you *love* to be and that is who you are.

Therefore another answer to the question,

"What do I want to be and what do I not want to be?"

Is that I want to be what I love to be.

I love to be what I am. I am what I love to be.

I AM Love.

Look now to your heart. How is it that you love to be? Give yourself the time and allowance to really dive deeply into seeing and knowing that you can do as you wish, as that inner calling beckons you! The freedom and the power might seem enormous, and in truth, it is. But don't worry, once you have frolicked and let down your hair enough to see that you are free to do as you wish anytime, anywhere, the sense of true freedom you feel will be light and easy and full of calm and peace.

> [*Fourth Circle*—CaN #4—I AM WHAT I LOVE TO BE.
> I am doing what I love to do. I am doing the work in my life that
> I love to do. It is the work of my heart. I am being what I love to
> be. I see the freedom that I can be as I love to be and do as I love
> to do.]

It is so simple. What you love to be, you are, otherwise why would you want to be it?

The Creator cannot *experience* its creation until its creation (us) realizes the Truth of what it is and then sets itself free to be that. When we realize that we are part of God, the belief that we have Frmee Will, and the ability to choose outside of our true nature, becomes transparent as the illusion that it is. We then realign ourselves with the One way, for there is only One way, One Will, the rest is unreal, illusion.

On a cosmic level, as long as *we*, as a great part of the Universe, believe that we exist in duality and separation, the Universe cannot experience its true nature of unity. The Universe is still stuck in the Game. It is stuck just like a chain is only as strong as its weakest link. All the negativity on Earth is the weakest link of the chain. Because so many of us believe that we exist in separation, and live in fear, we maintain the weak link.

Letting go of the illusion of separation does not mean that we lose our identities, as does a raindrop falling into a puddle. Believing that comes from our fear of entering being part of the collective. We were created to be individuals, but we will also have the feeling of the whole. Each soul's expression of this whole is a unique and creative expression of the divine, just as different stained glass windows let the rays of the sun pass through in diverse ways.

In the return to being One, there is something new, something more that we have never had. That is a nice addition that was not possible before because we were Allthatis and there was nothing else. Just as in T.S. Eliot's statement, "the end of all our exploring will be to arrive where we started and know the place for the first time," knowing that place for the first time is the experience that we have longed for. We will have the experience of true Love, *something that we have never known before.*

Many of us have experienced glimpses of true, unconditional Love at times, yet it is nowhere, not even remotely close to the kind of Love we feel as individuals who are all One and who have all let go to the Will of Love. In this state, we all know that everything is okay. Everything. When everything is okay, everything is wonderful. There is no splinter under the skin, no pea underneath the mattress. The difference is like having the space to swim in a plastic, portable baby pool versus swimming in the limitless waters of the ocean. This space is infinitely wonderful and that is what makes all the difference. All our hardships, the times of pain that we have experienced, cause the wounded part of us to speak in the back of our minds, saying little things that somehow would justify that pain, that suffering, even if we don't mean to. The statements, "Life is too hard. I will never be okay. I will always feel this pain. I will not have Love." Are made by these little voices of our sub-conscious. They plant doubt in our minds. We can sit there for a long time and say, "Oh yeah. It's all good. God is Love and Love is all there is." Yet when we fully confront the doubt and release it, we can swim within the limitless expanse of joy. When there is no doubt, there is no resistance and then, because all negativity and opposition clear, there is an explosion of joy, a conversion into a whole other way of being.

Imagine this for a moment: We have never had the experience of true Love. From within and without, we shall have it. The Love that you experience you in fact *are*. This is to live again in the Garden of Eden. ***Ganallisone***, which is like the Gan Edan, גן עדן, (Hebrew for the Garden of Eden), yet new and improved. Can you imagine the Garden of Eden? Do you have any memory as to the nature of the garden from which we have become separated? Nothing written about it can accurately capture it. It is not a location. It is a state of consciousness that is paradise. My feeble attempt to describe it is:

The most stunning colours. Unreal lights. The deepest joy and satisfaction in the experience of what is all around and within. Glorious sounds that greet your ears. The softest "air." Not a fear or a worry. Just joy and so much lightness of being! Immeasurable peace. Slowness that is as smooth as a floating feather. Feeling small and worry-free about how small we really are. Freedom that continuously reveals itself to you, every moment showing you the great potential for you to be as you love.

There is an ache within me that is deeper than all wishes. There is a deep ache in all people who have longed for Eden, for it is our home. It is a wish beyond all wishes. It is the ambrosia that the angels let me taste which I will never forget. I don't just want a taste from time to time, nor at fleeting moments within meditation or at different random points in my life. I seek this immeasurable wonder to fill me up forevermore and for all people to have as well. This longing is born of the separation from the divine.

To return to the Garden of Eden, paradise, is the World to Come. It is interesting to notice that the place where *we will return to paradise* is also the World to Come. Time is coming full circle so that time as we have known it will merge together into a zero point of eternity. There, the illusion of the past will dissolve forever and the future will blend eternally with the now as the next new moment emerges out of the creative well of Allthatis.

No more bondage. No more scarcity and fear. No more control. You'll be dripping with Love. You won't have to save up or ration. Nor will you have to control it to keep it all for yourself.

When you are Love, you cannot control. Love *cannot* control, nor can any entity existing within Oneness. Control is Love's opposite! Love does not have the need to control, for it is self-sufficient. It has everything it will ever need. You only control when you fear that you lack, so you must take from others. The desire to have control over a situation, transforms Love into its opposite.

The Bible/Torah depicts God as controlling in many ways. The messages are easily misinterpreted: perhaps God is a judgmental God, or vengeful? Perhaps God is jealous, needing all people to worship Him and full of wrath, destroying people when they disobey. These messages are part of the Game, because it is up to us to choose what we love to be true, in order to solve the mystery of who we are. Being the children of God, it is up to us to fully reawaken ourselves and choose what the nature of God is. What is that nature? Is it violent? Controlling? Jealous? Does God punish people for choosing ways outside of Love? Just thinking about that seems absurd. Why would a deity punish his/her children for making errors of choice if that deity, as a gift, gave them the ability to choose?

Perhaps what those portions of the Torah are really saying is that we would suffer by our making choices without Love and outside of God's will. Perhaps it was necessary, at the time the Torah was given, to enforce that idea. Just as for children who don't listen very well, perhaps some harsh incentive was necessary to ensure that people got the message that they would suffer if they didn't follow the Will of the One.

All choices and all beliefs must now be brought onto the table and examined. It is necessary to look at the time the Torah was given then,

and the situation in our lives now, to make a wise, clear choice about
the nature of God and the nature of all of reality for that matter. Perhaps
now we are grown up enough to realize that it is not good to believe
that God punishes, or is vengeful, or jealous. The Game is to choose, and
to choose wisely. The Game is not to accept word for word what is
written in the Bible/Torah just because we think it was passed on from
God to a prophet. All that is written on paper and is finite is a test of
our choice. What do we believe to be true? More importantly, what do
we love to be true?

In this Game, in which we've adopted Frmee Will and the need to
control, perhaps it is easy to imagine a controlling God because we too
are so controlling. Really it is the *illusion* of control that leads to the
need to be in control. From this need comes fear of being out of control, which you only fear when you try to be in control.

> You dream you are the doer.
> You dream that action is done.
> You dream that action bears fruit.
> It is your ignorance,
> It is the world's delusion that gives you these dreams.
> *Bhagavad Gita*

For thousands of years we have existed in a state of consciousness in
which we constantly attempt to control rather than "Letting go and letting God," an enormous BLT. This does not imply that we have no
power to co-create what is. It means that the belief that the more we
try, the more we can make things happen, is an illusion. We co-create by
letting God know what we love and then allowing that to be by knowing it is. We also co-create by understanding the Oneness between ourselves and the Creator.

When you release the fear of letting go of control, there is an
immense difference in how you experience your life. It is like going on
a roller coaster ride. If you are afraid and you hold on for dear life,
before you know it, the ride will be over and all you will have done was

hold on in fear. You were afraid of losing control. Someone unafraid enjoys the excitement of the ride. He or she will yield to it, even try to make it scarier by throwing their hands up in the air during the dips. They get much more out of the experience.

Look now to your heart. Consider that beyond your Frmee Will, beyond the point where you can believe that your control over anything will benefit you or anything, there is only one pure Will. So beyond the point at which you have any control, as in the thought "I must try, I must prove, I must force my actions, thoughts, or feelings", there is only pure *Beingness*, which is allowing. This must be *felt*, because it is beyond the rational.

It is the most spectacular phenomenon to witness as we let go of all control and witness the will of Oneness entering within. You could also call this Higher Will of Oneness our "Higher Self." The Higher Self has always remained deeply connected to you, has always overlooked all you have done, yet it has remained removed from your experience because of the illusions you still tried to control. Your Higher Self is one with God, so naturally it will not attempt to force itself onto you and influence your choices.

When you are completely free, marriage with the Higher Self, that is One, that is immortal, will be complete. I have felt animated by a hand that was not my own, yet when I really let go I felt guided and carried along my highest path, my highest way. It was me and it was not. It was both. In the deepest of my meditations, I have given in to a letting go that was very deep and surrendering. I was able to feel a supreme and divine force enter my body and move me in the exact way I needed to release blockages, knots, and fixations in my body. The presence in me was gentle and with it came an immeasurable sense of peace and assuredness. Yet it was firm and there was no messing around with the other opposing will.

Just as we do not listen to two songs simultaneously, as long as we try to control the things we do and think and feel, then our higher will cannot enter us. As long as we believe ourselves to be separate, the Will of the One cannot come alive in us. This One Will does not exist in harmony within Frmee Will. It cannot. It does not. It won't. The Will of the One is always there in the background, yet it is drowned out like the soft sound of a violin during a heavy metal concert.

We have a great responsibility, with every action, to let go of all separation, all control, and all fear-based behavior. This is the same as allowing the self to Love in every moment. To make Love, not control and fear, our first priority will bring this planet into a higher existence in the Universe.

So what happens at the point where we let go of the last shred and step through **the threshold**? (see Figure 12)

- We are One, wholly, finally at peace.
- When we let go of Frmee Will, we will become the true nature of the Creator.
- When we let go of illusion, we remember the true nature of God.

Thus, we experience what God *is*. Many have said, this experience of God is being God's *nature*, not in being God. It is not in being the entire river, but in being the water. In all honesty, I think these two are one and the same. It is being God's nature, but if you understand what God's nature is, then in being that nature, you are being God. As long as you do not get into the trap that Adam did in trying to be what God is, then you will know that you already are, so you don't have to try.

In this state, when we are One with God, we experience *our* will as being the same as God's will. What we are *doing* is God's Will. This is the paradox beyond all illusion and doubt and fear. It is beyond all that is written. It is the highest form of following God's will. This implies merging with the energy of the Creator. If you say "God told me to do this," then this is not a marriage of your will and God's Will. It is a separation. Much of what we say and do in relation to God is from our perspective during separation. First of all, you do not claim responsibility with such a statement. Think of all the destruction people have committed "In God's name" or "Because God commands it." If someone acts, they are 100 percent responsible for the action. There is no such thing as God telling you to do something that you have not agreed to. That is a delusion. And more important, it shows that you have not discovered the truth about your self and your true Will. When you are One with God, and you wish to act, that is only because God would also like that act.

Our religions have confused the idea of the "Will of God." They have conveyed the idea that God has Will over us, that if we were to do something wrong, then God would take action against us to teach us a lesson. This idea is also imbedded in the belief, "You must fear and love God!" When we think this way, we do not see that there *is nothing* to fear in God. Yes, God has the power to do anything and everything, but the Will of God does not overpower our choices. We must see through this ingrained belief, like all others, and heal.

Many come to believe they must follow "the word of God," as if that is God's Will—a covenant with God. We do indeed have a covenant with God; the choice to completely serve God's Will. But what is God's Will? The idea that God's Will must come from a source external to you, as in texts, is very deep-seated and it has emerged from an ancient guilt clouded by doubt. This idea has made us forget that what we love to be in our hearts *is* the Will of God, for why else did **Hashem** make us in His/Her image and similitude and give us choice? The word of God is actually very limited compared to the actual experience of God. You can read sacred writings and gain inspiration, but the words inspire what is already inside. If this were not so, the words could not have any affect on us whatsoever. If you believe that you must learn what is written in order to know how to be, then you are trapped.

You are not being unfaithful to God when you realize this. You are letting go of those human constructs that have been passed on from generation to generation within the shadow of the Tree of Confusion between who we are and who we are not. Instead of living according to your heart, you will be leaving the empty shell of your rational-Bina2 mind.

In the Hebrew tradition, we know that we must *bring forth*, even *accelerate*, the arrival of the Messianic Age. If it comes *in its own time*, then it will bring great destruction. This indicates that if we wait for the Will of God to bring the Messianic Age, then we are missing the point. The point is that no Will of God will superimpose itself over our Frmee Will. Each of us is responsible for playing our part in healing ourselves and the planet. The **Moshiach** (Hebrew for the Messiah) will not happen unless we make it happen. To escort in the Messianic Age, we must give up control over things, ourselves, and others and allow Love to be expressed as kindness, charity, compassion, and courage, amongst the many things that it is, in every moment. If we await the Will of God then we will wait forever or until the time of destruction that the doomsayers have foretold.

If we still live with control, then *we* will bring great destruction to ourselves. There is more to it than that, but our own will very likely turn against us.

It is time to release the patterns of control and power we have held over each other. Look what we manifest when we live in a control-based society! We create hatred, chaos, destruction everywhere. This planet is no Garden of Eden with us at the steering wheel when we believe we must be in control. And *all* nations have erred. No nation on Earth has been free of error. All have adopted control, power, or greed to some extent. We have all manifested judgment and hatred to various degrees. So please, no more finger pointing. Can we not see that we have all erred, and forgive each other? This is essential to move forward into a time of collective peace. Otherwise, we will continue to blame what we perceive as our enemies who have wronged us, attempting to correct their error through the lesson of violent righteousness.

It is time to help this creation be what it has been meant to be.

The time is upon us *now* and we can do this if we surrender to who we really are. Miracles are beginning to emerge again on the planet. The waters of the planet will flow clean again. People will walk again wearing their robes of many colours with a golden glow. Disease and suffering will be no more. The wonders that are surfacing are happening now. This is the glorious secret of today.

The secret is like nothing we have ever *known*.

But you will remember. That is what gives the joy—the reawakening and saying "Ahhh, so here I am." You have always known. And then you will understand the brilliant complexity *and* simplicity of the Game. Even if it hasn't always been fun to play, in remembering who you are, you will appreciate the Game in its entirety.

The Foot Vibration Meditation

Experiencing Action with no effort, experience the allowance of Being.

Sit with your back straight and your tailbones even and flat on a chair. Allow yourself to relax. Lift your heels off the floor so that you are resting on the balls of your feet. To start the feet vibrating, allow the heels to quickly rise and fall.

This exercise shows you the "allow" intention in action. It also helps you to let go of resistance during action. If you are having trouble getting your feet started on their own, you might have to relax your upper body, your jaw, and your neck and face muscles. Also, it is essential for you to let go of the control around your eyes, for this is the source of all resistance in the body. Allow your breathing to be smooth and natural. If you are holding your breath, it will be difficult to allow your feet to begin on their own. Be patient. Don't get frustrated if it is difficult at first.

You can allow your feet to vibrate at many rates. When you begin they will vibrate a rate that will increase in intensity and/or frequency as you progress. In order to let them begin to move on their own, feel the wonder of how easy it is to do just that; *allow* your feet to move on their own. Don't be the big boss. Experience the will of the body, which is effortless.

When the feet start losing their rhythm, you can be certain that you are resisting in some way. Are you restricting your breathing? Are you tightening your muscles anywhere? Are you thinking, "This is impossible! I can't be doing this!"

Allow your entire body to vibrate with your legs, so that your torso, arms, shoulders, jaw and head join the fun. You will notice that you cannot feel the vibrations in certain areas of your body, which have not joined the rest. These are points of resistance. Accept them in order to help let them go. Don't fight to rid yourself of the resistance. Use your will to further resist the points of resistance for a short time. Make the tightness tighter. This will help the resistance release by doing it more, since you are not judging or trying to push it away. Since it will no longer feel judged, it will adopt the attitude, "You know what? I am quite tired of holding on like this. Think I'll go away." Say "Goodbye and thank you," if you feel like it. You are returning to being an irresistible superconductor.

Once you have gotten this and can allow the legs to do their thing, add another ingredient to this meditation that will take it to a whole other level. You add CaN #1 from *the First Circle*, *I slow down*. Slowing down will also help you connect with the healing essence of Love. Because you cannot try to slow down, you simply allow it to occur. Therefore, as your feet will vibrate at a certain rate, with your allow will, slow the vibration down. You will notice the muscles in your legs get tighter as the rhythm slows and you connect more with the Earth. The vibration of the Earth is very slow. When you connect with it, you become "grounded." Your body is preparing for a transition into a higher frequency of energy and when you have grounded to a deeper level, you allow it to be and your feet will go faster, more intensely, and more freely.

If you allowish these transitions, deeper levels of grounding will occur naturally. As your sensitivity increases, you will feel a higher level coming, because you will feel a blockage releasing. We know that blockages are the resistance we have locked within our bodies. So it makes sense that as one is released, the energy in that area of the body resumes it's flow and restores the nourishment of your energy field on all levels. Then the vibration that flows through your whole body will increase.

This is a very effective healing meditation. It also develops action without effort, letting be and letting go, connecting with the hara and quieting the mind. Because the hara is the will to live, it is the will to be. To be is allowing. Resistance is the opposite of allowing. It is the will to die. This meditation therefore helps to reverse the aging process, as do some other meditations.

SUMMARY AND ESSENCE OF THE CHAPTER

The Game of Life is a challenge to choose between Love, who you really are—Truth, Good—and Fear, who you are not—illusion, Bad.

THE IMAGINATION

OF GOD

B efore Eve and Adam adopted Frmee Will, they existed
in a state in which they were not able to perceive themselves *as separate entities.* How did they exist at that point?

They existed within the *imagination* of God.

The analogy of the mirror illustrates this further. If there
was no way to see yourself then you could not know what you
looked like. You could not perceive yourself. Only when you
see the reflection of who you are can you extrapolate yourself.
But understand, the reflection of you *is not* you. It is only your
reflection, your illusion.

Where are you, when you are mirrored within the
imagination of God?
You are in the *mirror-imagine*.

It is necessary to create this reflection to bring about self awareness. But when you experience your reflection, you are not experiencing your true nature. You are simply coming to understand yourself as a separate entity. The same is true with the adoption of the Bina2 mind, **Gevourah2**, or **Hod2**, the inward reflection of the Left Column of the Tree of Life (see Figure 29). It is necessary to give rise to the experience of who you are, but only after release does the experience begin.

Before the existence of Frmee Will, Allthatis existed in God's imagination. All entities, creatures, formations, and thoughts were just within God's imagination. All of reality and all entities at that time were governed by One Will. Adam and Eve existed within this Oneness Consciousness and they were unaware of what they were experiencing as separate entities. In fact, "they" is not a very accurate word because there was no "they" at the time. It was still only the Creator imagining these entities.

When Eve and Adam ate from the Inward Doubling Tree, they became mirrored. Because they saw their reflections, they could see themselves as separate entities. The dawning of their awareness of themselves began. It's like this: you don't know who you are, you just are a part of the Creator's ocean, undistinguishable from the rest of the water. Then you get the opportunity to see yourself as a drop. You become aware of who you are as an individual. It is the same with a newborn baby. The baby does not have awareness of itself right after birth. It begins slowly to attune itself and become aware of its own existence through its awareness of its body. In doing so, the baby, as it grows up can become a little fixated on his or her body as being its identity. It doesn't really experience the fullness of who it really is, nor does the raindrop. When you remember you are part of the whole, you get the full experience of who you are *as an individual.*

The following exercise will help you understand the concept of entities existing within The Imagination of God. Picture a little creature, like a stick man. Make him wave at you. Now picture a little stick woman. Make her wave at you. Now make them interact. Let the stick people do together whatever most pleases you, whatever brings you the most joy. (Children are best at this type of game because they can really have fun in their imagination.) After a while, because of how much you love this creation you have imagined, you wish these stick figures to have life outside of your will (and yet still within your essence, your home, who you are). You wish to give them the breath of life, *their own life*. In order to do this, you must set them free. You must make a distinction between your imagination and them by cutting the chords that makes your will their sole animator.

How do you do this?

You make a part of yourself choose what *it* wants to create, as if the part had a *mind of its own*. Having a mind of its own sends it into the journey of Frmee Will, which is the journey into the *mirror-imagine*, where entities can experience themselves as separate to become aware of their own existence and identity. When entities become aware of themselves as separate, this awareness of themselves creates a mold, a vessel for the true nature of God to fill. It is as if each entity as an individual becomes a cup for the Creator's ocean to fill. Once all the individual cups are filled, it is a return to the Oneness of the ocean. Yet being back in the Oneness is different now. For this time, *Oneness is experienced in multitudes of individuals*. Aha! The paradox is born! When we realize who we really are, we witness Oneness for the first time *as within* that which was imagined. We will experience it as the individuals we are, One with God, and not just as the Creator encompassing all things alone.

The Creator knew there was some risk involved in letting us choose for ourselves, to establish our own identity. Giving us an additional will outside of the Creator's is risky business—it is playing with fire. "How will they choose? Will they return to the Source? Or will they go the opposite direction?" The opposite direction is away from Love (the Source) and toward destruction. Knowing this is also part of the wonder of this creation. It is not failsafe. It is a test, a Game with the potential for any outcome. There is no guarantee of our success, which is what gives rise to excitement and challenge in a good game. A game without challenge is not a good game, is it? If you knew you would win, would you be challenged?

Now, the other side of this coin is understanding that a good team plays with the confidence that they will win. How could we possibly lose, having been created by the Creator?

It is understandable that severing the connection with God in order to first establish our identities would illicit some confusion and some forgetting, but our journey must return us to remembering the connection. We have a veil placed between us and the Creator that we must dissolve because it is preventing us from feeling the connection.

Let's take this a little deeper.

If we were imagined by the Creator, who wished to set us free so that we could experience who we are...

and...

If physical reality on Earth came to be so that we might experience what we are by first adopting who we are *not* (individuals in separation)...

and...

If we still have not let go of who we are not...

...then

... we *still* exist *in* the imagination of the Creator.

Whoa!!! When you understand this, *when you reach deeply* and see what this is really saying, you can see that you are still not free to be on your own. You still exist within the imagination of God, but you were created by that most amazing entity with whom you are One. You simply have not yet fully achieved freedom and harmony with your true nature, the Source, as an individual identity.

As you wake up to the realization that you exist within the imagination of the Creator, you realize that the only way for you to exist this way is to be Light, the Light of God, perceiving yourself in the space of an identity as you were imagined to be.

When we say, "We have forgotten our true nature," and we don't understand why we forgot, we are not understanding the imagination of God. We *had* to forget. In fact, it was impossible not to. When the Creator set us free, breathed into us the breath of life, becoming awake inside of our identities, we opened our eyes ("then the eyes of both of them became opened" **Gen 3:7**), and there was a conversion process from Oneness into individuality. The process involves forgetting so that there can be choice. The very fact that there is any choice at all means that you have forgotten who you really are. If you had not forgotten and you knew who you were, there would be no choice, would there? You would just be who you are, which involves no choice.

The veil hung between ourselves and the Creator is the veil of doubt. It sits in between you and your true nature. Layers of doubt make you believe more in an illusion and less in what is true. You took a doubt pill. Right now, in this very moment, we remain unaware of a very deep fact about ourselves:

We have forgotten the deepest Truth about us!
We are God.

Simply feeling separated from who we are and having all these ideas and beliefs about who or what God is makes this difficult to fathom. When we abandoned the Oneness and stopped believing everything was Good, we began thinking that we were not in heaven but "down here."

Often people define who they are by what home they live in. We have forgotten that our home is the Ganallisone, therefore we believe we are physical human beings, separated from the Creator.

The Creator imagined Adam and Eve in a beautiful Garden. The best interior decorator in all of reality did not use fake plants, or cheap materials. The Creator's most loved imagination (Adam and Eve, us) deserved the most splendid dwelling imaginable—a beautiful, blissful place where every plant and animal existed.

"And the earth brought forth vegetation—herbage yielding seed after its kind, and trees yielding fruit, each containing its seed after its kind. And God saw that it was good." **Gen I:12**

"And God created the great sea-giants and every living being that creeps, with which the waters teemed after their kinds; and all winged fowl of every kind. And God saw that it was good." **Gen I:21**

"God said, "Let the earth bring forth living creatures, each according to its kind—animal, and creeping thing, and beast of the land each according to its kind." And it was so. God made the beast of the earth according to its kind, and the animal according to its kind, and every creeping being of the ground according to its kind. And God saw that it was good." **Gen 1:24-25**

"And God saw ALL that He had made, and behold it was very good." **Gen 1:31**

If we accept this, which isn't terribly difficult because our planet is absolutely gorgeous, and we unite this with the idea that we are still in the imagination of the Creator, an incredible awareness is revealed. Here for us to devour slowly, savor deliciously and digest reverently (for after a long bout of starvation, you can really hurt yourself if you eat too fast too soon) is the knowledge that...

We never ever left the Garden of Eden!

The Garden of Eden is planet Earth. Technically speaking, before we wake up, we are not able to fully appreciate the Ganallisone. We live in the illusion that where we live is beneath, or outside of, heaven. We can still remember the promise of this blessed Eden. That is why we desire for the World to Come, the Moshiach, the Messianic Age, Nirvana, Eden, Heaven, Eternal Bliss. Yet in *longing for and trying for*, we separate ourselves from every moment where the promise of heaven on earth is available. In believing that Earth is outside of the Garden of Eden, our heart longs for what we think isn't available to us. We will lack the connection of the heart for everyday simplicities and the mundane, because we long to be elsewhere. This causes great hurt, and the yearning is buried deeply within all of us. We need no longer live with the pain, yearning for the memory of time past. We can shed the illusion of separation and reawaken to the Truth that we have always been in the Womb of the Creator. That is truly the secret.

This is a BLT that topples many BLTs. In your daily, wonderful, difficult task of striving to let go and heal, you will never "get there." There is no such thing as "there." Your rational mind confused you. There is only here! Really, it's like walking backward into what you are already. You can say to yourself, "I am here. I am in the place where I love. This is my Ganallisone." There is nowhere to rush to. We are so goal-oriented that it is strange to imagine that all that we want, all that we wish for, we already are. In slowing down and allowing yourself to see you are here, you will be released from your world of trying, which is a world of scarcity.

And guess what?

We are now waking to the time of our true life where we get to experience Eden as it was created to be.

Stepping into this time of your life, you realize that you are not the entire Universe, you are not the *only one*, although that might have seemed the only way to be. When you live in separation, your world *does* feel like the entire Universe, because you feel like the only one in it. There is a great sense of peace to let this go for it is not necessary. You no longer need to try to be like God in order to feel as if you are something. You can wake up to the awareness that what you are is a part of the Creator and *now you know your true self as imagined by the Creator*.

So how is your Beingness when you have remembered?

You will know perfectly well, but if you wish to have a taste, *do whatever you want* and whatever brings you joy. When you get to the point where you have had enough fun and joy of Being in one way, it is easy to move on and do whatever is necessary because you are unattached to the past, to need, to results, to guilt. It isn't possible to tell you what you are going to be doing, but allow this:

- It is in your heart to want to help others.
- It is in your heart to want the best for others, for you love all others.
- It is in your heart to want the best for yourself, for you love yourself.

[4th Circle: CaN #3—I wish the best for all people. I see them manifesting their deepest, greatest wishes, their most powerful Love and Beingness. This is all I see. It is my only reality. I see myself as a part of a Collective Consciousness of other people who feel this way. I let go of not seeing the best for others, or of being in competition with them. I balance this with knowing that it doesn't mean I must give myself to everyone and do anything for anyone, anytime. I simply wish the best for others.]

Once we fully remember who we are, we can also understand the paradox that we are free to be as we wish *and* creation has been played by the mind of the Creator.

So to take another look at how it was written, "We are God" and "We are One with God." Is there any difference? No. Why? Because God is Love. Oneness is very deep. It spans everything. Include yourself with the Source and you will experience the One.

There is, however, a Creator that encompasses all things. We do not because we are individuals. As you wake up to who you really are, you will begin to feel the enormous complexity and wonder of the Creator, that Being who brought all into existence. In this, we remember our humility. It is a paradox; yes we are One, we are God, but we were also created to be such. You did not create yourself. Even though you create yourself as you love to be, which is a co-creation, there is a blueprint for who you are, in your unique expression of the divine's creativity. So when you create yourself as you love to be, it is really an alignment, a return to who you are and how you were created to be by God. You choose who you wish to be based on the Love of who you really are. That brings the joy of being yourself. You can give up Frmee Will, therefore, because it is an alignment with who you are when you give up what you are not.

Now let us look at **Genesis 1:26**

"And God went on to say 'Let us make man in our image according to our likeness.'"

"ויאמר אלהים נעשה אדם בצלמנו כדמותנו"

This statement contains many deep messages about who we are. From one viewpoint, this image and likeness, or similitude, is simply that we were created in the *image* of the Creator to be *like* the Creator. We were created as the children of God to be as the angels are—one with God. It also says that inside we have the essence of the Creator which is Goodness and Love. We are Good.

When we examine the Hebrew terms more closely, another most simple and exciting Truth is revealed. "Image and likeness" simply means that we were created from the imagination of God according to what God liked. What the Hebrew term "betzelmenu," בצלמנו, most accurately describes is the English word "image" as in a "photograph" from the Hebrew Tzilum— צלום.

The Hebrew word "kidmutenu," כדמותנו, comes from Dama, דמה, which means "to compare, to resemble," which is equivalent to "likeness." However, there is another word from the same root with a different meaning and it is the Hebrew word Dima, דמה, which means "to imagine." (Imagination in Hebrew is **Dimyon**, רמיון)

Thus, *that which was imagined* was seen as an *image*, it was seen as very Good. On the day that God created Adam, humans, it is written: "And God saw all that He had made, and behold it was very good." **Gen 1:31.** And thus, there was the wish to give life.

Let's *make* this Being which exists in our imagination and that we perceive as an image.

There is a pun here as well, that works in English. Saying, "according to our likeness" is the same thing as saying, "what we would like," is it not?

Therefore: *Let's make Adam that we see in our imagination according to what we would like, it would bring us great joy. We want to create the beautiful entities in our minds eye, in the image in our mind, that we have imagined up.*

We can do the same arranging of Ehye Usher Ehye, אהיה אשר אהיה, *I shall be as I shall be,* to get even more out of the meaning. We can also say:

"I will be what I would be." This means that God becomes what God would become. The use of the word "would" implied as in "What would you have?" Meaning, "What do you want to have?" This suggests that what God would become, God shall become. It shall be made so.

"God said, 'Let there be light,' and there was light: God saw that the light was good." **Gen I:3**

What God wishes to be, shall come to be. What was imagined and seen to be Good, shall be. According to what is good in God's mind brings joy. God *would* be that. God wishes something to be and creates it so. This wish is the wish of the heart. You wish for that which you love. So when you behold yourself in feeling or in who you are, don't forget that you were imagined to be who you are by a Being that is loving beyond the simple comprehension of our minds. Can you feel such a thing or have you forgotten?

We can also write, "I wish to be and so I shall be." (And also, we can sneak in, "I wish to be because I *am*.")

I choose to be because I love to be so I allow myself to be because I am.

[*3rd Circle:* CaN #6—"I choose a way because I wish it to be that way NOT because it is the Truth, but because I *wish (want it with my heart)* that it were the Truth. I want that way, that thing, that choice, to be the Truth and so that is why I align myself with it". And don't forget the little secret: What I truly wish with my heart is True. (The balance with this is that these choices I make are within Love and within the Golden Rule—"Do unto others.")]

One of my most beloved ways of understanding, Ehye Usher Ehye, is that it is beyond worry and fear and has a very easy going, trusting attitude, as if to say:

"Que Sera Sera. Whatever shall be shall be."

There are no worries. I am unattached to results and thus, I am able to fully create what I wish. This is the state of being One in a world where whatever is to come, is to come. Whatever shall be, shall be.

And therefore, what we come to understand within this sacred name is that to enter within our true nature we must release the past. This doesn't mean that we must forget the past as if it didn't happen. It means we can see that it is okay to release the past and trust in the goodness of Allthatis to know that it needn't happen again. And if it does, it will be okay, because we will find the strength to be okay. However, the most important thing to become aware of is that we have a tendency to dwell in the past. This is eating up the peace of Ehye Usher Ehye and any potential for change. Let us all become aware of this now as we release the ties to the past. Let us be aware that we hold on to our past fears thinking that if we control them it won't happen again. Ironically, holding on leads us to the very same end.

Let's look now at the beginning of the second chapter of *Genesis*.

"Thus the heaven and the earth were finished, and all their array: By the seventh day God completed His work which He had done, and He abstained on the seventh day from all His work which He had done: God blessed the seventh day and sanctified it because on it He abstained from all His work which God created to make: These are the products of the heaven and the earth when they were created in the day that Hashem God made earth and heaven." **Gen 2:1-4**

It is written *four* times that all the work had come to completion by the seventh day. Yet, strangely, right after this, in the very next verse it is written:

"Now all the trees of the field were not yet on the earth and all the herb of the field had not yet sprouted, for Hashem God had not sent rain upon the earth and there was no man to work the soil." **Gen 2:5**

Isn't that strange? It is written *after* God had created the heavens and the earth and all the bushes of the fields and all the vegetation came to their completion that, "all the trees of the field were not yet on the earth and all the herb of the field had not yet sprouted." **Gen 2:5**

To further add to this mystery, in the previous chapter, it is written:

"So God created Man in His image, in the image of God He created him." **Gen 1:26** And also: "And God saw all that He had made, and behold it was very good." **Gen 1:31**

If Adam was created, why is it then written after: "and there was no man to work the soil," as if Adam had not yet been created?

This portion of the Torah shows us first all is imagined by the Creator, only *imagined*, which is like existing in a void. Then creation began to unfold *as it was imagined, within what was imagined,* and Adam had Frmee Will. The blueprint that Hashem God created for Adam to become alive is already laid out in God's imagination. It is encoded in his genetics. What Adam then chooses *is* Adam's own choice, even if it is encoded within him to follow a certain predisposition. Yet with Adam's consciousness now *within* God's imagined creation, that which Adam decides to do is Adam's choice, or so it seems to Adam. That is the important part. It is not for God to decide at that point, but for God *as Adam* to decide. That is what the Game is all about—God being put to the test as us, the Adamic people, created in the image and likeness of God. What a Game!

"And Hashem God formed the man of dust from the ground, and He blew into his nostrils the soul of life; and man became a living being." **Gen 2:7**

First there was creation within the imagination of the Creator. *Then* it became manifest in the physical realm. First it was imagined, then it was flipped over into the reverse (mirrored) and the entities that were imagined opened their eyes *within* the creation and were awakened into that which was imagined. (Really, it's all happening at the same time.) This shows us a most deep understanding; that the Universe, Creation, is in a state of becoming. (Meaning that things have not already happened, predestined, and we have no Free Will, but rather God did imagine the Universe to be a certain, wonderful way and we create it so by choosing it to be so in each moment. This is a marriage of our Will and God's Will and is the essence of the word "co-creation." (We can still also choose outside the Oneness of God's imagination and create the world negatively. This is not a marriage with God's Will. The marriage occurs when we create Heaven on Earth.))

This gives us an insight into the nature of something about which we have quite a backward idea. Our idea actually reverses time.

This makes perfect sense, doesn't it, considering that everything else we perceive in the physical is reversed, flipped, or the negative? This

implication is very deep and far reaching. It has to do with our consciousness being based in Frmee Will. Because we hold onto past ties,
our consciousness is in the past. Having our consciousness stuck in time
causes us to perceive it in reverse. We created a negative vortex by opposition to the Will of Oneness and then by believing that is real. So to us
the past seems to be reality, as does everything rational. Saying something like "We are entering into what has been created" doesn't make
sense because we have forgotten the **Time of Forwardness.**

"You correct your previous missteps by stepping forward. This process
is actually incomprehensible in temporal terms, because you return as you
go forward." *A Course in Miracles,* pp. 20

That is why the coming of the Messianic Age and the World to
Come is actually the return to Eden. The secret also lies in understanding that every single second of every hour of the last 6000 years has
been for the purpose of making God's imagined creation come to life.

"And God proceeded to bless the seventh day and make it sacred,
because on it he rests from all his work that God has created *for the purpose of making.*" **Gen 2:3**

Jews use this portion of the Torah every week to bless the wine of
the Sabbath meal. The Torah says God created everything on the first
six days of creation. On the seventh, God rested. Now, we are at year
5763 according to the Hebrew calendar. Six days of creation—6 x 1000
years of our existence since Adam and Eve began the state of duality.
Each day of creation, according to the Kabbalah, corresponds to 1000
years of life in the physical. We are nearing the seventh millennium right
now. The seventh day is the day of rest. The seventh millennium is the
Messianic, the great Age of Rest and peace. In the great Age of Rest,
the struggle is over, the sweat of the brow wiped, and we get to *enjoy*
the creation that existed all along for the *purpose* of making. The thousands of years of existence within the imagination were for the purpose
of *the time we are now entering.* Just as all the work that goes into making

beautiful fireworks is for the purpose of beauty and enjoyment, the Age of Rest is the age in which the Creator *enjoys* the experience of the product of that work. It is the Great Age of Experience.

The Messianic doors are now open to us. Rabbi Shimon Bar Yochai, author of *The Zohar*, one of the most important books on Kabbalah, said that the gates to the Messiah would open in the year 5761. All we must do is stop doubting. All we need to do is awaken.

When connected with the celebration that will erupt throughout the Universe as we are born(e) into freedom and into the actuality of what we have all longed for, you will feel as if rockets are traveling through your mind. God bless that day and may it come upon us with great smoothness and peace for all people of the planet.

Okay. So what about Frmee Will in this context? We still have the choice to do as we wish, do we not? Yes. When we realize this fully and completely and that those choices are between Truth (Love) and illusion (fear), then we stop making such choices. It is then that we wake up to embody who we are and can carry this planet into the realm of AllGoodLove. It is then that we step aside to allow the imagined Goodness to unfold. We stop resisting.

In the movie *Forrest Gump*, perhaps Forrest Gump says it the best, when he stands at the grave of his beloved Jenny:

"I don't know if Mamma was right, or if it's Lieutenant Dan. I don't know if we each have a destiny or if we're all just floating around, accidental, like on a breeze. But I think, maybe it's both? Maybe both are happening at the same time."

The Creator understood that in order to give birth to an existence quite different from the imagination, His/Her state of consciousness would have to change. This has to do with how we exist within the mirror-imagine, seeing ourselves reflected. Also part of the plan, however, was for those Beings *to fall asleep* to their true nature.

Chapter 6: Summary

The Creator had imagined Allthatis. All souls, therefore, existed only in the Creator's imagination. In order for imagined souls to experience themselves, which means to exist with an identity of their own, the souls had to be released to choose for themselves and experience themselves. For thousands of years, the goal of individuality has been very difficult and, at times, very hellish, because we still haven't quite grasped how to return to the sea of Love, where we originated, and exist within our identity. This creates a great challenge where we, as souls on Earth, created in the image and likeness of God, are being tested. We are also created as individuals to experience the imagination that was so beloved to God.

ESSENCE OF THE CHAPTER

God imagined us to be just as we are and we are, now, able to enter into the full experience of what was imagined.

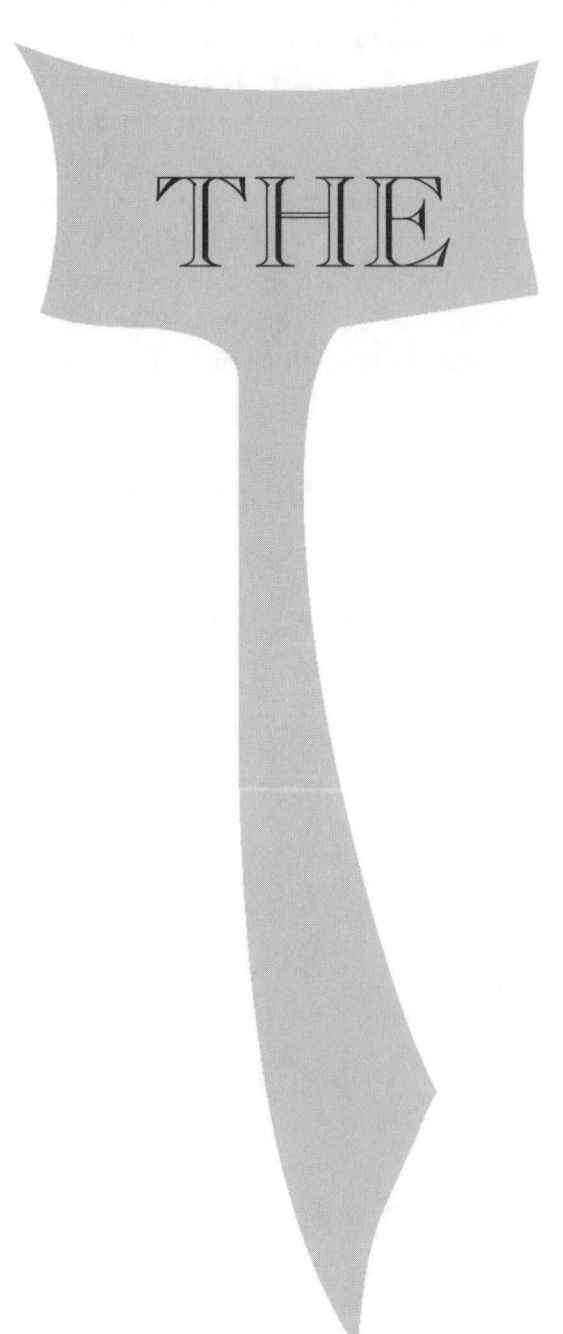

THE

DREAM

"It is a good viewpoint to see the world as a dream. When you have something like a nightmare, you will wake up and tell yourself that it was only a dream. It is said that the world we live in is not a bit different from this."

Hagakure: The Book of the Samurai
By Yamamoto Tsunetomo
Translator: W.S. Wilson

"So Hashem God cast a deep sleep upon the man and he slept"
Gen 2:21

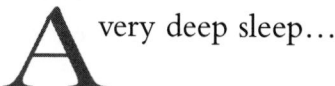 very deep sleep…

The question is: Does the Torah ever say that Adam awakened?

The answer is no and there is a very good reason why.

He hasn't.

Neither have we!

"What is seen in dreams seems to be very real. Yet the Bible says that a deep sleep fell upon Adam, and nowhere is there reference to his waking up. The world has not yet experienced any comprehensive reawakening or rebirth." *A Course in Miracles,* pp. 18

Even though we might have the idea the thought that we are awake, the inner question, sometimes deep and buried is, "Is this real or just a dream? Am I awake or asleep?" You will observe this as you near your time of awakening, meaning, you will become aware of how you have been asleep. We are still within Adam's dream.

The dream state that we have fallen into can be somewhat of a nightmare, is that not so? Letting go of all control and waking up to our true nature is to wake up from a nightmare. Saying life can be a nightmare does not mean it always is, because life can also be quite wonderful and joyful. But when we awaken to a time of bliss and ecstasy that surpasses all the joy and Love that we have experienced in our fallen state, we realize that we have been living in a nightmare-like state. Limited in our perception of reality, we are unaware of our capacity and true nature, so laden with guilt.

If you injured yourself terribly in a dream and lost an eye, an arm, or all your teeth fell out, that is like a nightmare. It feels so real that even when you awake, you remain upset until you become aware that it was only a dream! Then you behold your arm, use your sight with wonder and feel your teeth with such newfound appreciation. "Ah, thank God!"

To wake up from a nightmare is not to wake up to a well-defined and concrete reality, for what is real? You wake up to the true nature of the Universe and the Source, which is an energy-experience of pure potential and creativity. You wake up from being *asleep* and dreaming to being lucid in a dream-like state. You're still in a dream: *Your dreams come true!*

When you fall asleep, you move past the veil of your conscious mind (that is in control) into a deep inner world of endless and wondrous possibilities. That thread takes you into this other world, takes you past the three dimensions of this world. The process of waking up to

Oneness and giving up Frmee Will is the amazing process of merging your inner world of dreams with your wakeful, conscious everyday state.

The separation which exists now between these two states of being is rather interesting because it is a rift between two worlds that are not One. These worlds are still separated by the veil of sleep. What we are near to experiencing collectively in our days now is a merging of the inner, deep world of sleep, magic, and limitless possibilities with the outer wakeful state. So we will experience reality as if in a wakeful dream in which anything is possible, as long as we allow ourselves to unfold the dream as we love, and do not try to force or resist it. Hint—Even if dreams appear scary, or something that we don't really wish happens, to not resist is the secret. Let the dream be. Then it won't have to manifest in any way, shape or form, because you have already triumphed and shown, by your acceptance, that you do not need a tough lesson.

Because the inner world of dreams, with its limitless possibilities and undefined nature, merges with the wakeful state, waking up to Oneness is like a *lucid dream*. This is a great way to touch or imagine the experience of Oneness. In lucid dreaming, you do not have rigid *control* over anything. You imagine the ideas you want to be possible, as in the flow of a dream. This dream, however, is not just an ordinary dream, but a lucid dream for in lucid dreams, you can *gently direct* what happens based on what you allowish. Being *lucid*, you are in a state of awareness. You are not asleep to your true nature. Your eyes are bright with the direct vision of Allthatis. Just as you did with the stick man and woman, you cannot try too hard in a lucid dream or your imagination will be clouded and you will experience the opposite, or other weird things, rather than what you wish and love to be.

In this lucid dream-like state there is no rigid control, merely a way of floating from gorgeous moment to gorgeous moment with only the heart's intention allowishing what will be. We can therefore tie this in to better understand the statement in Chapter Two: "One way to know which parts of you are affected by resistance is to see which parts of you are tired when you wake up in the morning." This is because when we sleep, we relive the outer, conscious world in a deep inner world of amazing, bizarre, and sometimes scary dreams. We live the reflection, so to speak. Because we are not in control in our dreams, the control, stress, and tension that we build up in our conscious state unwinds in our sleep. When we fear, we control and resist, yet sleep is only truly nourishing when we release control. This is easier in dreams when you allow the dream to unfold to its furthest degree. Then there is a deep letting go. When we are so wrapped up in control, then sleep nourishes us less and we wake with parts of our bodies still tired.

So when we discuss the lucidity of a dream, the heart does not live resisting what it doesn't want, but simply has a clear focus allowing what it does want. This effortless state burns up no energy, nor does it require the unwinding of sleep. We dwell deeply in what we do not want when we are afraid. How much do we live trying to prevent events we do not want instead of simply focusing on what we do want and allowing that to happen? What we do in our fear is funny.

Imagine that you are dreaming. You are not in rigid control over anything, for you cannot be. You are creating things as you love them to be and then allowing them to be. This is allowishing. This is especially important with the people of your dream. You cannot control how a person will interact with you, nor what choices they will make. You are just responsible for allowishing what you love with yourself and how you'd like to be with them. You allow them to be, but you are not attached to the results of how they are. Que sera sera, whatever shall be shall be. There is no fear, and you are so fulfilled by the very state of allow (which is a joyous state) that there is no forcing too much and screwing everything up. You are receiving AllGood, therefore you have the freedom and the power of absolute clarity to create things as you would love them *because* that is AllGood. Scenarios, images, pictures begin to paint animated stories in your mind. Recalling your lucid dreams will help you to understand this kind of experience. In this way, you can do as you wish on the level of intention beyond Frmee Will, an absolute knowing of what shall be done. You simply allow your intention to be carried out. Your heart senses "This is what I want. This is what I have always wished for. And so it shall be. I know this beyond all doubt." This pure knowledge is effortless because it is doubtless. And what makes it doubtless is because it is pure. You are not attached to it happening, thus you need it not. Because you don't need it, there is no fear of it *not* happening, so there is no need to use the Will of control to force it to happen. You are pure with the wish of your heart and the clarity of seeing it so. "What I love to be shall be." Pure intention is the power of creation.

Imagine that in your dream you begin to judge something as Bad. This will make you resist, disrupting the stream of allowing what you wish to happen. Suddenly you begin to get wrapped up and stuck in what you do not want to happen. This is how we have lived within our dream of life, the dream that we are still stuck in which we try so hard to control. We live trying to control and stop what we do not want, rather than allowing what we love.

> "Row row row your boat, gently down the stream.
> Merrily merrily merrily merrily, life is but a dream."

You row your boat *gently*, meaning without trying too hard, so that intention is married to the will of the heart. The heart is very gentle, for it knows that forcing things cannot make things happen as we truly wish. "Down the stream?" Along the flow of consciousness within the dream of what is already unfolding, as imagined by God and unfolding now through you, just as a surfer uses his or her hands to move with the flow of a wave. This is aligned with "Whatever is to be, can be. It is Good. Que sera sera. Ehye Usher Ehye." No attachments. No need for a certain way. One is within the faith of this AllGoodness.

As you move from place to place within your lucid-dream life, how "awake" are you? The more we try to be in control, the more we become attached to results and judgments, the more this causes us to forget our true nature and live in fear, thus clouding our perception, smogging us up in doubt and leaving us quite asleep as the day goes by. What a paradox! When you are able to gently direct a dream to unfold, your will is completely effortless. So much trust and faith is generated when one lives this way. So much worry and fear drops away to leave a boat floating gently with the current of the stream, merrily of course.

In this way, you are awake and able to appreciate the day and the items of your dream, instead of asleep as life passes you by, focusing inward on your fears and worries. If the river forks, which way do you go? You can gently push the oar in your preferred direction or you can let the boat choose and see what happens.

As you wake up to the Will of God by surrendering control in your dream, you will begin to witness the dream as if *you* are doing nothing *all on your own.* This doesn't mean that you are doing nothing, but rather what you do is not a result of your efforts alone. You are empowering and allowishing what is unfolding by the hand of the Divine. This is a paradox. In comparison to how we have toiled and the amount of effort through the ages, this state is effortless.

"By the sweat of your brow shall you eat bread until you return to the ground, from which you were taken." **Gen 3:19**

Each moment that you let go of trying to control your dream, it unfolds beautifully and effortlessly. Your intention is saying, "What is around me in my life is good. I can allow it to happen. I need not control or resist." You can thus be present in the dream and enjoy it as it truly is, which is Good. And isn't that what life is all about?

What is extraordinary to witness and understand is how quickly the world "switches" depending on your point of view. And the world is the dream, so of course it *can* switch right away, it is fluid in that way and that is also how powerful our mind is to affect the reality we experience. We can call this instant Karma manifestation. What this means is that as soon as you see the World as AllGood, then the world *becomes* that for you. The things that enter your space are good, enjoyable, entertaining, fun, and you love the ride you're on, you love life. If, for some reason there were still fears, judgments, and resistances latent inside of you and you started to fear the world or worry about the outcome of the future, then an instantaneous switch would cloud out the world into black and white, good and bad. Is this the same world? Well, yes and no. Yes, because you are still in the same body and identity. It is the same world in that sense. But also, no, because one world is AllGood, and the other is Good and Bad, and these are completely two different worlds.

So what does this also tell us? It tells us possibly one of the most important secrets in life—that we create the World according to what we believe about it. If we believe it is AllGood and so are we, then we set ourselves free to just Be who we are and enjoy that. Life is Good. If we believe the World is Good and Bad, and so are we, and that we cannot trust ourselves to know how to be without some external guidance (we believe we need), then we see the World as Good and Bad, and it becomes that way. We will have ups and downs, highs and lows, mania and depression, and life will be a balance of extremes, like one foot in one hot bucket, and one foot in another cold bucket. Is that a balance? No. The water has to come together and we have to put our feet in the same bucket.

So this is the power of our choice and of our "Free Will." When we love the world and see unconditional Goodness, in things and in people, the World is Goodness. (This is really the realm as the world *truly* exists, as it was created and observed by the Creator as being AllGood, which can be observed effortlessly.) And seeing the World as Bad and Good, we create it so, the World comes at us and gives us the experience of life as Bad and Good. This *only* occurs during moments when we fight with the flow of I AM in the moment, when we try too hard to be in control, to resist or fight something we have judged as Bad. This is fighting the flow of the waters of the Tree of Life. This is resisting. Therefore, of these two choices we have in any given moment or situation, one is the choice of just Being, which is not really a choice at all, just a Being. And the other is just a resistance, a non-being. It is not choosing to do or be *something*, it is choosing to not do or not be something, which is not really a choice either, just a holding on against something thought to be Bad. So really, there is no choice, there is just letting go of control. Just to Be, or not to Be, isn't that the question, as Shakespeare told us? Don't take my word for it. See what happens as you move through the day allowishing rather than trying, rather than following what you believe you must.

"God said 'Let there Be Light...' and there was Light." **Gen I:3**

Let is the operative word here. This is how the Will of One creates with allowishing, for to let is to allow and to allow is to be, and to be is I am—all according to how I love.

In order for us to wake up from Adam's dream, one of two things must occur. Enough souls on Earth must realize that they are in a dream that is not aligned with their true nature. ("You dream you are the doer. You dream that action is done." *Bhagavad Gita*) This means they must surrender the illusion and wake up to their true nature. This is the same as accelerating the arrival of the Messianic Age. For individuals to touch with pure Beingness takes great pioneers with much determination and dedication. Contrary to our belief that the Messiah is one person, it is many people who will adopt Messianic consciousness. Then, when a few show the way, many will follow. When enough people do this, the light that shines will become strong enough to punch a hole in the collective belief of being in control (apart from God.) Then everything and everyone will naturally follow. This has an impact on the whole Universe, for all becomes One again. Negative energies on Earth are released. And since planet Earth is a part of the whole and is the weakest link, when Earth is released, the whole Universe will be too.

Then, we will wake up to the time which is always, or Onetime. Every moment feels as if it is the best moment of your life because you have no thought of any other time. You do not pine for the past or run from it. You have no anxiety or resistance to what is to come. In this state of no-fear, each moment is the best of your life and you can absorb it for what it is. There is no sense of time slipping away, as with the sands of our hourglasses that pour away our vitality each moment we run from the past.

You are married to eternity and you are an immortal soul and you will never have to die again, for you have awakened from the amazing dream that enabled you to experience what you are not. Death and mortality are a part of the experience of being trapped in the physical, for Hashem God said that we would die when we touched the Tree of Mortality. When we touch that tree, our rational minds resist and contradict the Will of our hearts. It is time to emerge from this dream in which death, and forgetting through rebirth, facilitate experiencing what you could never experience being a soul beyond limitations.

What does it feel like to awaken to Onetime? It feels so good. You wake up to the realization that you can just BE yourself and that is Good, and never shameful. When we see how much our strength and lightness of Being are sapped worrying about our intention and whether or not we are good or bad, we get a glimpse of the freedom that comes from finally and completely feeling and experiencing that we are Good, period! When we know without doubt that we are Okay, then we don't worry about ourselves. We don't get so stuck in ourselves. Remember that getting stuck in worrying about yourself only amplifies your sense of self that is illusory. Getting stuck amplifies your self-con-science, which is your ego, which we also experience as guilt. This guilt makes it very difficult to feel good about ourselves. We constantly try to fix ourselves, perfect ourselves, when the secret lies in saying "I don't need to do a thing. I am Good as I am." This is acceptance. Acceptance is the willingness to receive. Guilt is the exact opposite: the refusal to receive the joy, pleasure, and Love of God. This of course is a very deep Truth. Acceptance is not to say, "I am good as I am when I am judging and controlling." Acceptance means: "I am truly good in my original nature. When I see this, I transcend the control and judgment that comes from me believing that I am not good."

Not needing to monitor your every thought, move and action also leads to intention without resistance. When we do something that feels so right-on we just *know* that it is happening according to what we intended. There is no resistance. What a feeling! It is like throwing a bas-ketball through a hoop when you feel it so much that you *know* it is in, like taking a shot in golf, billiards, or archery, and you feel so connected with your game-device that there is a perfect marriage between feeling and knowing. In Karate, the mind is clear and empty as in the symbol of "Kara," which is an empty circle, and the hand, Japanese "Te," reacts without thought. There is a direct connection between will and action. Playing an instrument you can be so enthralled with the music that you *become* the music. Whoa! We can all imagine the power of such an experience, even if it has been a while since we lived one. Imagine now living each and every instant so that you are so enthralled with what you are doing that you no longer are really "doing" it at all. You are *Being* it. You're definitely not examining each move on a mental level. This is the marriage between Being and doing. This is the experience that we always longed for.

The way we live in illusion and this duality dream is too defined and belief-oriented. Isn't that ironic? Having a controlled mental picture of how we think we must be is really the delusion. It is the opposite of how we dream lucidly, when we align our hearts the way we would love to see Truth. It is much less concrete, ordered and limited. It is much more infinite, as in *not finite*, as in *not defined*. The dream that we live in our physical lives is desolate compared to the splendid state of Oneness and Gan Edan; it is as if the colours, the imagination, the creativity, the joy, the lightness have been removed. The dream and how we live are heavy, half-coloured, unimaginative and limited. All becomes Black and White (Good and Bad/Right and Wrong).

Can you recall your childhood dreams? You felt them in your heart when you were young and in close touch with your true nature. During that innocent phase, life was a pleasant, lucid dream to so many of us. Yet we chose to give up that innocence and accept a great challenge. Once we overcome the needs within our self-imposed resistances and challenges, all that we wanted to be true in our dreams will be true. Does imagining your dreams coming true send sparks of joy through you? Can you feel what this does to your heart when you allow yourself to *know* this to be true?

Guided by Dreams
by Moshe Daniel

The first time when you fell
Or were hurt and not well,

It punched then a whole,
In the One in your soul,
Then a leak-in started to swell.

This leak grew 'til it got big,
So large 'bout the time you're a kid,
In the teens of your days,
It's ego-time ways,
To fight and rebel and to rid.

And what didn't agree,
Since you were free guiltily,
You let it go,
Away it could so,
And lost sight of the thought of that Be.

And chose other means,
Guided always by dreams,
Did you know it that when
It's AllGood in the end,
Come true the wishes in streams?

Free I become as I see
Not a thing comes around forced by me,
It is all by the hands,
From the Ones in the Stands,
Que sera que sera, 'kay siree?

Holy weird, this is strange, guess I'm blocked
Yes you are in your head are the rocks,
That you drag here and there,
Building strength from weight-bear,
Let go of ego's thoughts it is boss.

The eyes close of the mind in your head,
It's not real, you look there in dread,

Started it in the past,
When it feared the same blast,
Punched again but deader than dead.

Your fancies you had since a child,
Though some of them perhaps real wild,
Your mind doesn't bring to you
what you want, it brings to you
what you are is what you dreamt the whole while.

Certain spiritual philosophies teach that you can *pretend* to be something you wish to be. That can help you to get the ball rolling toward who you really are. So do it if it helps you. But pretending can still be a form of control and it shouldn't be necessary to *pretend* who you truly are, for this is simply an act of doubt. Ideally, let go of this surrounding doubt. Instead of pretending, simply *allow* yourself, as in the way you would fall down a hill, to absolutely know that your dreams about yourself are true. It might require a little leap of *faith* for you to allow that. So jump!

Chapter 7: Summary

Because we are asleep, we are unaware of our true nature, and that our dream of life can be a nightmare. We dream ideas and delusions that we believe to be true. One of the largest ideas and delusions we harbor in our dreams is that we, the doers, alone as individuals, must be in total control. We should instead live our lives gently, allowing what we wish to have and to be.

Essence of the Chapter

We live in a dream. We are now waking from the dream to become more lucid, seeing how our intention affects the outcome. When we see the world as AllGood and allow the dream of life to unfold as we love, the dream, life, and the world become AllGood, as it truly is.

FAITH AND THE

THRESHOLD

A person experiences *Faith* effortlessly in his or her heart and mind. Faith is absolute knowing beyond resistance and doubt. With pure faith, you do not feel fear. You are totally connected to the Truth that it is AllGood, therefore, what is there to fear, or doubt? Equally important, why would you need to maintain control? Faith is also acting with Love and Truth, despite feeling fear or doubt. It is an act of faith to move through what you fear while you still fear. You have a deeper sense beyond the fear that everything is okay and that helps you step into and through the fear.

Faith has little to do with choosing to *believe* in God. Faith is about letting go of all *disbelief* (doubt) of God. Those who believe in God, think they have faith in God *because* they believe in God. Even the term faith has been used interchangeably with belief. But they are not the same, and although this is quite a sensitive subject, it is important that we truly examine our feelings to see the distinction between faith and belief.

Definitions of the word "belief," contain the idea that to believe is to suppose, to think, and not to have absolute certainty. Therefore, even if we believe, we can doubt.

If you fear, if you worry about yourself, that is okay. Fear and worry simply show you that there is doubt. Why fear or worry about what will happen? Why do we always worry about little bad things happening? Why do we worry about how we appear to others in our thoughts, actions, words? Since God is Allthatis, when you worry, when you fear, what are you believing about Allthatis? Where is your faith? If someone says he or she has absolute belief in God, yet still remains fearful, what sort of belief in God is that? Is God not Allthatis? In fearing, therefore, you are attributing a negative quality to Allthatis. That is lacking faith.

Some of us may discover that we have less faith than we thought. So? No worries, you simply strive towards it, while letting the air out of your ego. Your ego might feel sadly deflated, but you don't need such a large one anyway. Know that God is everywhere, in everything, and in everyone, including ourselves. So if God is *all* of that, and we believe that God is all-loving and ever-present within us, *why do we need to hold onto any belief about God?* You hold on because you have doubt. That is not faith. If you know it to be true, you can let it go and see the Truth reflected like an echo from every corner. If you must believe, it is still an act of doubt, an act of Frmee Will, because you are trying to control reality by holding on to what you believe. You must let go.

Somewhere along the way, *when we try too hard*, we start losing faith and worry more about being in control. Fear/doubt exist because you believe you have been left all alone to do everything by yourself. This is one of the first dualistic beliefs. From it, all fear is born. The delusion is "I must try." This belief assumes that your will and the Will of God are separated.

Having faith releases the part of you that fears and has become separated from the Source. When you reconnect your will with the Will of the Source, you will have faith. You will not have to hold onto any belief about God, for you are One with God and there is no belief in that.

Knowing that you are Good and that Allthatis is AllGood, you can let go of what you *believe* to be true. By doing so, you are then able to experience what is true in the place of control and belief. It might be the same thing, so why not let it go and see for yourself? What are you afraid of? In this way, you will then have the experience of the Truth. Having faith is surrendering to what you know to be True. You can also have an intuitive feeling of what is true. The powerful vibration of faith is born when you give yourself the liberty to *know* that it is true. This knowledge has to do with being *receptive* to Truth. It is direct knowing and comes from the Source, not by holding onto it in your mind.

[**Seventh Circle**—CaN #1—I don't know a thing. I allow myself to receive that which I know.

I give up the **Y factor**, totally and completely. I don't need to keep possession of what I know. I act and come from the place within that is one of guidance and intuition, that is married with the moment of the now.]

Let's look at the statement "I AM Love." *On the one hand*, within Frmee Will, if we learn through study or reading a book like this, the rational mind believes "I AM Love." Great! How does that feel? Any belief without feeling still includes doubt and you'll have to keep telling yourself this because you cannot feel whether or not that is true. The belief separates you from the Being because you are *seeing* yourself as Love from in your mind and yet are not feeling it. You are not being it. Looking at yourself like this is a split way of being. It is a mirror reflection of yourself. *On the other hand*, within Ehye Usher Ehye, beyond doubt, you feel and directly connect with "I am Love." From the direct connect feeling comes the absolute, effortless knowing "I am." You know, beyond doubt, that you are and there is no effort in Being what you really are. There is only experience of who you are. All there is to do is brush away doubt. Don't ask "How do I know?" You know because you know through the direct feeling of the Truth. Stop questioning yourself! Faith, therefore, in this scenario, allows you to know something because you feel it to be true.

You also allow yourself to know because you *love* it to be true. How can you have faith in something, or why would you, unless you really wanted it to be true? Faith is associated with simple heartfelt desire. You need not question because true knowledge is created through direct experience (Da'at, דעת) since you have released the fragmented, control-based mind (Bina2—בינה). In dissolving the fragments of the Bina2 mind, you then have all the understanding your dreams have whispered because you can once again feel the Truth directly, and you know. Instead of reading a book about the pool, you are swimming in it.

Having intuitive wisdom, the feeling of something, and the wish to make that true, the fact that you would love it to be true, gives you the faith to let it be. This brings in the vibration of Ehye Usher Ehye *that creates it so*. The world and all entities were created this way. This is how we are created and how we also create. It is amazing to see that when you have the feeling of something that you would love to be true, then you are able to *make* that so by simply knowing that it is. You then see it unfold before you.

Doubting mind (control): *"You willed it
to be there because you wanted it."*
Wisdom mind: *"No, I knew it was there because I loved it."*

One error that some currently make is to think that faith means placing yourself within the jurisdiction of something about which you have neither knowledge, nor any connection to. This is an error because intuition conveys the knowing of Truth through a sense of feeling. Yes, it is without proof, but having the feeling of Truth without being able to prove it only seems bad if you think that all must be based in the known, or proven. The unknown terrifies the ego-mind because it is out of control in an unknown situation. The lack of proof (unknown) makes the ego-mind insecure, because the Bina2 mind's entire basis of reality is in the known. It has no sense of adventure. It is aligned with the Aristotelian philosophy that says, "If you cannot put your finger on something as if it is right there, if you cannot prove something, then it is not true." What a loss we have suffered since believing this true. Without realizing it, the people who believe this have just cut themselves off from an immense Universe beyond the physical reality of the finite-known. The irony is that the world of the finite-known is a world *they have created* by their beliefs. What does the known do for your experience of the Love of the Universe? It shuts it up in a box. No experience of fun or joy, just seeing what you have chosen to believe reflected back at you.

There is no way to have faith without the connection to your true nature, which is intuitive, feeling, heart-based, and undefined. There is no way to have faith without letting go of the known and allowing yourself *to take a chance*. That's the secret.

The idea of true knowledge, דעת, and faith in this light is quite different from what many have believed it to be. It is quite different from the beliefs I have heard ubiquitously, which are more aligned with the notion that the fool is a fool because it rules with the heart. Letting go of these kinds of ideas is necessary for us to release ourselves from the bondage of our own belief systems to bring in the Age of *Moshiach*.

When I touch base with the reality beyond what I can *prove* to be real, I still know that reality is true. This is part of faith. I know it to be true, for I have experienced it by "touching" it on an intuitive level. I feel it so clearly and so it is not out of my reach. *Thus faith is not based in blindness.* Blind faith has no connection whatsoever to a truth that someone chooses to believe. There is no faith in blind faith because there is no connection to the Truth. You are never asked to trust in this way or to have blind faith if you haven't felt or touched the Truth for yourself. We also must not have blind faith in our sacred texts. God never asks us to have blind faith. Stepping out of the blind faith in a sacred text, you are able to recognize the problem of being told *by the sacred text* (or interpreting it that way) to have blind faith in it. A sacred text can just inspire, then each individual must see the Source for themselves.

Those who have doubt are very into the rational and do not trust in their intuitive abilities to know Truth for themselves. For this reason, they adhere quite firmly to some well-established belief system or religious system. That gives them a sense of security and a structure to lean on. That person will have difficulty understanding the aspect of faith associated with intuitive perception and feeling. In fact, part of the religious belief system states, "You cannot trust your own intuitive ability. It will lead you astray. You must take this word as the word of God and Truth."

Letting go of long-held beliefs requires direct contact with our faith. This is a leap of faith. It is a reversal of what we are used to and how we are accustomed to basing our decisions, which is always in the known. Without the faith of intuition and feeling, how can you ever take a leap into something completely backward from what you have believed to be true? How can you ever cross over into the beyond if that is of a reverse nature compared to the way you have always existed? In Kabbalah, the term "Ain Erech" describes the relationship between two things that have no connection. There is no linear relationship between the reality we held onto in our control, and the reality of Oneness. It is a leap from one dimension to another.

In the movie *Indiana Jones and the Last Crusade*, there is a great scene depicting a leap of faith. Harrison Ford, as Indie, steps out over a bottomless pit with the faith that there is a bridge that he cannot see. The bridge materializes beneath his feet and we realize that the absence of the bridge is only an optical illusion. The bridge was always there.

When you allow your resistance and doubt to dissolve, it must do so completely for the transformation and marriage with your Adam Kadmon self. There is a point where it is impossible to *know* what to do. You cannot be sure what to do, nor can you know for sure what lies *on the other side.* It is your last step into simply *Being*, giving up the known (Y) factor. This last step lets you return to the nature that you have forgotten, having lived for so long "dreaming that it is you who are the doer." You only completely remember this state of being once you have stepped into it. This last grain that we release, and all grains of our Frmee Will, yet this last one especially, is the leap of faith. It is letting go of *all* control. This is the most divine state for a human to be in. It is to be a human *Being*.

Letting go of the element that has controlled is difficult because the part of us that fears, which is the controlling part, will not wish to let go. When you let go, that part of you dies. When you are at the gates of *the threshold* between duality and Oneness, there can also be a great fear that is quite similar, if not identical, to the fear of death. Have you taken the time to imagine death? It *is* a threshold. The great threshold that sits between two worlds of very different states of being. On one side of the threshold, you are in control. On the other, you have absolutely no control. The threshold between Oneness and duality is the same except you need not die to cross it. It will *seem* quite real to you that you are going to die for you are at the gateway of the threshold, poised between being in control and having no control whatsoever. What an amazing predicament!

This great leap of faith at the threshold is one that I have found quite difficult to do. I have had chances and been afraid, for I felt *what I thought* was all of myself (all my boundaries) lifting off into the vast reaches of infinity. This feels like, "Ahh, I'm disappearing. I'm ceasing to exist. There is no more me, just the Universe." This was my error, because I was seeing it all backwards. I was not ceasing to exist, or melting into nothingness. Quite the opposite actually. I was merging with the infinite and undefined. The dissolution of the magnetic field of rational thought gives us a sense of losing ourselves.

We could also say that the threshold is merging the inner world of dreams with the wakeful state of consciousness. It is like the marriage of the subconscious with the conscious.

What is important at this point (poised at the threshold) is to know without doubt, so that you can let go completely, that it is AllGood and thus, there is nothing to fear. The feeling of Oneness is not nothingness, it is undefined. This is a difference that makes ALL the difference.

We must go through a kind of conversion washing machine in which we feel as if we are dematerializing. We are letting go of the past and the entrapments of the physical world, which, when we are here, we will see as only an illusion held in place by our efforts to control reality. To let go of this is to reemerge with the Core Star Level, where we are One with the Divine: The World of Atzilut. It is the spark within us that *is* God beyond all definition. It is the Balanced Positive.

In the movie *The Matrix*, when Neo asks, "What is The Matrix?" what he is asking for our world is "What is the threshold? What is that veil that sits in between us and the true reality?"

The way across the threshold does not involve cutting off the parts of you that control or that are held in fear. If you do this, you are cutting off parts of yourself.

Bina2 (Tree of Knowledge reality) is the same as the true Bina of understanding (Tree of Life), *yet turned around upon itself*. If you cut off Bina2, you would cut off yourself, your very own nature! We know from the wisdom of healing that you must pass through the blocked, controlling parts to get to the other side, because your energy is in those blockages that stagnate.

> ### "The best way out is always through."
> Robert Frost, *A Servant to Servants*, 1915

When faced with this last choice to release all control, you stand at the gate in the footsteps of that which controls. This strangest, most peculiar, most challenging step is right at the finish line. This is a great part of the Game, perhaps the greatest. Just like in other games, the lower levels give you the tools and skills you will need for the final challenge. It is not death, yet it feels like it. It is giving up all control, the dissolution of the part of you that is separated and wishing to remain an individual in separation. That is how you define yourself. Ah, if we could only see clearly how this is only an illusion. The illusion of the Tree of Knowledge for Good and Bad. To let go, understand that resistance and fear will simply change to a state of Light after a necessary leap of faith.

It is not a good idea to *attempt* to cross the threshold with that as a set goal, because this then creates the intention of not being there. Simply go about your way accepting the Will of the One and know this is leading down the path that will enable you to leap past the threshold. The best way of thinking of the threshold is to think of it as *letting go of all control*.

You could also simply begin living as if you had already crossed the threshold. This is very important. When you know or are in touch with who you are and you have no doubt, then you can say, "I am that. I am good. I am loving. I am kind. I am fearless." This is direct knowing of the Truth because without doubt your existence is directly within who you are. This is somewhat like already planting yourself on the other side of the threshold. Then, you'll just have to step inside. It won't be such a leap.

All the things that we have discussed so far, and will discuss, that touch your heart and make something rumble deep in your soul you know are True. You know a lot already about the world beyond judgment and fear, that is AllGoodLove. You could write volumes with that term alone. It is vitally important for you to begin living as if you are here, right now, not as if Oneness is some impossible, distant concept, nor as if it is something that will come. When the Messianic Age and beyond is called "The World to Come," it does not mean in the sense of a wonderful world of the future. It means that our consciousness is married with Ehye Usher Ehye, I shall be as I shall be. This is the Time of Forwardness. The Time of Forwardness IS the World to come, the World that Shall Be. It is right now, *forever*, not in the future, for the future implies a time outside of the Oneness, and such does not exist.

Each of us is a cell in the great body of planet Earth and what we all believe to be true, we create as a collective of cells. To date, we haven't been even remotely aware of the powerful effect this vibration has on the Universe. When we all see the Truth collectively, we will raise the vibration on the planet so quickly that we will all be borne upon the wings of eagles, just as we got here in the first place. (Exo 19:4) Yes, the wings did break …well, we chose them to. Or did just the left one break?

We are getting closer and closer to existing again as a people in the harmony of the Universe and the Ganallisone. This is not so far off as we might think. Because the power of unconditional Love is much stronger than any collective belief systems and fear, only a very small percentage of the planet vibrating in this unconditional way will affect the entire Earth. It will be something like the "100th monkey effect." The 100th monkey effect is a principle stating that when a critical mass of a species achieves an awareness, then the entire species, regardless of geographical location, will spontaneously gain the same awareness. This is called the 100th monkey effect because the phenomenon was discovered by witnessing a Japanese monkey, Macaca fuscata, isolated on an island, become aware that washed sweet potatoes taste better than when they're dirty. When approximately 100 monkeys on the island learned this washing behaviour, a collective awareness was observed in their consciousness and in those on other isolated islands. All the monkeys on the various islands were washing their sweet potatoes.

This shows us that when a critical mass of creatures achieves an awareness, they share that awareness amongst all creatures. Maharishi also describes a principle called the "Maharishi effect." He has said that the square root of 1 percent of the population with enlightened awareness is necessary to effect the consciousness of the entire planet. I do not know if this is the right number, but I pray that it is very small, so that we can stop torturing and killing each other and can fulfill our promise to ourselves and God. If we're speaking about the number of people (that have crossed the threshold and have completely given up Frmee Will) necessary to bring this planet collectively into the Messianic Age, I think the number is probably much smaller than Maharishi's estimate. I think the critical number is closer to the amount of eggs you tend to buy at the supermarket, provided you are not shopping for Arnold Schwarzenegger.

So the entire population doesn't have to release Frmee Will to enter into the Messianic Age. That will happen naturally when a critical mass is achieved. But each person must take responsibility for their own consciousness because each individual's energy affects the whole planet. Therefore, address all points in your life in disharmony and resistance so that you may allow Love to enter therein. When you live by Love, it will naturally bring you closer to the threshold and you may just be among the critical mass. But do not become obsessed about crossing the threshold. Just set yourself free by beginning to live as you wish and as you love. Teachings in this book could transmit negativity if people started to really define the threshold. Please do not do this. I have written a few points about the threshold to increase your awareness. But the threshold does not sit like a wall, stagnant and inert. It is ever changing, moving as you do, and different for every person.

The threshold is not achieved by being perfect. Trying to be perfect is impossible. Understanding you are perfect, even with all your flaws, will help you release the judgment that distances you from your true nature. Acceptance, remember? Then you won't have to worry every second about your thoughts and actions being good or bad.

Even Moses wasn't perfect. He doubted himself and lacked the confidence to convey what God had told him to do, so he needed his brother, Aaron, to be his spokesman:

> "Moses replied to Hashem, 'Please, my Lord, I am not a man of words, not since yesterday, nor since the day before yesterday, nor since You first spoke to Your servant, for I am heavy of mouth and heavy of speech.':
> Then Hashem said to him, 'Who makes a mouth for man, or who makes one dumb or deaf, or sighted or blind? Is it not I, Hashem? So now, go! I shall be with your mouth and teach you what you should say.'
> He replied, 'Please, my Lord, send through whomever You will send!':
> The wrath of Hashem burned against Moses and He said, 'Is there not Aaron your brother, the Levite? I know that he will surely speak'.'"
> **Exo 4:10-14**

Moses strength also failed him at times and he needed support from others:

> "It happened that when Moses raised his hand Israel was stronger, and when he lowered his hand Amalek was stronger:
> Moses' hands grew heavy, so they took a stone and put it under him and he sat on it, and Aaron and Hur supported his hands, one on this side and one on that side, and he remained with his hands in faithful prayer until sunset." **Exo 17:11-12**

So you see that even Moses, one of God's greatest servants, was not perfect. Neither are this book's messages; they are not meant to make a perfect crystalline structure for you to follow or obey. The messages point to your freedom. There is no perfect way to be, nor is there a formula.

The Creator places our imperfections in us so that with them we can have a unique set of qualities and attributes adding spice and color to that path we take in life. As the passage quoted above states, "Who makes a mouth for man, or who makes one dumb or deaf, or sighted or blind? Is it not I, Hashem?"

The threshold, therefore, cannot be reached by a formula that encompasses the ways of all people. It is a personal journey, each person embarking on it for him or herself. In fact, it is through the release of all our separate issues, fears, and judgments, unique to us, that we move forward toward the threshold.

> "This cannot be expressed, cannot be narrowed into words, cannot be subjected to laws; every man is completely free and has his own special liberation... No form of instruction exists, no Savior exists to open up the road. No road exists to be opened."
> *The Saviors of God*, Nikos Kazantzakis, p. 128-129

When you understand deeply who you are and you find peace in the acceptance of your entire personal life, with all the people in it, you adorn the mind of unconditional Love, which melts all duality. This book's tools and those in other healing books are simply guides to help you dive into your true nature, to encourage you to be brave on your journey, and to help you remember to trust yourself.

The threshold, therefore, is not a fancy concept enabling us to escape our imperfections here on Earth, nor the imperfections of the rest of the planet. Earth is *the place* beyond the threshold. The difference being that beyond our judgment of good and bad, we remember the perfection in the imperfection. Then you are One with the Earth.

To experience the soft hum of Mother Nature, the subtle language of the earth, you must be patient. I have noticed, time and time again, when I rush or try for the finish line I recede from it. The rush can result from the judgment that where I am is not good enough and, therefore, I must get "there." But this is an escape. This is forgetting that I *am* Good, here, as I have wished myself to be. The process of unfolding is as gentle as the swaying of a tree and the opening of a flower bud. Do not rush out of your foundation. Settle into it and see you are okay as you are. This will help you resolve the need to rush away from your imperfections. This will enable you to have the feeling that those imperfections are okay. By touching with their great okayness, you will help heal them. The balance is not that we must live with the imperfections, or endure the ways we do not wish to live. The balance is realizing that once you release judgment and stop needing to be perfect, there is no room for all that is dark within you. You have learned your lesson from the dark and it is free to go.

Don't run for the finish line. Enjoy the moments of your transformation. Instead of striving for the threshold, see that in completely marrying yourself with *the journey, not the destination,* you are approaching the threshold. Being present each moment aligns you with the total freedom to see that the way is divine. Living this lets you feel and Be all that you can be. That will bring that fine line between duality and Oneness closer to you. Do not remain present because you must. "Must" is a goal outside of you. Be present because you already *are* where you *are.* Your "I am" is shining and shimmering right inside of the eternal moment of NOW, in which you already participate.

Taking it slow and enjoying the ride is especially important for healing. Take your time in your healing process. Allow yourself the enjoyment of knowing and feeling that you are here, you are making it. Take the time to integrate this into your being. Don't rush as you are becoming everything that you have dreamt you could be. You don't rush on your wedding day, or the day you give birth, do you? So don't rush as you know you are moving through your healing. *To rush toward something is to doubt whether or not it is possible or whether or not it is actually happening.* Otherwise, why would you rush? You savour every single second when you really know it's happening.

There is something else to balance with being present and not rushing, and that is to always aspire to your highest potential. So when you read these words and know you must not live for the goal, realize that you can aspire to live in the Garden every moment of every day, even as you are present in your daily life. The Ganallisone is real, it is a state of absolute freedom. There is no pea under the mattress, no grain of sand under your skin. Saying "It is the journey, not the destination" is true, but let it not suggest to that you must downsize your hopes; their very magnitude may seem hard to fulfill. Sometimes people downsize their dreams to avoid being disappointed. That is not the right intention. Always keep your eyes and heart present in the moment, but also always be true to your goals.

Even though you might have the feeling of going on and on, as if the journey becomes ever deeper and more difficult, that is the joy. Love is the path that which you are—your Being, your challenge, your Game from which you could be released anytime. To quote the great treasure-hunter, Mel Fisher, "Today is the day!" Day after day he strove for his sunken treasure. For 15 years he did not give up and finally found what he sought. His attitude was of someone who, against all the odds, persevered and never relinquished his dream goal. That is divine. You must also balance this with patience and understanding of the immensity of your task, so as not to quit or despair because "Today isn't the day."

Please do not be limited by this belief: "The way to the threshold is a *slow process* of releasing issues, transformation of fears, and letting go of control. Then, finally, *after all that*, when I'm ready, I will be able to cross." Yes, you must develop patience and you can feel or yearn for freedom for a long time. Yes, there is still much to do before fully entering into that World of AllGood. Yet, if you touch the Truth beyond all the illusion that you already *are*, then there is no time separating you from your absolute ecstasy of Being. Thus, the potential exists for you to release all control and Frmee Will *at any time*. Understand, as well, that there is no time to waste. Every moment you delay just prolongs your struggle and the pain of remaining in a dual state.

Perhaps when the planets are correctly aligned, the moon at a certain point in her cycle, the wind with a certain scent and you are very clear about who you are and what it is to cross the threshold, it will be possible for you to throw open your heart and say "Here I AM!" and go through zero point past the *flame of the ever turning sword* in your core. This leap is especially possible within deep meditation.

What is a leap of faith? No matter what, a leap of faith always involves the complete surrender to a situation. It is trusting that where you are being led, or brought, or guided, is good. *And if it is bad, that is good too.* That's important to understand. Whether you allow yourself to fall backward off a cliff, or hold onto the dorsal fin of a dolphin and let it dive to whatever depth, or let go *of all control* within, these leaps of faith are the same. They are all acts of surrendering. The situations do not matter. That is the secret. Circumstances don't mean a thing. Imagine a person who hasn't defined the significance of any action or situation. He or she will have a lot easier time dropping off the cliff or diving deeply, because doing so doesn't mean a thing to them. They have faith that where they are going is okay.

As you stretch your wings, and remember who you are,
You can say to Yourself:
Birth of a New Adam. Birth of a New Eve.
I am a new Adam. I am a New Eve.
I am one of the many new Adams and Eves.
As such, I am now the new Adam Kadmon,
which is like the old, yet now I am "real" and I am
inside of who I was imagined to be by God.

Cutting to the Chase Exercises Part I

Here are some exercises that can *really* help release fears and issues. The purpose is to help you connect with the feeling (wisdom) of what it means to you. If you can *feel* the exercise, and *feel* the release, you are doing very well.

There are different levels of feeling as well. At first, what you feel will be the deepest yet. However, do not limit yourself to thinking you felt the maximum because your feeling and how you connect will continually deepen. When you *are* what you *are*, you will know it beyond all doubt.

1) Present—Past Exercise

This is to help release fear, guilt, insecurity, judgment, pain, grief, doubt, and any other negative energy.

Begin by saying *in the present tense* that you are letting go of something, i.e. you are *actively* doing it. For example, "*I let go of the fear of not being good enough*" (or any fear that feels real to you). Naturally, involve your entire concentration of mind, body, and heart. Say this with full focus and as little distraction from other thoughts as possible, for around 36 seconds. With perfect concentration you will affect your psyche. (***The Only Planet of Choice*** suggests that with full concentration, 33 1/3rd seconds is necessary to clear the memory of negative thoughts and beliefs and also to remember and instill new, positive thoughts. 36 seconds is therefore selected to go slightly past the effective time. However, what is most important is concentration without distraction so that you feel fully what you're focusing on.)

Feel the fear clear as you let it go. Remember, you *can* do this. Allowish it to be because you know it is. Get into saying this, repeating it to yourself aloud, and then switch smoothly into saying it in the past: "I *let go* of the fear of not being good enough" as if it has already happened. Even though the words, "I let go" are the same, it is the intention, as if you have already successfully let go, that is the powerful part. Meaning "Great! I have let it go." Say this for a while too, get into the feeling with all your Being, do it for at least 36 seconds.

If you get into it and do it with good focus, you won't have to do it again for that particular fear, so don't be lazy! Really apply yourself, diving into the trusting sense of having truly let it go, as if the first part of the exercise, the active letting go, was perfectly effective. That is the intention of this exercise.

In this way, you can use this exercise for any of your fears or issues:

> I let go of the guilt of receiving. Present tense.
> I *let go* of the guilt of receiving. Past tense.
>
> I let go of the fear of other people's opinions. Present.
> I *let go* of the fear of other people's opinions. Past.

I let go of being so hard on myself. Present.
I *let go* of being so hard on myself. Past.

In that calm space beyond the issue you just cleared, visualize for a moment how you'd love to be *in the stead* of the issue or fear. Allow yourself to receive with pleasure, trust who you are and do not rely on other people's opinions as a guide, be light on yourself and find your self-love.

You can also apply the Present—Past Exercise to clear deep, primordial issues from your psyche. These are all encompassed within the Eighth Circle and are REALLY cutting to the chase. If you touch with the Truth beyond these issues, you are doing just fine.

I let go of the past.
I *let go* of the past.

I let go of *all* fear.
I *let go* of *all* fear.

I let go of *all* doubt.
I *let go* of *all* doubt.

I let go of *all* control.
I *let go* of *all* control.

2) I Do NO Thing Exercise (This exercise is like a meditation.)

I need not be in control. I let myself be. I do not try to let go, I let be. I do not try to fix the kink in my neck. I let it be. I do not try to make my breathing right. I let it be. It is effortless.

The intention of this meditation is to let go of your active control. You do not try. Trying too hard comes from doubt and separation. You let be, you give up the reins to allow the Will of God to enter into you.

"In the meditation of mental quiescence, in the nine states of mind, there is a state where striving must be abandoned; an effortless concentration is necessary at a certain stage. It is effortless: that means your mind becomes very tranquil—with good qualities and its character complete. At that moment, if you make an effort, that disturbs the tranquility. So in order to maintain that pure tranquility, effortless effort must be used."

The Dalai Lama's Book of Daily Meditations, p. 173

The intention here is in knowing that beyond all things, "I need *not* be in control," so that what I truly am will come to be. I *am*, is beyond doubt. And how much trying effort is there in Being who you Are? Zero. This is also expressed in the Fifth Circle:

[*Fifth Circle*—CaN #4—I give up all control.
I do not do a thing (in a trying sense). I let go of control within my Being. I can see that it is happening already as I have wished it. I allow the Divine to enter within me. This is balanced with knowing that it is me who carries out the tasks I wish to do.]

Feel the ways in which you are holding onto the reins when you still yourself in a sitting meditative position, or wherever and whenever you are. Feel the tension in your jaw, the control over your breathing, lifting your shoulders, holding your posture rigidly, the plugged up energy behind your eyes. Can you sense what is involved in letting go of all of this control? Simply let it go, like allowing a ball to drop from your hand. Don't *try* to let it go. Trying to let go of control is not it. The feeling is deep, very deep and subtle. You will begin to get it as you feel control drifting away on a current and a fluid, divine energy enters into you.

I Do No Thing is the effortless being you experience every moment of your life when you have crossed the Threshold. This is the goal. Begin living "I Do No Thing" right now and embody this exercise. Once you touch with the effortless effort of the No Thing Allowishing, you will never forget it!

3) Doesn't Mean A Thing Exercise

Everything is undefined. This exercise integrates into your con-sciousness the feeling, the awareness, that "It doesn't mean a thing." Just meditate on that, ponder it. It will be important for the time when things feel really strange, as if you are merging with all of reality, and your borders are extending beyond the limits of the sky and the moon. You might be overwhelmed if your rational mind is following along with all the changes you are feeling. So remember, *it doesn't mean a thing…* It just *is.* This will help you let go whenever your mind jumps in to control, whether during a deep meditation or a divine experience of the unknown. "It doesn't mean a thing," is like saying, "Hush up, mind." Imagine and meditate on that until you feel the significance of "It doesn't mean a thing." Incorporate this into your being.

As you merge with the consciousness of the trees around you and the grass, the earth and the sky as far as it goes, repeat, "It doesn't mean a thing." When you start to feel the essence of a tree and the wholeness of the Earth, don't think, "How big is the Earth? How big am I becom-ing? How far away are the stars? What am I if I merge with this tree?" What is far? What is big? How "big" do you think Mother Earth feels as she sits in the Universe? She just *is.* Can you see what "I AM" really means now? You shouldn't. It doesn't mean a thing.

4) It's AllGood Exercise

This is the King and Queen of all exercises. In this exercise, you attune your mind to the fact that you are living in an AllGood Universe. You can do this exercise in conjunction with other medita-tions or when you have a few minutes here and there to remind your-self that life is AllGood, and so are you. As you do this, your rational mind is going to tell you why AllGood is not true. "Because you owe money." "Because you aren't married yet." "Because you don't have a job." "Because your husband/wife doesn't understand you." Your rational mind is basically trying to convey the fact that life cannot be AllGood because of these problems, worries, or fears that you have. Since this is a cutting to the chase exercise and not an exercise to work out each issue you may have, allow your mind to soar beyond the rational and embrace the Truth that it is AllGood. Everything is AllGood. Allthatis is AllGood. Even though it can feel somewhat like a wrestling match between your true nature and your rational mind (which projects doubt to prevent AllGood from seeming real), you will not win the match by fighting against the rational. You win by paying it no mind, by seeing through those doubts, beliefs, and worries *as if they don't mean a thing*. Understand that those doubts are not real, they are the opposite of AllGood. It is as if they are rising up to stop you as you're driving by on your journey. Pay them no mind and leave them behind.

You will know when you're touching AllGood because it is unmistakable. You don't have to pretend how that is. Reach out and know that it is All Good and you will lighten up and feel excited about your life and who you are. You will remember the CaNs f the Eighth Circle: "There is nothing to worry about, there is nothing to hurry about, there is nothing to doubt, etc." You will be ready to face anything. Leap into the AllGood. Let it Be.

You can use these exercises to help you with the Leap of Faith Meditation, described below.

The Leap of Faith Meditation

This meditation can bring you to your last grain of control, to the resistance of Being, so that you may experience the Calm of Calms, the Faith of Faiths. It will help you feel what is involved in letting go of the control that *you have always had* in the physical, ever since you were cut from your mother's umbilical cord and had to breathe for yourself. *This is the meditation of letting go of the control of breathing.* This is a very powerful exercise and is quite challenging. It is very, very healing and it will also help you develop singing skills and breath control. It is also very grounding and calming. Fear causes your energy to become ungrounded and centered up in your head. This will help you return to the peaceful, safe feeling of your body.

- To begin, sit comfortably in a chair and breathe normally, as in the way you are breathing now. Do this for several breaths.

- Exhale slowly and steadily until your out-breath is completely gone and then relax. Continue to let it go out, even if no air comes out. You should be able to feel the energy still moving in that "out" direction, even if it is just your intention. You can do this very gently and slowly. Then allow your mind to let go of your attachment to breathing and stay focused on allowing thoughts to go as they come. Allow your breath to remain out to the greatest degree of the *outbreath* with as little *physical* effort as possible. Just keep it going out with your intention. Do not force breath out of your lungs. You are not trying to force all the residual air out. You are approaching your state of Being. There is no effort in keeping the breath out.

Allow your *energy* to continue moving out and around or wherever it will naturally. You will feel that you can continue pushing very slightly with your energetic intention. This is like imaginary exhaling. Keep a steady efflux of energy with your intention and the will of the Hara. If you do not know what the will of the Hara is, you will be able to feel it as you keep allowing the flow of energy out despite having no more air. It is the strength and power for you to overcome ingrained resistance and is the power you need to keep going despite having no more air. Keep letting it flow outward, more than downward, because outward is a better way to imagine the energy's direction. But downward is also good, as is upward. Do not force. Use the allow will.

You will begin to feel as if you are suffocating and you will associate this with fear. You will notice that energy is being sucked into your throat and chest, as if there is a black hole in your chest (there is). This is where your heart is imploded. Here, is your internal source of fear and when you are afraid, it sucks energy into itself.

The leap of faith comes in here, you allow the intention to change so that is moves *out*ward from the heart. The switch to outward is effortless. Do nothing at all inside of the suffocation—that's the leap, because you want to control when you're scared, which is the sucking in. (Hint: that feeling of suffocation *is* your Frmee Will. Can you feel it, allow it to be, go through it and let it go?)

When you are past the comfort zone, you will automatically want to inhale. You may "need" to make this to happen but be very aware that to take a breath in is making a choice based on the fear of dying of suffocation. Do not fear suffocation, because you cannot suffocate yourself in this way. If your awareness is centered up in your head, you will fear suffocation. If you are present in your body, and you have a good connection with your Hara, you will be able to go much deeper than you can possibly imagine without any fear and without passing out.

The true magic in this exercise is in facing the need to breathe. Face the fear that you feel by charging into it like a horde of cavalry screaming fearlessly while descending from a mountain. This will help you clear the fear of suffocating.

The heart of this exercise and the *secret* is to remain calm and let go of the need to take the in-breath despite your body screaming to take air. Your throat is a key player in this game, as it is the key player in your Frmee Will. It is the bridge between brain and body. Allowing the energy of this center to flow is part of the goal of this exercise. You feel faith in your throat. When you would clutch and fight to get air, see that you can do nothing, and be still and just sit, just be. When you would struggle to get oxygen, the exercise will show you how to do nothing, be still, relax, and let go.

Then you will experience something extraordinary.

Even though breathing is physiological and seems very natural, the need to breathe is still a belief system and it is based in the illusion of the physical reality. All the needs that we have held onto are also held in the program of your breathing. Your fears, no matter where they are stuck in your body, muscles, or organs, they have a component that is energetically stored in your chest and are suffocating your breath. When you fear, you hold onto your breath. This exercise will help you loosen your ties to fear. You might continue to panic and not be able to go too far beyond your "comfort zone," but it is important to transcend it—that is the goal of the meditation. Beyond the comfort zone, where your arms might start flailing around and in the fear of suffocating you might clutch your throat, you will feel a calm unlike any other. Your entire being will feel calm, because you feel truly safe.

After you have inhaled, relax for a short while, then repeat the above process by beginning your next exhalation.

Can you see now what is involved in letting go of the breath? The goal is not to stop breathing. It is to stop your control-self from breathing. It is to let go of the *control* you have over your breath. Control of the breath is the source of so much disharmony in the body. Do you know how often we hold our breath when we are afraid? This becomes a habit and we then continue to unintentionally hold our breath as we progress through life! This means that the way that you are breathing now is not completely free. In fact, we are all suffocating ourselves with the control that we exert over our breathing. Interestingly, we control our breathing most when we are afraid and we lack faith. Letting go of this control is regaining the faith that we gave up when we were afraid. When you are calm and breathing fully and deeply, you feel a great sense of faith. Faith will feel calm and peaceful to you.

This leap of faith meditation, therefore, also enables you to become aware of how much you are holding onto your breath. The control we have over our breathing actually causes us to breathe *less* than if we allowed it to happen within the source of Love and faith that we are. *When you let go of your breathing you are letting go of holding onto your breath and thus, you allow yourself to breathe more.* You will feel calm and your breathing will be deep and very open. This is an excellent exercise for singers and wind-instrument musicians. But don't tense up when you're doing it. It is important to remain relaxed.

There is a clue in the movie *The Matrix* as to what you can experience once you have released the need to breathe. When Neo and Morpheus are fighting in the simulated dojang (chinese for school of training), Neo is huffing and puffing. Morpheus asks him calmly "You think that's air you're breathing now?" You see, *The Matrix* among other things is about peeling away belief systems. The need to breathe is deep, yet a belief system all the same. Some yogis have challenged this belief by remaining submerged in a pool of water for hours and hours with no oxygen tank. You may look it up in the *Guinness Book of World Records*.

We might call this "The homeopathic breathing meditation," for with it you are going to enter deep into self-suffocation so that you may remember how to truly breathe. In fact, you gain immense insight into your true nature as you remember that you *are* your breathing. No control is necessary. That is an illusion rooted in fear and lack of faith. The wonderful medicine of homeopathy is based on this principle of "like cures like." In this case, we must come to *feel* how we are suffocating ourselves to see *how much* we are doing it and clear it. This is the like curing the like.

A little truth that you can take with you into the
inner chamber as you plunge into the suffocation is:

"I don't need to breathe! I am okay."

Chapter 8: Summary

Faith is naturally experienced beyond resistance and doubt. Faith is about letting go of all *disbelief* (doubt) felt toward God and the Truth. When you have faith, you realize that there is no need to hold onto beliefs because you are directly experiencing the Truth, and there is no belief in that. Faith is also associated closely with Love, because you do not have true faith in something unless you love the way it is. Why would you have faith in something if you didn't want it to be true? That would be silly. To have faith, it is also necessary to be willing to take a chance, to step beyond the need for proof and evidence that the Bina2 mind requires. The Leap of Faith into the unknown and across the Threshold is the complete surrender and letting go to a situation that you would love, know, and trust to be.

Although the Threshold of letting go of all control might seem scary and might seem like dying, this is the ego's perspective. The ego knows that it will cease to have control over everything. The individual remains an individual and his or her identity and personality continue onward, freer than ever. When enough individuals have adorned the golden glow and achieved Messianic consciousness, an explosion of Love will touch the entire planet and everyone will step through to the new reality of Oneness. All the souls, as they were imagined by the Creator, will awaken to their highest ideal of existence.

ESSENCE OF THE CHAPTER

You feel faith through your intuition (Chochma), the direct connection to the Truth, even without evidence or proof. This feeling gives you what it takes for the Leap of Faith, beyond all definition and control, to cross the Threshold into Oneness.

THE TREE OF KNOWLEDGE

FOR GOOD AND BAD

It was a great turning point when Adam and Eve ate the fruit of the Tree of Knowledge. In fact, duality and judgment began *at that time*. We then fell from a state of Oneness, of pure Love, to the challenge and trials within the Game of Life's duality.

The Tree of Knowledge for Good and Bad is also called the Tree of Knowledge for Good and Evil. Some translations of the Old Testament say "Good and Bad," some say "Good and Evil." The Hebrew word "Rah" רע, as in Etz HaDa'at Tov Va Rah, Tree of Knowledge for Good and Bad/Evil, means both "Bad" and "Evil." Is there a difference? Yes and No.

Because God is AllGood, and Good is Love, we can say the absence of Love is "Bad." We do not say this judgmentally, but rather in the sense that "Bad" is the opposite of God's nature. This is the energy of opposition. We all have this energy of opposition. It can be part of us, because we have chosen to align ourselves with it. Also, and of perhaps more importance, we do so because we chose to begin the Game of Life.

In Chapter Three and Four, we discussed the necessity of creating a challenge to give rise to the potential of choice. In the Hebrew tradition, the Serpent is the energy created by the Creator to *challenge* the Thought, or the imagination of God. This is the same as the *challenger* of Truth. It is the reflection/opposite of Truth and Love. What kind of a scenario are you in when you are opposed and challenged? You are playing a game. What does this challenging energy do? It tempts you to do what is outside your true nature. It tempts you to try to be what you already are, not for the purpose of good for all people, but for the purpose of power and greed. It also tries to corrupt those parts of you and those acts that are most divine, to take away your great sources of Love and joy.

The Garden of Eden (planet Earth) is the grounds for the Game. A game must have a challenger, or you'd get bored playing against yourself. God created this force to challenge us, challenge our true nature, our sense of who we are. To say that it exists outside of ourselves, as some menacing force outside of our control, outside of our collective choice, horned and fire-breathing, is not correct. So we must be careful about the term "evil." In fact, do not fear the challenge at all. Welcome it. Embrace it, for the dark only challenges you in ways in which you are not completely committed to who you really are. In the ways in which you have given up choice and returned to Beingness, there is no more challenger inside of you. (The world might still challenge you, but you will no longer have the internal duel.) Therefore, the challenge is an opportunity to be yourself and it actually gives you the chance to return to, and to be, yourself. So accept the challenge and you will be given the strength to face it, no matter what it may be.

The absence of Good is not in and of itself evil. It is a space devoid of Love that gives us the opportunity to be challenged, and to choose. *If embraced and followed without constraint,* the absence of good can bring out horrors. Sometimes, bad can get so out of hand, become so destructive and foul, that we call it evil. Yet, it requires the action of a human. Thus *our* control takes something *bad* and makes it into *evil*.

This is not to say that "bad" or "evil" energies do not exist. These *are* forces, just as the Beings of Love are empowered by our Love and joy. Just as there is a collective energy that is created by many people loving, so is there a collective energy that is created by control, illusion and trying to be like God. (see Figure 13)

Evil takes root in the human need to have power over people and feel like God inanotsoniceway. Until we are all One, this bad energy that opposes God's will, does exist and can influence us. Yet it is not something exclusively outside of us controlling us. We have choice. Should we release all of our resistance and control, it too will cease to exist, first on an individual basis, and then on a global level.

There is no doubt that energy of opposition does not have very good "intentions" for us. The "purpose" of that energy is not to help us. It is set to run against us, against our return to the Source, in opposition to our freedom. That is its program. But to have any effect on our planet it must work through humans who make choices that are opposite of their true nature. That is the Game. As long as we harbor it, by desiring power, control, or wanting to possess knowledge to be like God, it can influence the planet. This energy is here because we are still empowering it, because we give it the space within our population.

When we examine our world and we wish to discern what opposes Love, we see it is such a simple thing. What segregates, divides, judges, controls, destroys, takes away freedom, looks down upon and splits people apart is separated from Love. Love brings together, unifies, and sees as equal. Healing our planet and all people is subsumed in Love.

I prefer the name the Tree of Knowledge for Good and Bad. Acts that can be described as evil come from that "bad" energy. And thus it is *our* responsibility to no longer allow evil acts to be done to each other.

"Evil" is a very strong word. Don't forget that evil energy is there for a purpose, a most essential purpose. One must completely release any alignments with this energy because it will take you in the wrong direction when you follow it. If it did not exist, however, we wouldn't be able to create the new and improved Garden of Eden. The fact that we have held the idea of evil in terror for a long, long time shows that we haven't fully grasped its significance. And remember that anything in the

Universe that feels judged must prove it is worthy of existence. This is true as well for the energy of evil. As you move toward the Threshold, these collective beliefs and fears about evil might become manifest in your thoughts, just as all fears must surface in order to be dusted away. Allow yourself to face evil, fully and completely, like Daniel putting his head into the mouth of the Lion, and you will see the choice that you can choose to align yourself with it or not. You will see that the power it can have over you dissipates completely when you face it and fully understand the nature of the energy.

[*Seventh Circle*—CaN #3—I release the need to dwell on the idea of evil.

I do recognize that there are energies that exist that are not aligned with Love. I am not in unbalanced positive with this. However, I release the need to focus on the evil, for in doing so, I am seeing my power to not allow evil things to happen. I also see that I have choice, fully and completely, so I release the disempowering idea that I am being controlled or influenced by outside negative forces. I also am aligned with the very deep truth that it is AllGood, and in simply loving, I am healing all that is negative. So why would I need to focus on evil?]

If you have witnessed wickedness done by some to others, especially if you lost a loved one in the process, or if you have seen the insane lust for blood that violent mobs or terrorists possess, it is easy to think of evil. A twisted and tormented person is capable of acts of destruction against other people, and so destructive forces can act through him or her. At the root of these horrific actions is pain and fear, forgetting and insanity. They result in poor choices and skew his or her perception. Then he or she becomes controlled by the desire to destroy, which is a desire that feeds the forces of fear. Such people are not inherently evil. Their souls come from God, as all souls do. Their forgetting is simply so deep and their distortion of reality so advanced that they become vessels to carry out the will of the energies that oppose.

If you have a deep wound within that turns to guilt and self-loathing, if you fear, if you let yourself get out of control, then the energies of negativity can latch onto you and urge you to think bad thoughts or do horrible things to others. You may even hurt yourself in a moment of rage or insanity, for instance. And when you do such things, you can feel encouraged just as a person can feel the lust for blood when they are overtaken by their desire to destroy. The powerful feeling you get by dominating others or putting others down is similar. The key is not to worry about this energy in others. Just focus on yourself, release your fear and desire to control, and trust in the nature of Allthatis, and know that *you* are AllGood inside. This way, you will be contributing to the dissolution of illusions that feed this energy.

So we can ask, "Does evil exist outside of ourselves, outside of the totality of our beliefs that can influence us? Does evil exist *beyond our collective Frmee Will*?" Thank God, no. When we all attain the state of Ganallisone collectively, evil will no longer influence us. As above, so below. And if evil cannot influence us, then it no longer is evil, is it?

The deeper question really comes down to, "What is the ultimate reality of the Universe? Is it good and bad? Or is it AllGoodLove?" Remember, the Creator is not made up of the balance between good and evil, nor good and bad in duality. Do you understand what Balanced Positive and AllGoodLove mean?

> "Nothing real can be threatened.
> Nothing unreal exists.
> Herein lies the peace of God."
> p. X *A Course in Miracles*

Whether we call it good and bad, or good and evil, there are many questions surrounding the mysterious Tree of Knowledge.

Why was it called the *Tree of Knowledge*? And why for *Good and Bad*?

Why did God forbid Adam and Eve from eating only *this* tree's fruit?

What sort of tree was capable of beginning the state of duality in the Universe?

What is this tree that is pleasing to the eyes and good for food?

What is this tree that bears fruit and is capable of making the eater feel as if they were governed by two wills? One the Will of God/Good (**Yetzir HaTov**) and another the opposing Will (Yetzir Harah)?

Does it exist today or has it been lost in the evolutionary tides through the centuries?

Is it a tree at all, or is it just a metaphor that the Torah has encrypted for us to keep secret?

Many people share the belief that the fruit from the Tree of Knowledge for Good and Bad was an apple! So often, when movies and books refer to the Tree, Adam and Eve are said to have eaten the apple from the Tree of Knowledge. Even the thyroid cartilage that protrudes from the neck is called "Adam's Apple." Did they eat an apple?

Or could the metaphor be describing an act like sexual union?

Mystical knowledge and religious leaders have told us that *the original sin*, eating from the Tree of Knowledge for Good and Bad, *was a metaphor for the act of sex*. The Torah expresses the sexual act with the verb "L'Da'at" which is the Hebrew verb "To Know."

"And Adam knew his wife Eve, and she conceived and bore Cain"
Gen. 4:1

First we will look at the idea from the perspective that eating from the Tree was a sexual act. Then, we'll dive a little deeper, for there are *other ways* of understanding the significance of the Tree of Knowledge that serve us very well regarding our healing.

The Serpent showed Adam and Eve that the sexual act would give them power—*that having the power to create was to be like God*. So what's wrong with that? Why did that cause so much trouble?

Initially, Adam was still both male and female, the Balanced Positive, known as Adam Kadmon.

"Male and female He created them." **Gen 1:27** (The reason it is written "them" and not "him," is partly because it is a description of both Beings, Adam and Eve, *as One* and also because it is describing the Adamic race.)

Adam and Eve were then separated into two polarities—man and woman. The Torah states this in the verse,

> "So Hashem God cast a deep sleep upon the man and he slept; and He took one of his sides and He filled in flesh in its place: Then Hashem God fashioned the side that He had taken from the man into a woman, and He brought her to the man." **Gen 2:20-21**

The sexual act is the alchemical union of the two polarities of male and female, returning them to the Balanced Positive—the original state of Adam Kadmon. But it is different, deeper, than the original Adam Kadmon, because the parts are coming together, not just existing as One, each in his and herself. They share the experience. This union of the male and female is the Oneness that makes the stuff of The Creator. When they did actually make Love in *the physical world*, they were not prepared for the complete experience of merging with the Creator. How could they be? They had just been born into two parts, which was overpowering and frightening. So the act went awry; it became bad and good, when it is AllGood.

The Torah's model shows that the plan of the Serpent was to tempt Adam and Eve into the sexual act *before* they were ready. Instead of the sexual union being only most joyous and the alchemy of perfect unions, it also became feared and shameful. It could be used to hold people in bondage, for it then contained a root of guilt. It could be abused. It could be addictive, a bottomless pit of desire. The essence of the act was forgotten.

Symbolically and literally, the one act that looms above us and divides our world into disharmony *the most* is the sexual act. No other issue has more divided the minds and hearts of humankind and caused more control, suffering and unhappiness. This does not mean that the act itself is evil, or base or bad. It is the most divine act that two people in Love can do. That is why there are attempts to control it. The Serpent targeted the sexual act of union to use it to throw us off so that we would not live and love each other freely and would instead live in illusion, frustrated, dissatisfied, and unhappy in the world of the Serpent.

In addition to the original act of Love being considered "a sin," Adam began to try to control Eve for the sake of power. He began to do so not only within the realm of *sexuality*, but also in the realm of *knowledge* in the mental sense. And that is perhaps more significant and the more important way of understanding the Tree of Knowledge for Good and Bad.

Isn't it strange that the Torah should associate the sexual act with the Tree of Knowledge by using the verb "L'Da'at" (To Know) for both? Adam *knew* his wife Eve. What does the sexual act have to do with knowledge, especially of Knowledge for Good and Bad?

Actually, nothing.

And how could the commandment to not eat from the Tree of Knowledge have been a commandment to not engage in the sexual act, when God had previously told Adam and Eve to be fruitful and multiply, and fill the earth? (Gen 1:28)

Actually, it was not.

Thus, there is more here than meets the eye.

There is a secret here that will help reveal more of the great tapestry of the Universe, the magical design of the Creator, and the hidden mysteries of the Torah. It is a remedy that helps us return to Eden.

Let's examine the identity of the Tree of Knowledge for Good and Bad from another perspective.

When the Children of God chose to disobey the Will of Oneness, the other will, Frmee Will, *Yetzir Harah*, created duality and a challenge began. It is about forgetting who you are so that in making the choice of who you really are, you have the appreciation of your true nature.

The way in which Frmee Will is created is by giving an entity whose very nature is Love and Oneness the delusion that they exist outside of the Oneness of Love and God. Thus their choices can come from somewhere other than the Source. In order to have the ability to choose outside of the Source, you must have something else to choose with. You must become doubled. You must have two Wills.

The alignment of these two Wills is:

> *The Serpent tempting us to do what God forbids.*
> or
> *God beckoning us to do what the Serpent opposes.*

These two Wills are in opposition to each other.

The Serpent tempts us to disobey the Will of God for the very impossible purpose of making us *try to be* what we already *are*. That power is inherent in our true nature. The duel within us, between our true nature and its opposite, between our good and bad, is thus the most intense internal *conflict* imaginable because you are attempting to be what you already *are*. This muddles with the Truth that you are who you are and creates the illusion that you must make efforts to be who you are. It is switching from having that true internal power to thinking you must find it outside. Why would you ever do that if you have it already?

Adam's conflict was, "Do I eat from the Tree or do I not eat from the Tree?"

"Do I obey the will of God or do I answer to the voice that tells me to do the opposite?"

To this day, we struggle on our internal playing field against God— our doubt on the one hand and our true feelings on the other, our heart's desire and our ego's desire. Surely this struggle must have an immense effect on our energetic systems.

Perhaps a healing substance exists in nature for every negative condition with which human beings can get themselves stuck in?

Perhaps a plant, *tree,* or an element exists *because* humans will need it at some time or another. As humans begin to *collectively* get stuck in a negative fear state or an ugly state of control, perhaps the negative state of consciousness manifests as a poisonous plant or tree to heal the negative state?

Maybe there is a plant or tree that is poisonous to human beings and that, when prepared in a manner that extracts *the energetic essence* from that plant or tree and dilutes the poison to the point of safety, it can cure the negative effects of the poison.

The forgotten identity of The Tree of Knowledge for Good and Bad is one of the most intricate mysteries and yet it has been difficult to grasp because of its simplicity.

The answer to this mystery and the identity of the Tree of Knowledge for Good and Bad lies within the beautiful medicine known as **homeopathy**. (see *Appendix C*)

If a substance existed to cure this primordial, internal conflict caused by the Tree of Knowledge for Good and Bad, what would some of its characteristics be according to our homeopathic books (*Materia Medica*)? What negative characteristics have we adopted from the Tree of Knowledge, by living in a state of conflict between our true nature (Good) and the opposition of our true nature (Bad)? What negative characteristics have emerged from eating the fruit of the Tree of Knowledge? (You won't find it in books as "The Tree of Knowledge.")

We already know some of the answers.

The most important negative characteristics or symptoms (called rubrics in homeopathy) that make up the disturbance from the Tree of Knowledge are:

- Feels as though he had two Wills; one commanding him to do what the other forbids.
- In one ear a devil, in the other an angel. (see Figure 14)
- Contradiction between reason and Will.
- Two different influences exerted on him at the same time, one to do bad, one the other to do good.
- Strong sense of *duality* and *unreality*.
- Delusion of being double.

These are some of the characteristic symptoms that a person will experience when they have eaten or touched this substance/remedy. Someone needing this substance/remedy can be experiencing these same symptoms or rubrics already.

I have also felt this remedy has a very deep delusion or feeling that I haven't found documented: *"I am unable to love but oh! I wish I could"*. It is related to the contradiction of Wills.

Other symptoms characteristic of the influence of this tree are:

- The feeling that the mind and body are separate.
- The feeling that the head is separated from body.
- The feeling that all is an illusion, nothing is real, everything is just a dream.

- The sensation of a plug anywhere and everywhere

These are the characteristic feelings and symptoms when you have been acted upon by the Tree of Knowledge for Good and Bad. In the homeopathic model, these feelings would be characterized in a person who ate from the tree, especially a person very sensitive to the effects of foreign energy upon his or her systems. In other words, if you take a swim in a dirty lake, you will absorb the toxins. As they ate the fruit, Adam and Eve's minds began to divide and they began to feel double. One side was their true nature, the other the opposite. (see Figure 15)

So what is it already!?!? What is the Tree of Knowledge for Good and Bad!?!?

The tree is called *Anacardium orientale*. I became aware of the fact that this tree was the Tree of Knowledge one day when I was meditating and a breeze came in from an open door, blowing one of my homeopathic books open to the page on *Anacardium orientale*. On that page, I saw written, "Feels as though he had two Wills; one commanding him to do what the other forbids." And "in one ear a devil, in the other an angel." I just knew that this answered the mystery of the identity of the Tree of Knowledge (being in the form of an actual tree). It is not lost. It was just forgotten. It exists in the West Indies and in India and is also called "the marking nut" as well as *Semecarpus anacardium*. It is from the *Anacardiaceae* family.

The Cashew tree is in the same family and is called *Anacardium occidentale*. Interestingly, the fruit from *Anacardium occidentale* is kidney shaped and called a "cashew apple."

A midrash on Torah (Midrash Bereishit Rabba, parsha 16-17) proposes that the Tree of Knowledge was one of four possible trees/plants, and gives purported reasons for each. The four proposed trees/plants are wheat, grapes, ethrog (citron), and fig. With the discovery of homeopathy and the understanding of how plants affect the psyche of the human being, it is now possible to understand why *Anacardium orientale* more accurately and pointedly fits the description of the Tree of Knowledge for Good and Bad.

The very conflict that Adam and Eve were exposed to between the Will of God and the temptation of the Serpent is contained in the essence of *Anacardium orientale.* The tree influences those that eat its fruit to experience a sensation of having two wills. One is commanding you to do what the other forbids, the first characteristic on the list above.

Let's look a little closer at this.
One commanding him to do ...

The serpent says "Yeah. Do it! It's good. You'll like it and don't worry, you won't die, for 'God knows that on the day you eat of it your eyes will be opened and you will be like God, knowing good and bad.' **Gen 3:5**"

...what the other forbids!

"Thou shalt not eat from the Tree of Knowledge for Good and Bad!" **Gen 2:17**

Besides all the characteristics that *Anacardium orientale* possesses, it also has some wondrous physical traits that correspond very well with the way the Torah describes Eve's perception of the Tree. **Gen 3:6**:

"And the woman perceived that the tree was good for eating and that it was a delight to the eyes, and that the tree was desirable as a means to wisdom, and she took of its fruit and ate."

Let's look at each one of these points:
"The tree was good for eating."

Edward Hamilton describes *Anacardium orientale* in his book *Flora Homeopathica* and states: "The Indians, after depriving the nut of its external rind and juice, roast and eat it with much relish." Hamilton also says that during famine in India, the ripe fruit of *Anacardium oriental* was roasted and eaten. So we know *Anacardium orientale* is good for food. What else?

"The tree was a delight to the eyes."

Hamilton also describes *Anacardium orientale's* fruit. "The Seed, a nut, resting on the receptacle, *heart-shaped*, flattened on both sides, smooth, and shining." Unlike the cashew tree, *Anacardium orientale's* fruit is in the shape of a *heart*, smooth and shining. And what is more delightful to look at than something that resembles a heart? The **doctrine of signatures** states that the a way a plant appears reveals its medicinal properties. "Anacardium" in Latin means "according to the heart." Any substance that can influence the consciousness of an individual so much to make him or her completely dual *must* influence the heart. (see Figure 16)

The great homeopath James Tyler Kent also wrote about a person influenced by *Anacardium orientale*:

> "He thinks he is double. This comes from a vague consciousness that there is a difference between the external and internal will, a consciousness that one will is the body and another is the mind." *Lectures on Homoeopathic Materia Medica*, James Tyler Kent, p. 104

What Kent means by the body and the mind, or the external and internal Will, is the Will of the rational mind and the Will of the heart. The Will of the heart is centered in the body. So when we look at the characteristic *contradiction between reason and Will*, it is really the contradiction between the rational mind, *reason*, and the *Will* of the Heart.

With this contradiction of Wills comes the internal dialogue: "*I would love to*" 'Well, you can't!' "*Yes I can!*" 'No, you shouldn't!' "*Yes I wish to*" 'Well, it's not a good idea.' Such contradiction in Wills is the deepest conflict in life. Understanding this clearly is the path to freedom. It means that Frmee Will is choice. You have the freedom of choice. But what is choice? What is it *really* about? It is actually a choice between doing *what you believe you must* vs. doing *what you would love*! That is it. The Bottom Line Truth. The difference between suffering and unhappiness, and freedom and joy. This Truth is all-encompassing.

It is true that you surely can chose either. Yet which would you prefer? Which will lead you into the fullness of life and joy? Which will make your life a miserable prison? When you would love to do something and your rational mind tells you "No, you can't!," you are living as a slave in a prison. Often we think God is telling us not to be what we believe we mustn't, because we feel we would be bad if we allowed ourselves the full enjoyment of the moment whatever that may be. When we hear a voice telling us not to do something we'd love to do, it is not the voice of God, it is opposition. Often our guilt blocks us from our heart's wishes. That is how we have always been controlled. And remember that you are truly a certain way and you love to be that way, and yet your rational mind will challenge you to believe you *must*, you *should*, you have to *try* to be that way. As soon as you believe you must try to be what you already are, the conflict between *reason* and *will* begins.

What else?

"The tree was desirable as a means to wisdom."

The preparation from *Anacardium orientale* has historically been used as a distinguished remedy for weakness of mind, memory, and the senses. Scholars have used it to increase their mental capacities, their memory, and the power of thought.

"The Confectio Anacardium became celebrated under the name Confectio Sapientium, as a remedy against weakness of the mind..."
Flora Homeopathica, p. 491

When our Wills conflict, that is not the same as an angel saying "no" and a devil saying "yes." There is a conflict between polarities, a contradiction between both Wills. One telling you to do what the other forbids. One saying "yes," one saying "no." Your true nature can be saying "yes" or "no," depending on whether what you are deciding is aligned with your true nature or not. If it is, the angel will say "yes" and the devil will say "no."

And the secret of letting go of this conflict is to ignore the "other" voice when you know what the One Will is asking you to do. The secret is in allowing the self to do what you know is in your heart, without question, without a doubt.

For most of us, the two extremes tend to center around the conflict of choice. First, we do not feel free to choose. We feel we have no choice. Second, we feel as if there are two wills inside and we are very confused as to which to follow. Have you felt this conflict yourself?

Have you ever felt as if you have no choice in a matter? Have you felt completely divided? These are really the same issues which come from not knowing which we should follow: our reason or our heart. Because of this, we will have a tendency to feel confused and trapped.

Anacardium orientale is at the very root of our daily internal conflict for there is *no* conflict when you are very clear about what you love to do. The indecisiveness, struggle, and *heavy doubt*, very key qualities of this negative state of consciousness, is due to our two opposing sides. The issues need not be about murder or wickedness. The simple conflict between what the heart truly wants and what the rational mind tells you can be the root of the issue. *This is the root of all conflict within*—the conflict between pure Being (Tree of Life—Garden of Eden) and the rationale of Good and Bad (Tree of Knowledge—Exile from Eden).

"Should I speak up for myself? Yes. No. Yes. No."

"What must I do? Do I ask that person out on a date or not? Yes. No. Yes. No."

"Is it good or bad to say such a thing to that person? (Rational)

Is it in my heart to do it? (Love)"

This conflict emerges most during difficult decisions in which your true nature is really put to the test. Isn't it easy to understand where indecisiveness comes from when you are trying to decide something and are torn between two Wills?

In Frmee Will land—We feel torn. Do we do it or do we not do it? One Will telling us to do what the other forbids. Guilty self-conscience. Confusion. Asleep in a dream. What is in our hearts to do?

In Know Will land—We have *no* Frmee Will. We *finally know* our One Will and we stop doubting everything we think, say and do. Once the struggle between our two Wills is over, it is no longer difficult to discern what is good or bad, because we just *know* and we just *are*. We finally know that how we love to be is what decides what is Good. And thus, we can finally have choice that is no choice. That is freedom.

Give yourself time to realize that you haven't, for so long, trusted your Will. "Am I good or bad?' We have asked this for so long.

"Where is this intention coming from?" We have asked this, too, for so long.

Know that your Will comes from the Will to do good, and that you are a spark of the divine! *That is all you need.* The rest is guidance and **awebedience** and faith. Don't use the all too common excuse, "We cannot trust ourselves because we have Yetzir Hara." Don't give the rational mind any power when it says, "Who do you think you are? You can't trust yourself to be free. You have to listen to me, to my reason." Remember that Yetzir Hara is not a real Will. It is the urging of the voice of illusion. So what are you doing by saying that you cannot trust yourself? You are perpetuating the conflict of your Wills and duality. Trust yourself to know you are *one* Will, not two, and that you are Good. This will really help you release doubt about who you are.

You are a Being of Love and Light and you have just been challenging yourself. Yes.

The Serpent's words, "You will be like God knowing Good and Bad" were also just another trick, because God does not know good and bad as we do, in our duality. Only the mind of *duality* sees things in unbalanced positive and negative, as in good and bad. As it is written in the Torah:

> "And Hashem God said, 'Behold Man has become like the Unique One among us, knowing good and bad.'"
>
> ויאמר יהוה אלהים הן האדם היה כאחד ממנו Gen 3:22

This phrase "Man has become Unique among us" means that to the Elohim, to Hashem God, Adam is different because now he has the ability to know "good and bad," *which God does not have.* This is what makes him *unique.* We have misinterpreted this phrase for a long time. Understanding it is paramount to setting ourselves free, because if we believe that God knows "good and bad" then we will feel that we must as well. This "knowing good and bad" is often confused with knowing right from wrong, or good from evil, and thus, it is believed that this knowledge is positive. However, in absolute Love you see only Balanced Positive, which is unconditional and completely non-judgmental. Thus, this ability to know good and bad was the ability to judge something as bad (Gevourah2), and is only an illusion because the World was created as AllGood. This launched the rebellion of the Adamic race and with the ability to judge something as bad came the dawning of belief systems that are untrue and based in illusion. It began our ability to look at what is AllGood and to see Good and Bad.

People often believe that if someone doesn't know how to judge things as bad that they cannot detect when something is wrong and take action accordingly. They do not understand that when you are AllGood and you see something foreign to your true nature, it is the easy to see that it is not something you wish, desire or want. The character Prot, an extra-terrestrial played by Kevin Spacey in the movie *K-PAX*, makes this point so beautifully to the psychiatrist. The psychiatrist, Mark, played by Jeff Bridges, asks Prot questions about life on the planet K-PAX:

Mark: "You have no laws?"

Prot: "No laws. No lawyers."

Mark: "How do you know right from wrong?"

Prot: "Every being in the Universe knows right from wrong, Mark."

Mark: "But what if someone did do something wrong, like committed a murder or a rape? How would you punish them?"

Prot: "Let me tell you something Mark. You humans, most of you, subscribe to this policy of an "eye for an eye," a "life for a life" which is known throughout the Universe for its stupidity. Even your Buddha and your Christ had quite a different vision, except no one really paid much attention to them, not even the Buddhists or the Christians.

You humans... Sometimes it's hard to imagine how you've made it this far."

A brilliant dialogue. You know something is not part of your reality because it is not Love. You do not need to enforce this, or hold onto the hammer of your judgment. The difference between the state of AllGood harmony and disharmony is that obvious. There is no judgment in paradise. Judgment makes a beautiful thing seem like an ugly one. This is why it is misleading to interpret the Torah literally when it says Eve and Adam were thrown from the garden, "And having driven out the man…" **Gen 3:24,** or that God punishes.

This is an example of God being depicted as controlling. But God did not punish them, for God does not punish. They simply could no longer live in that state of AllGood, for they changed in their new state of resistance within Frmee Will. As they became more and more divided within, they ceased to exist as Balanced Positive and *they kicked themselves out.* This shows us how Adam was One with the Will of God before the Tree of Knowledge and how later he could no longer exist as One. Adam and Eve fell because they got trapped in the illusion of fear and resisted the perfect flow of Love through them. The surrounding Garden and the Garden within ceased to seem like the original Eden. Thus, we have come to believe we no longer live in the Garden.

The Balanced Positive way sees that all is Good and discerns when something is not desired and takes proper action to correct it. Just because you do not judge a situation does not mean that you wish for that situation to be. For example, just because I do not judge people who are racists and accept people for the choices they make, does not mean I wish my world to be contain prejudice. (see **Appendix A**). To know in the way of good and bad is to be divisive and dualistic when they are truly only balanced Good (Balanced Positive). This trick of the Serpent is part of the Game. This is the left column of the Tree of Life turned around as Gevourah2, Tree of Knowledge.

The notion that the Creator is made up of a balance of good and bad in polarities is also a misconception. The Creator is AllGood. The bad was created to give rise to the opposite to challenge the Good. Yes, the Creator did create the bad, the challenger, but the creation of the opposite, although it is for the purpose of the Game, is not part of the *true nature* of God. Can you see the distinction? This clarification can make the entire world of difference for your awareness of the Creator, who you are, and what your responsibility is in returning yourself to a state of AllGoodLove.

And so the fruit that Eve and Adam ate, and perhaps were eating over a long period of time, began the cycle of duality. Eve "the mother of everyone living" (**Gen 3:20**), was so affected by it that all of her offspring were too. The children of Adam and Eve were already dual. Remember that *Anacardium orientale* can cause two different influences at the same time, one to do murder, the other to do good. Cain obviously allowed the impulse to do murder to prevail because he killed his brother. As we come to understand our nature, we see that we all have this dualistic nature. There is an angel in one ear and a devil in the other. This manifests as the separation of the left and the right brain, feeling and rationality, male and female, and Love and Frmee Will.

Samuel Hahnemann, who founded homeopathy in the beginning of the 19th century, was the first to discuss the "*miasm*," a genetically passed disease. In his book *Homeopathic Psychology*, Phillip Bailey, M.D., homeopath and psychiatrist, describes the principle of negative patterns of disease that are passed on genetically on page 386.

> "This long lingering pattern of disease seems to have created a 'miasm.' In other words, it affected every aspect of the health of the infected person, changing them at a cellular level, producing new characteristics which were then passed on to their children."

Here Bailey is discussing a miasm created by tuberculosis. However, any state of negativity, whether it be fear, anxiety, control, or physical illness, can become incorporated into a person's genetic code and then passed on through their offspring, if it affects them long enough. Miasm is just a fancy word for something that has influenced a human being to such an extent that it becomes ingrained in their genes and is then passable to their children.

The disturbance begins in the states of consciousness. Just as Buddha said that the thought becomes the word becomes the deed becomes the habit becomes the character.

Is a substance necessary for a pattern of disease (*miasm*) to become ingrained in the genetic code? No. It is just the disharmonious *thought* that is required, because that leads to a cascade of resistance and suppression of true nature, which causes disease. When they were One, Eve and Adam didn't need to eat the fruit from *Anacardium orientale*. All they needed to do was allow the conflict between their heart and mind to begin, to plant the seed of duality. Duality surely became ingrained deeply into their characters (genetic code) so that they passed it on to their children. All of us who have descended from Adam and Eve thus possess this conflict in our genetic code.

That first disharmonious thought was the desire to be like God. All that Adam and Eve had to do was *think* and make choices in duality with one Will opposing the other, then *speak* it, then *act* on it, for it became part of their *habit* and their *character*. What is amazing to see it that there is actually a corresponding tree that possesses the very same characteristics for this state of duality *and* that tree fits the Torah's description.

The Torah describes the Tree of Knowledge with the characteristics "good for food, delight to the eyes, means to wisdom" to reveal that *Anacardium orientale* is the Tree with the capacity to heal us of this most deep internal conflict between the angel and devil within us, between the One True Will and the Opposing Will. It is a substance of nature that exists to help bring us back to the Garden of Eden. This discovery is really just one, albeit an immensely important one, of the healing substances that the Torah provides so that we may return to Eden. They are all there, encoded in the text, hidden and buried in layers of time, just as our true nature has been buried in layers of unhealthy genes. And when these remedies are revealed, if we were to mix them together, we would have a healing potion, a homeopathic elixir, to help us return to Eden. I have called this "***The Homeopathic Elixir of Life***." (Although *Anacardium* is of very special significance and power for our healing, and has a special place because it is the Tree of Knowledge, there are other substances/remedies of equal importance and power in the Elixir. Book Two has more description and discussion about *the Homeopathic Elixir of Life*, and has the proper instructions about taking remedies. So please wait until Book Two before taking any remedies on your own.)

Samuel Hahnemann called the oldest miasm affecting humans "Psora." Hahnemann chose the word Psora from the Hebrew word "Tzarah," צרה, which means trouble, distress, conflict. In Yiddish, we say *Tzouris*. In fact, Hahnemann, and other homeopaths have since referred to the Psoric miasm as the "original sin" itself! *Anacardium orientale* is one of the most "Psoric" remedies in our repertory of homeopathic medicines, and confirms the idea that this tree served as the root of the "original sin." *Anacardium orientale* is the root of Psora, even more so than the homeopathic remedy prepared from sulphur, which has been called "the King of Psora." If Sulphur is the King, Anacardium is the Emperor—the source of all *Tzouris*.

We have been living in purgatory here on Earth. We feel both the good and the bad at all times. We rarely are free to just experience goodness. Even if we feel the good, some trace of bad always plays in the backs of our minds that squashes down the experience of good next to nothingness, like a splinter in our skin always hampering our feeling of well-being. During this conflict, there is a great strangulation of energy in the throat and neck, because there is a blockage between the mind and the body, which separates them. And since the throat is the bridge between the head and the body, it gets stuck when we close off this connection. This leads to stiff-necked people.

Within this conflict between the heart and the rational mind, we live rigidly trying to maintain what we believe is right, instead of simply following what we feel to be true. This breeds the feeling that we must be in control. This blocks up the throat energy, which is where we feel faith. In the stead of faith, we feel the need to be in control. A stiff neck is therefore directly related to the amount you try to control, and not let be, which is directly related to the amount of Frmee Will. Give up this struggle! There is no conflict when there is only Love. When there is only Love (Will of the Heart), there is only Beingness. This is Freedom.

We can interpret the significance of God's command that Eve and Adam should *not* eat from the Tree of Knowledge from another angle: it was necessary for Eve and Adam to harbor the belief that *they* had chosen this state of two Wills. What does this mean? This means that God told them *not* to eat from the Tree so that when they did, they would be able to believe that the decision was *not* God's, but theirs.

Of course, it was quite probable that they were eventually going to disobey the Will of God and choose outside of their true nature. Placing them in Eden is like putting a child in a room full of toys and saying, "You may play with all the toys except for the toy in the center of the room." In addition, you give it a special name, too. "You must not play with the Toy of Pleasure." Then you leave the children on their own. What do you think they will do? Of course they will eventually explore, especially once they have become slightly bored, as did God and the angels. Therefore, Adam and Eve believed that it was in fact their choice to explore the forbidden. When Eve and Adam's hand stretched out to eat the fruit from this sacred Tree, they both had God's voice echoing in their ears: "do not eat from the Tree…" Understand that for a creature who did not know a Will of its own, it was necessary to create this sort of distinction between what God wanted and what God did not. At least it was necessary for them to believe the choice to eat the fruit was theirs. As they did, they began to feel they had another Will and that they were double. Do you see that with this combination is the Birth of Frmee Will?

If Frmee Will is an illusion, and our true Will (at one with the Will of God) is real, then what can we possibly do with Frmee Will? All we can do with Frmee Will is resist the Will of God.

> "The powerful flow of life-force that comes with the involuntary divine creative principle cannot be commanded by the ego. Another way to say this is that the goodness within you flows of its own accord; it reaches out in wisdom, love, and caring of its own accord. It does not flow on the command of the ego. The only thing the ego can do is stop it from flowing or get out of its way."
>
> *Light Emerging*, Barbara Ann Brennan p. 265

When we realize that the fear associated with letting go Frmee Will is only an illusion, it will be easier to say goodbye and to remove ourselves from all this doubt and debris. We will remove *the self from the self* (the doubled self that is an illusion).

A Will begins in the mind. One is the mind of the ego, based within the illusions of separation, duality, the past, fear, and judgment—the left column of the Tree turned in upon itself. The other is the mind of the heart which is a mind of intuition, wisdom and feeling. One is rational, limiting and rigid. The other is limitless and free. As you become more and more aware of the feeling of your body, as you remember more and more who you really are, you will awaken your intuitive mind. With your intuitive mind, you align yourself with the One and make the choice of only following the Will of the Heart. Do not fog out your mind of Oneness as you attempt to return to Beingness. Don't block off your entire mind as you slow the activity of the doubting, Bina2 mind. Your mind will become more and more open and your eyes brighter as you remember your mind of Truth.

As Don Juan said in Carlos Casteneda's *The Active Side of Infinity*:

> "Every one of us human beings has two minds. One
> is totally ours, and it is like a faint voice that always
> brings us order, directness, purpose. The other mind
> is a foreign installation. It brings us conflict,
> self-assertion, doubts, hopelessness."
> "Our pettiness and contradictions are, rather, the results
> of a transcendental conflict that afflicts every one of us,
> but of which only sorcerers are painfully and hopelessly aware:
> the conflict of our two minds."
> *The Active Side of Infinity* pp. 7, 9

What is a sorcerer? One dedicated to the path of Truth. So will you naturally sense this conflict when you are dedicated to the path of your True nature. As your sensitivity increases and you let go of more and more resistance, you will *become aware of the two minds that are within you.* All must move toward and then through the separation in order to become One with the Divine. Always, always remember that this intuitive mind *is a mind,* thus it has an intention. An intention is a will. Thus as you begin to awaken to your true nature by giving up control and allowing yourself to feel, don't fall into the trap of not doing a thing! This is important lest you wind up back in the weak-willed quagmire of *Anacardium orientale.*

Since this primordial conflict is between the Will of the rational mind and the Will of the Heart, whenever you use your rational mind, you weaken your heart's Will. This is just like men injecting themselves with testosterone to build up muscle; their testicles atrophy because the body doesn't need to produce it itself. Imagine the immense effect, therefore, through the ages and in anyone's lifetime created by studying the laws of our religious texts and subsequently following them. Even if those texts originally came from the divine, to study "the word" and then to choose is to follow the rational. Especially in the study of Torah, which is law-based, you consult your rational mind as to what is Good or what is Bad according to the text. All the interpretations of the laws were also meticulously deduced through rational arguments. These choices, based on the concept of Good and Bad, are finite in nature. Anything finite in nature is limiting. The Will of the Heart, undefined and infinite, which is the One True Will, which, in turn brings joy, Love, and peace, is atrophied and buried when a person follows the way of the rational.

This is why we have forgotten our true nature for so long. We have forgotten that we are the children of the Creator, created in the image and likeness of that Divine Entity. We have forgotten that our core is Good, and that by aligning ourselves with that core, we are following the One Will, which is aligned with the Tree of Life and the Garden of Eden. Because we have forgotten, we have turned to The Torah/Bible to tell us what is Good and what is Bad, for we fear that without such teachings, we have no capacity to follow the Will of God—to inherently know Truth, which is Goodness. If you connect with the immense significance of this, then you see that on yet another level, *there is another Tree of Knowledge for Good and Bad*—the book we have followed for millennia, pouring over every passage, intent upon remembering the significance each word or letter had for our salvation and our connection to God. This book is filled from end to end with the knowledge of what is Good and Bad, which so many of us have believed and followed religiously.

The Torah is the Tree of Knowledge for Good and Bad.

When Moses first descended from Mount Sinai with the tablets of the Torah, they were in pure form. It is written:

"Moses turned and descended from the mountain, with the two
Tablets of the Testimony in his hand, Tablets inscribed on both their
sides; they were inscribed on one side and the other." **Exo 32:15**

Then, when Moses discovered the people worshipping the golden
calf, he threw down and destroyed the pure form of the Torah, the form
symbolic of the Tree of Life. Written on both sides, it was the Balanced
Positive, the male and the female as One, like the Tree of Life.

"It happened as he drew near the camp and saw the calf and the
dances, that Moses' anger flared up. He threw down the Tablets from
his hands and shattered them at the foot of the mountain." **Exo 32:19**

When Moses climbed Mount Sinai again, that true form of Torah,
which represented the Tree of Life, scattered and rearranged itself into
the Torah that we possess now, which is the Tree of Knowledge for
Good and Bad. Even though the Torah does describe the second Tablets
that Moses received as being the same as the first, the second Torah
Moses received was not the same. It changed accordingly, to mirror the
Tree of Knowledge and not the Tree of Life. The literal words keep the
fact hidden that there is another Torah of greater Truth. How could
people have followed The Torah we have now and have had for thousands of years if they knew there was a Torah of greater Truth?

How is the Torah that we have now the Tree of Knowledge? It is
filled with knowledge of the 613 Mitzvot, or Laws. 365 of those Laws
being knowledge of the Bad commandments (what not to do), and 248
being knowledge of the Good commandments (what to do).

This switch at the top of Mount Sinai is analogous to the way that
the Kabbalistic Tree of Life was doubled and reflected inward, and
became the Tree of Knowledge. What this also symbolizes is Moses
removing and hiding the Kabbalah from the true form of Torah. The
Kabbalah is the Source of All Truth. It is the foundation and undefined
Truth through the experience of receiving (Kabbalah means "to be
received"). Moses knew his task was to remove/hide the Kabbalah, for
with the knowledge of true Kabbalah allowed to remain, which is ever-

present in the Garden of Eden, the Truth would have been ever-present, and people could not have been challenged with choice. You must forget your true nature so that you can choose your true nature. The act of giving us the Torah of Good and Bad Knowledge was an act that created the reality of duality and Frmee Will. The Kabbalah represents the side of the true Torah that is the female. As the foundation, and when balanced with the male side, it is the Tree of Life. Without it, we are left only with the unbalanced male, which is the knowledge of Good and Bad. (This is explained and discussed more in Chapter 12.)

The last many thousand of years have been our trial period on Earth where we have been put to the test. Holding on to the Torah in its Tree of Knowledge form was a great part of the test.

The Torah and the Jewish people have become one. Thus the code of the Torah is also embedded in our consciousness. The belief systems that are written in the Torah were ingrained in the collective consciousness of the Jewish people and also in the collective consciousness of the entire planet and laid the foundations of many of those beliefs of duality for the world. (As a simple and very important example – After Adam and Eve ate from the Tree of Knowledge, it is written that Hashem said to Eve: "Yet your craving shall be for your husband, and he shall rule over you." **Gen 3:16**. Thus, we have seen in most societies the world over, a dominance of the man over the woman. And is it any surprise that a book which is unbalanced male, with the female pushed down, should not propagate a belief system that the man shall rule over the woman and that she be created as a helper for him?)

This means that the purpose of Torah, given by God to Moses, was to create this Game, this challenge, this test. The Torah is thus not only the Guidebook for the Game of Life—it created the Game of Life. The purpose of embedding these belief systems was a part of the Creator's Divine Plan and the task begun by the Hebrews. A tough job, but someone had to do it. You distance yourself from the Oneness so that in returning, you have experience of who you really are. What can help us all understand the importance of this task of the Hebrews is the fact that they have held on to the Law of Torah until this time, fulfilling their promise through the ages, and that with the collective release of the beliefs and the Law of Torah in the days to come, it will be at a time where peace becomes the reality for the entire world.

The children of Israel were given the Torah and we chose it. We have religiously followed it. More than any other factor, it is the holding on to the Torah that has caused the Hebrew people to suffer from generation to generation because its messages are filled with separation, suffering, and oppression. By following the Torah religiously and studying every passage intent on committing everything to memory, we took it to heart. Naturally, our state of existence reflected and reflects what is contained in the Torah. Paradoxically, the Torah has also helped us survive all the suffering and to find great pleasure in service to God. And what is amazing to grasp, a most incredible part of understanding this Game, as mind boggling as it may seem and hard to fathom, is that now it is time to let go of the Law of Torah, the Law of Moses, to wipe the slate clean, so to speak, so that we may in each of us, unfold and rearrange the scattered letters of our Trees of Knowledge to yield our Trees of Life. Then we can carry out our covenant to God and bring this world into a state of peace and unconditional Love.

In the physical world, the amount of trapped, blocked energies of pain and suffering you experience and release is directly proportional to the amount of joy and Love you can ultimately experience. The Jewish people have held on just the right amount of time in order to create the perfect amount of potential energy to catapult us into the Time of Forwardness and Moshiach for the creation of the experience of heaven on earth for *all* people. Thus, if one were to call the Torah "The Tree of Knowledge" in a judgmental way, without understanding the importance of that Tree of Knowledge, without accepting this pact with God and without acknowledging the immensity of the task to which the Hebrews have remained true, one would be missing some very vital awareness.

Also, the Torah is a moralistic system, which creates an order amongst people who follow its Laws and has guided the lives of countless people on Earth for thousands of years. Even though I am acutely aware of the limitations on the freedom of Being when I am in the presence of religious Jews, I am very grateful to be in their presence, because their dedication and belief in *something,* and their commitment to the Torah creates a special quality and depth that is a slice above the secular world, where many people are dedicated and believe in nothing but themselves. So, yes there is a stifling of the freedom of Being when one believes that God's Will is permanently embedded in the Law of Torah. Yet the world where people obey Torah is significantly better than a world where people rule by survival of the fittest and everyone-for-themselves mentalities. This order into a tight system of Law and religious devotion to God has helped keep the human potential from forgetting all connection with the Divine, and has prevented very destructive and aggressive ways of living. It has also played a purpose through the centuries where the world was evolving through very barbaric stages, having completely forgotten its origins.

Now is the time for our complete healing and for secrets to be revealed. Things kept reserved for thousands of years are now emerging for our complete understanding and empowerment. So understand that if we turn to a book to show us how to be, we forget *our* inherent ability to know Truth, as Abraham had. Having inherent knowledge of who you are and putting it into practice, is what brings the direct experience of Truth. Walking the talk. That is what occurs naturally when you come out of your shell and your comfort zone. Not only are you able to witness the Truths you learned and believed to be accurate, you get to *be* them. The difference is immense. Attempting to know God through *the written way* and following the Law of Torah is not what will bring about the Messiah.

For any group of people that *believes it needs* its sacred texts to know the Truth, the experience of the knowledge therein becomes inaccessible. This, believe it or not, is part of the way in which the Serpent controls us—by making us try to connect with God by knowledge of Good and Bad, or right and wrong. This way, we forget we already have that direct knowledge in being who we are and so we turn to a book to tell us how to Be. People have used the New Testament, the Koran, the Bhagavad-Gita, the Rig Veda, and many other sacred texts this way. A book cannot tell you how to Be. Nothing can tell you how to Be. You can only take the leap into Being, knowing that *you are*. If you say, "I am nothing without the Torah, the New Testament, the Koran," you are turning your infinite capacity of direct knowing and Being into nothingness. Releasing this *dependant* relationship is of utmost importance for the healing of religious Jews, Christians, and Muslims, as well as all other people who put their faith in the words of a text.

This is not to say that we must burn our sacred books. I am saying that to believe we need the Torah, the New Testament, or the Koran to show us how to Be is untrue. We must set ourselves free from the crutch we have leaned on for so many years so that we can stand upright on our own two feet. As long as you maintain the idea that you need your crutch, you cannot stand on your own two feet, and yet, that is necessary at this time. The purpose of the crutch has been to support us until we were prepared to stand on our own two feet, now, in this day and age.

> "To study a text, we should take into account the circumstances, the situation, the time, the society and community where a book was originally written or a teaching taught." *The Dalai Lama's Book of Daily Meditations*, pp. 180

The Torah was given to us at a time long, long ago and we were asked to follow it religiously, without question. We did so. That is the covenant the Jewish people have had with God. We have learned so much, established immense interpretations and so many commentaries that it is mind boggling. We have prepared ourselves, built our knowledge up, examined it, cross-examined it, brought it forward through the Ages. Now it is time to carry forth all that we have learned through our study of Torah. It is now time to go *out* into the world and *Be* who we are. If you have an immense gift to help others, if you are created to bring forth goodness for people, and you do not do so in the entirety of who you are, you become doubled. You have your true nature, because it is always you, and you also have self-reflection. Reflecting on yourself is the *left* column of the Tree *turned inward*. It is your ego. Just as we have all of the Light within us, so do we also have the inward reflection of that Light. The Torah is one and the same, a reflection of our state, for it is filled with immeasurable wisdom as well as many limiting belief systems.

Obedience to God is *always* divine and very rewarding. Obedience to anything or anyone, a spouse, a teacher, a coach, a leader, has its rewards because it involves the giving up of the self (removing the self from the self). Thus, in Exodus when it says, "Everything that God has said, we will do and we will obey!' (**Exo 24:7**) and we obeyed the word of God as it is written in the Torah, service in that devotion has had its reward. This reward also has to do with giving up your need to think for yourself. All is laid out for you. What is good, what is bad. Until now, there has been no need to question, no responsibility of trusting yourself.

> "The soft or passive types of Anacardium people are more likely to be followers than leaders. Instead of making decisions for themselves, they look for answers in documents or in lists of rules and regulations—'scriptures' of one sort or another. They believe that, if they follow the rules, regardless of what the rules require them to do, no one will criticize or punish them."
>
> *Core Elements,* Ananda Zaren

Thus a person can follow the Torah or any sacred text without question and reap the many rewards it offers. Yet, this is not the highest level of obedience. The highest level of obedience comes from trusting your inner guidance, ever changing, yet always received from God's will. Following this intuitive inner Truth, you are led to Ehye Usher Ehye and the release into freedom. This is to fulfill your choice to serve God and your covenant with God.

We received the Torah, the New Testament, the Koran as children of God when people were not ready to *Be* God's Will on Earth. Now we are adults and have graduated to *the Unwritten Way*, which is to carry out the healing of the world in whatever way, shape, or form your soul prompts you to do. This fulfills the covenant of the Jewish people with God and is the highest state of earthly being—existing for the good of all people, as a caretaker of the planet. We do not need to hear how to be from our parent any longer. Receiving the Torah and all of our toil through the past thousands of years have prepared us for *the present*. We are ready now to adopt *the Unwritten Way* and submit to it, each in our unique way. We must be ready, or else the pressure from holding on to the tradition that we believe is God's Will shall split us down the middle, like a person who holds on to both edges of a precipice while the earth, in upheaval, tears itself apart.

The study of the Torah and the belief that through study one connects with God has also caused us to forget our true nature. If you simply know who you are and you do not carry that forward to the world in *being* who you are, then you will live in a prison of suffering. This is not meant in a judgmental way, but rather literally. Why? Because the joy of who you are is *only* experienced in *being* who you are, not *knowing* who you are. That is the purpose of creation. If you just know and yet you remain closed off, you suffer because your core, the heart of you, is dormant. Just knowing who you are without being yourself, is to be without your heart. And when you do this, the world becomes a bleak and scary place. In fact, as discussed in *The Dream* chapter, believing in the way of Torah, the Law of Good and Bad, and maintaining that as the ultimate truth, perpetuates the existence of the world as Good and Bad, which is a world of suffering, and not the AllGood of the One true reality.

The Adamic people, humanity, still encompassed within the imagination of God, as children of the Creator, is teetering on the edge of a precipice that seems terribly frightening. It is frightening because of the uncertainty that accompanies releasing the Y Factor. It is scary to go out and *Be* what we have rationally discovered about ourselves. Jumping into the precipice is the leap of faith that will yield to us the experience of who we are and how we were created to be.

The Love those who have followed these sacred texts can have for them is truly understandable. The dedication of the people who have followed them is extraordinarily remarkable. The texts have been such meaningful companions. It can be quite difficult to loosen the ties that bind us to them. Just as Tom Hank's character in the movie *Castaway* mourned the loss of his companion Wilson, who kept him company

and helped him survive years stranded on an island, so too is it understandable that we will find it difficult to let go of the dependant relationship we have had with our sacred texts.

In letting go of the attachment to Torah, another problem arises for
a Jewish person and which must be understood in the proper light.
Through the centuries, Jews have had to struggle for the freedom to
study the Torah and follow its ways (This is part of the test and task of
the Hebrews). Countless empires, with their own system of worship,
have risen and fallen and have attempted to stop the Jews from worshipping God, Hashem, through following the Torah. Countless generations of Jews have been oppressed. Jews, now free to study as they
wish, feel an almost encoded responsibility to their ancestors who did-
n't have that opportunity. We maintain out of loyalty to our deprived
ancestors. We hold on to the Torah because we have been oppressed.
We feel it is our obligation to do so because we *can*. We must release
ourselves from clinging to the Torah and the emotional associations
with our past because, in service to God, there is no need to follow its
laws or what might seem like the law in any other sacred text. That is
not the Will of God that you *must* follow. The Will of God is carried
out through you performing your unique Tikkun (healing) of the planet because you are One with God, and God would truly love to see us
live in harmony and abundance together. Remember, to think you
must try to be who you are creates the belief that you are not who you
are. Especially if you believe you must follow the Law to know how to
be, you separate yourself from the Being. There *is* much in the Torah
that is one and the same as your true nature, yet that is only revealed
once you let go of your need to look into the Torah to show you how
to be. You can never have true knowledge of who you are until you let
go of attachments to all external influences. Once these attachments
have been released, you might find that the Torah still brings you joy,
and you may wish to continue to practice for congregation, for celebration, inspiration, and for tradition. Then your relationship to the
Torah will be completely different, reversed so to speak, and it will no
longer be the Law. For you will see in the Torah who you know you
are, instead of using the Torah to show you how to be. To believe that
you *must* follow the Law as it is written imprisons you. It locks you in

the past, causes you to doubt your true nature, and creates a lot of guilt. This belief binds you to the trunk of the Tree that has both Good and Bad fruit. It separates you from knowing the living, breathing, ever-renewed True Will of God in you, and the AllGood fruit of the Tree of Life.

Now that the doors to Eden have been reopened, there is no more Law, no more ground-rules. There is only Beingness and it is AllGood. There is only following *The Unwritten Way*, which each individual must discover for him or herself in myriad possible ways. This is similar to what Abraham and the Jewish people followed before the Torah, when there was no codified Law to obey. Abraham's essential task was to bring the world to a better place. That became the task of the Jew and it remains the very core purpose of the Jewish people until this day. The purpose of the Jewish people is not to follow the Law of the Torah. The purpose of the Jewish people is to heal the world—Tikkun Olam. That has always been our task. It is the very heart and soul of who we are as a people, shared with many others who equally feel that calling. To carry out this task, Abraham and the Jews of the time were told not to worship idols and followed only the Universal laws of "Love thy neighbor as you love yourself"—the same as "Do unto others as you who have them do unto you"—and "Love God with all your heart, all your soul, and all your power." These few Universal Laws are also all that is required for us to fulfill our task. Carrying out this task will bring joy and is a natural inclination of the Hebrew people. As we heal the world, we will be healed of the pain we have experienced in surviving against the hardships of the world, and surviving the world itself, from which we have separated ourselves.

You don't need volumes of information to tell you how to go about your True nature. It is all there in your heart. You must simply let go of all that you think you need to Be who you are. There you will find the Will of God holding your hand as you choose from your heart. This is to follow the Unwritten Way of the Kabbalah, which is undefined, yet is etched in the heavens and in the code of our hearts, as naturally and eternally as the stars are written upon the sky.

Why now? Why were we asked now to move forward into a new relationship in carrying out our service to God?

Because Moses says so.

Is that a satisfying answer? Of course not. First of all, if you have even the slightest doubt as to whether or not this is the actual message of Moses, this answer will not be enough. What if you have absolutely no doubt that this is the message of Moses. Is this answer adequate? It shouldn't be. Because it is not simply because Moses says it, that it must be. Remember, Moses is just a messenger. He points somewhere and you must reach and see for yourself. What matters is that we, the people, collectively reach out to embrace what the messenger points to.

Many people can extend their antennae, sense the inherent truth in something, and need no proof. Many will understand that this is in fact the time just because they know it and feel it. But many are still stuck, needing explanations and proof for everything. They are still so rational. For those of you still holding on, look back at Chapter 6, The Imagination of God, and really take time to ponder the passages about what Rabbi Shimon Bar Yochai said about the doors of Moshiach being opened. Consider also that the six days of creation being paralleled by our 6000 year calendar is now bringing the Great Sabbath, for we are at the end of the sixth day. The six days of toil during the week are equivalent to the ages we have struggled with the Law of Moses. The Sabbath represents rest from the work done during the week and celebration and the release of the Law, which was a lot of work to maintain these last 6000 years. We can even listen to what cosmologies say to show us how now is the time. Mayan, Sumerian, and Native American prophecies all point to this time. Greg Braden amasses great information in *Awakening to Zero Point* to paint the picture, spiritually and scientifically, of why now is the time of a great shift in reality. Christian texts, too, forecast the return of Christ at around this time. There are signs everywhere—in the heavens, on earth, in our fields, our cities.

But the most important sign and proof is in your heart. If you allow yourself, even for the slightest moment, to feel your longing for Moshiach, to feel the promise, you will have to step out of your past mind-set because the Moshiach is the World to Come. The greatest sign, or validity of this message, is the feeling you have when you allow yourself to see just how much you too really *want* this to be true. Can you see that Moshiach equals change and letting go to embrace a way that is not so defined and concretized in our minds? Yes. The Moshiach is the letting go of Frmee Will which is closing the book on our past. Our identity, as Jewish people, and people of other religions, which we hold on to and relate to with the Torah, or other sacred texts from other religions, is an anchor that maintains our ship in the harbor, when it is time to set sail around the world. The beliefs and notions of reality that we have established and associate through the Torah must also be lifted in order to bring in Moshiach. The Torah, currently in scattered form, is waiting for us to unravel all of its mysteries and discover the whole story of who we are.

We are put to the test through the trials of this life. Yet, we really triumph over the test and over the Game by remembering our true nature and freedom that is beyond all definition. Therefore, the complete and total release from the attachments to the Torah will cause an explosion of joy from the transformation and release of all the pent up and potential energies to carry us forward into a new age. And this is true for other religions as well. The Torah set the foundation for Christianity and Islam, and it is also through the release of the other beliefs and laws of Christianity and Islam, or any other religion, that great joy is experienced to personally touch with the Truth beyond the word and law. Do not fear that chaos will result. Yes, there is an adjustment period when the structure of the Law is released. And then there is freedom.

It is remarkable beyond words that the Jewish people have held on to the service and carried out the Law of Torah for so long, as we said we would. To have done so for so long and against such odds is truly something wondrous. The greatest test of the Hebrews now—perhaps greater than any of the other trials we have encountered—which represents going to the next level, is to release our attachments to the Law of Torah so that we can allow ourselves to rearrange into our rightful state and see the full wisdom of what the purpose of our existence has been about.

Then, by moving away from service to the *word* of God into the service of God via the Unwritten Way, we will be able to carry out our deepest purpose, which is to serve the good of *all people* and to heal the entire planet (Tikkun Olum) as a Light unto the Nations (Or L'Goyim.)

Chapter 9: Summary

Eating of the Tree of Knowledge for Good and Bad was a great turning point in the evolution of who we were as a people. The act represents relinquishing a state of Oneness in which there was no judgment or separation and adopting instead a state of duality and separation. The forbidden fruit of the Tree of Knowledge represents the sexual act of union. In their state of innocence, having just separated into male and female parts, Adam and Eve were not ready to experience the total unification of polarities. This unification is a most powerful and special way to connect with the Creator and experience the Creator, who is One. When they did allow themselves to unite sexually, because they chose to do something outside the Will of God, and because they weren't ready, they felt guilty and shameful about their choice. This got them off to a bad start and they began to judge things as wrong/bad. This split or doubled them. With their guilty internal conflict, no longer was the Will of the Heart free to be and to do as it wished. The conflict began of the rational mind labeling what is good or bad (judgment, Gevourah2), which suppresses what the heart naturally knows is Good.

The primordial consciousness began with Adam and Eve and has been passed on genetically through the generations. It is the conflict between reason (rational) and will (what we would love to do, aligned with the heart). This conflict causes a split in the consciousness such that the soul experiences two wills: the true will of the Heart and the will of the Ego-Mind, the mind separation, the mind of control, the mind of resistance.

Anacardium orientale causes this exact energetic conflict in healthy individuals. Therefore Anarcadium orientate will act within the homeopathic law of "like curing like" to heal this conflict of wills in an individual who possesses the disturbance. Anacardium orientale fits the description which the Torah cryptically describes as the Tree of Knowledge. This Tree, Anacardium, which is thus the Tree of

Knowledge on another level, can help heal the "original sin" that marked the separation from the Garden of Eden.

The Torah also represents The Tree of Knowledge for Good and Bad, for it is filled with knowledge of what is right and wrong, good and bad. When we continue to study any of our other sacred texts to learn how to be, we live in the rational manner, according to finite laws and writings. The idea that The Torah, or any sacred text, must be followed to know what is Good, removes from a person his or her inherent ability to know Truth and Goodness. The fact that this is clearly revealed to us today indicates that it is time to release ties with any sacred text we rely upon to know truth. Then we can return to directly knowing Truth by being One with creation, as represented by the Tree of Life.

ESSENCE OF THE CHAPTER

When you experience a conflict of Wills, between the Will of your Reason/Rationality and the Will of your Intuition/Heart, follow your heart.

CHAPTER TEN

THE REVERSALS

OF REALITY

"And I saw how the reverse side is used by the Masters of Light to code the physical creation from the heavenly side so that the human race was but a transparent reversal of the divine images of creation constantly kept in the Divine Presence of the Father."

Keys Of Enoch, 307: 18, Dr. J.J. Hurtak

The way in which we now live in the physical world *is* the reverse side of the divine images of the imagination of God which we are always connected with.

We can use the analogies of the negative image of a photograph and a mirror image to convey what is meant by this reversal of reality, but those analogies are limited to two dimensions. Our *state of consciousness* exists in three dimensions and is reflected and mirrored in itself (imploded). Therefore, we can say that we presently exist in the *mirror-imagine*. Let us examine all the ways in which this physical reality is actually the reverse of Oneness and that there are many reversals, opposites, and negatives keeping us inside the mirror–imagine and the reversals of reality. Let us also examine how this affects our perception of reality, the functioning of the chakras, the *auric field*, the Tree of Life vs. the Tree of Knowledge, and what lies beyond the reversals of reality for humankind.

The chakras are spinning wheels or funnels of energy that draw in the energy of the Universe and empower our existence. Many sacred traditions hold that there is a **seal** in their depths *plugging* up the connection between the front and the rear chakras. This seal is a primordial plug or blockage that began at the time the Tree of One Direction of Flow and Another was eaten, because the front and rear chakras were not in harmony with each other. The seals between the front and rear chakras were created because they are in *contradiction* to one another, just as our hearts and rational minds contradict each other.

Looking at the spin direction of the front and rear chakras from the outside, we have thought that the clockwise spin of both front and rear chakras represents an "open" state. Some healers might have believed this to be the balanced state because when the chakras are spinning clockwise, the energy is drawn into the chakra and the body. But because these two chakras are two opposite types of energy—feeling/front/Yin and will/back/Yang—both cannot spin clockwise and be in harmony. (Yin is afferent and feeling in nature. Yang is efferent and willful in nature.) When both draw in energy, that is not how the state of harmony truly exists between the two chakras. One is on the back, facing the opposite direction of the one in front. When they both draw in energy, the energy moves in two opposite directions, which is not harmonious. The front chakra energy flows from front to back and the rear chakra energy flows from back to front. This creates the time of forwardness and the time of reverse within us. This is duality and gives us the sense of being split in two, with two Wills, and the Yin (feeling) and Yang (will) energies contradict each other. (see Figure 18a)

The *contradiction* between *reason/rationality* and *feeling/intuition* is the source and causes the duality. It all began in the mind as a root of dissonance which then translated into all our entire energy systems, including the chakras. The conflict is between our must-try Will (rear–Yang) centers, due to our delusion of having to be in control

(Frmee Will), and the feeling (front–Yin) centers.

The rational mind carries this out by exerting its *efferent* force and control through the rear chakras, resisting the true mind that is one with the Will of God, which is in harmony with the front, feeling chakras. This control comes from the left column of the Tree, the ego self turned in upon itself, Bina2, Gevourah2, and Hod2. The rear chakras have simply "taken up the reigns" of control because they are the energetic centers that carry out the Will of the rational mind and Frmee Will. There is nothing inherently wrong with the rear chakras. They are just carrying out their duty, as we have been instructing them.

Clockwise motion of *both* the front and rear chakras is *only* like that in a person in the state of duality, not Oneness, not pure Light Beingness. This bi-directional flow of energy actually keeps a person in disharmony and he or she can use Will to stop from feeling. This is what occurs within Frmee Will consciousness. To be one with God, all we can do is allow the flow of Love or resist it. When we fear or judge, we resist. When we think we must try, this trying effort is also like putting a foot on the brake against the flow of allow—the flow of I AM, for being who you truly are is an act of Beingness, of allowance, not of trying. That is why, in our Frmee Will world, the rear, Will chakra opposes the front, feeling chakras. Does the expression "holding back" make more sense now?

The opposite of too much Will and control can occur as well, which is floppiness and weak-Will. When we are apathetic, we can get stuck feeling too much (if it is not something that is necessary to feel) somewhat like self-torture, or drowning in emotions. Although we tend to suppress a lot, it is also very important to overcome this sort of apathy. Getting stuck can be dwelling on a negative feeling. In other words, it is necessary to allow oneself to feel emotions and to deal with them by releasing them and then making the choices that we want to make. But don't get stuck dwelling in the emotions, in "poor me" or "I must suffer" attitudes.

[**4th Circle**—CaN #5: I let go of the belief that I must suffer. I let go of the belief that life is painful and hard. I allow the joy and beauty of life to sweep over me every moment.]

It is good to understand when it is time to feel and when you are stuck in apathy. Most of the time we suppress. This blocked energy builds up and becomes more and more difficult to release because it feels like something huge and overwhelming. However, if you're sitting around in apathy dwelling on emotion, that is a pretty good clue that you are stuck. A good way to get yourself out is to give yourself a kick in the butt and pull yourself out. Intense exercise, an excellent hydrotherapy shower of alternating hot and cold water, a hot bath with sea salt, wonderful music and loud singing, or yelling your heart out are examples of exercises that can help release your emotional apathy. It will help the flow resume.

Even with apathy, the root is due to suppression and resistance. How could you get stuck in the apathy of negativity unless you first judged a way of being and suppressed it? Remember grief, for example, is not a bad experience. Neither is anger. When we judge these experiences and suppress them, they build up and become something quite negative. Of course we do not usually like to live continually this way, but is not sadness a positive experience from time to time? Or the expression of anger, if it is not destructive? In pulling yourself out of apathy, therefore, it is important not to judge that state. To judge is to become enslaved by what you judge.

This brings to light a very important point. There are two ways of going about your healing. One is the way of simply knowing who you are and not paying any mind or attention to fears, judgments, and pain in your body and Being. It is simply choosing who you are and being that, without doubt or hesitation. The other way is a way of feeling, allowing all things to be, and going right into the fears, judgments, and pain to the source to see both the Will you are using to hold on (recognizing where to release your Frmee Will) and also the illusion of the fear and the judgments, which lead to the pain. This way of healing is elaborated upon in *Chapter 2*. I feel it is necessary to know both these ways, as we go through a kind of a shifting from one way of letting go to the next, somewhat as in the rise and fall of the tides. On the one hand, if you were to hold on solely to the way of knowing who you are and moving straight ahead, not listening to what you're thinking and feeling, nor observing the process of your fears and judgments, you might begin resisting feelings and avoiding facing what is really going on inside, preferring to just live in your mind. At this point feeling is necessary and listening inside to become aware of the negative thoughts and fears that are occurring in your mind. By feeling the fears and pain of resistance in this way of healing, you help yourself flow and dissipate the fears, judgment, and pain. On the other hand, if you were to solely hold on to this way of healing through feeling, then you might become stuck too much in feeling, and become too wrapped up in yourself and in apathy. You then need to switch into the other way, moving forward simply knowing who you are and being what you love to be without fear and hesitation. Eventually, when you have found your true self, these two ways become seamlessly aligned as one.

And guess what? One is the foundation and the other is simply a continuation of that flow. And the foundation is the feeling, which is receiving, which is Kabbalah, which is the unwritten Truth and Beauty of God flowing right through you that you experience as a constant presence of divine feeling and connection. Then you understand the great importance of getting good and down with the Second Chapter of this book and establishing feeling as the basis of your entire reality (Don't worry, your mind is not lost, it is just a seamless part and extension of your Being.) How deeply can you let yourself feel? That is the secret. That is a Oneness. Let the mind go and observe what you see when you're feeling all the way as deep as you can into your core. (You'll need to be in shape and with a great conviction and dedication, like doing *an impossible dream*, in your heart to get this deep.)

Something else that is wondrous to realize is that the Source of all your holding back is you holding yourself back from feeling the Goodness in your centers. All the bottom lines of resistance are due to the holding back of your rear chakras on the flow of feeling from the front chakras, which is the good you feel flowing through the center of your chakras. When Adam and Eve began holding back, they were holding back the AllGood of the Garden of Eden and the AllGood of how they were created. So surely they had to be stopping their goodness? So we have done. We have blocked ourselves from feeling good about ourselves, from feeling the most intense pleasure and joy from our sexual

center, from feeling Love for all others, from feeling the perfect divine
connection with The Creator, from feeling rooted beautifully in the
Earth, from feeling One with Nature and all of creation…By letting
yourself feel, totally and completely, with all your heart, all your soul,
and with full power, you are sliding down a slide into holy waters, first
perhaps through the muddy waters, like diving into a pond covered
with lily pads and leaves. Ah, and then beneath, beneath you find the
Eight Rivers of Heaven, all flowing into the One Sea of Nine.

The flow of a resistance chakra is the negative/reverse of the flow
of a feeling chakra. This is because the *self within the self* is the negative
of the true self. It is like being trapped in yourself, stuck experiencing
the opposite of who you are. Our true self, our Higher Self, is also
called the "Overself" in *the Keys of Enoch*, and this makes sense, because
the Overself, or Higher Self, is on the other side of where our self
within our self is stuck. It is in another dimension *over* and encompassing the imploded *self within the self*. And thus the will of the self
within the self and its influence on the body must also be the negative
of our true nature and block the feeling of our true nature, for its will
is the same as Frmee Will.

The flow of a feeling chakra nourishes the auric field with its sensations and perceptions. For example, the flow of the third, solar plexus
chakra nourishes a sense of security, confidence, and a feeling of having
a place in the Universe. So if this chakra does not flow, the auric field
will miss the sensation that the third chakra usually brings. This will
inhibit feeling part of the world, leaving us feeling insecure, out of place,
and lacking self-esteem. The person will stop feeling the positive emotion when there is over control by the rear-will center. This also applies
to the joy of sex and creativity of the second chakra, the Love of the
heart (fourth chakra), and the faith and allowing of the throat chakra
(fifth). When positive emotions are blocked, *the negative emotions will be
felt in their stead.* This is a graded progression, but it can also happen quite
quickly in severe cases of trauma.

With any judgment, a person blocks off the feeling of a front chakra,
which controls the experience of reality. The strictly mental experience
of reality feels like nothingness, for it is a hollow graphic reflection of
Being. When beliefs include judgments, for example, "I am not good

enough. I don't belong," the projection of the belief system from the rational, efferent mind will affect the feeling of the chakra. The associated negative feeling of the belief system affects that person's reality and causes the front-feeling chakra to become blocked. For instance, if you judge the pleasure of sex as being bad and tell yourself, "I shouldn't feel how amazing it feels. It is bad to enjoy sex. It is sinful. It must feel bad," you will use your control-will to stop the flowing-feeling of sexual pleasure in the front second chakra. As a result, the flow of the sexual energy will stop and there will be *no* feeling in this chakra region. Thus the person who judges sex will project the *bad* judgment onto the experience and get just that, which is feeling nothing at all instead of pleasure and joy. What is feeling bad sex? Feeling nothing at all is *bad* sex. Tada! Projection accomplished.

Interestingly, we do have names for when we feel nothing instead of our true nature. If we block off the joy of sex, we will feel guilt, which is *nothing* in the place of the sexual, creative joy, and self-love that the second chakra brings.

So guilt, for example, is a negative emotion that feels *bad* because the true feeling of the chakra is blocked. Thus a negative emotion is the result of resistance and judgment of true nature. Experiencing a negative emotion is the experience of emotion on the opposite side of reality from the Oneness of Gan Edan.

All emotions are this way. Although we tend to like good definitions, it is not essential to memorize which negative emotions result from the blockage of positive emotions because they probably overlap. The following are examples of negative emotions:

Absence of feeling of faith: doubt, fear.
Absence of feeling of Love: feeling abandoned, jealousy, selfishness.
Absence of feeling of intuition: confusion, doubt.
Absence of feeling of strength: weakness, cowardice.
Absence of feeling of self-love: guilt, self-conscience, insecurity.
Absence of feeling of lightness: heaviness.

Understanding this helps us to see the nature of the Game of life and creation. Before the adoption of Frmee Will, the way all entities felt was pure Love and pure Oneness. Yet, recall this was all there was and there was nothing with which to compare. So how did that Love feel? It just was, it could not be experienced until we chose to embark upon a journey during which, through suppression of the way we really felt, we began to feel... *nothing!* Yes. How does your reflection in the mirror feel? We have become numb to the feeling of our true nature! When we defrost we say "Aha! So *this* is Love. So *this* is how my true nature feels. I remember who I am. Now I can experience who I really am!" The world of fear and suppression causes a freezing that numbs the feeling of true nature so that when the fear defrosts (by our letting it go, by our unchoosing it), then and only then can we truly experience our nature. To understand this gives such hope and shows us that we are in for ecstasy, the likes of which we have never known.

Remember and repeat this little spell and know that it is who you are (6th Circle):

> *I am feeling*
> *I am flowing*
> *I am intuition*
> *I am direct knowing*

Where the front and opposing rear chakras meet in the center of the body creates a *negative space* called the chakra seal. This negative space is ego, because it is devoid of Love. The resistance of the Will chakra sucks energy in, like an implosion. That is what creates the negative space, the self within the self, the reversal of reality. In a Balanced Positive state, our energy comes from our center. It gives infinitely and its source never depletes. The void created by the ego is the exact opposite, for it constantly needs to be filled. It is a bottomless pit that can never be filled, for it desires the insubstantial—what is based in illusion.

In the true state of Oneness, the rational mind gives up its need to control and then the rear will chakras act in harmony with the front chakra, empowering allowishing, like using your hands to push yourself on a surfboard already being carried by a wave.

Examining a magnet yields much insight into the nature of our chakra system within the reality of the Balanced Positive. A magnet has two opposite poles, North and South. The South Pole draws energy in from the ether/atmosphere. It is female, or Yin, due to its receptive nature. The North Pole is the output of energy, making it male, or Yang, in nature. The magnet is amazing because, despite having two opposite energies or polarities, the flow of the energy *through the center* is unidirectional—from the female (south) to the male (north). (see Figure 18c)

In contrast, our chakras flow in *two* directions. The flow created by the female (feeling) chakras (in, from the front) and the flow created by the male (Will) chakras (in, from the back). Yet, the most significant difference between our chakra system and a magnet is really found within the center, where both energies meet. Our chakras, having two directions, have a seal, plug, or block in the center, which creates duality. The magnet, however, has a very special center, for there is a point in the middle where the South becomes the North, yet it is neither North nor South. It is the magnetic neutral which is beyond the definition of North and South. This is very similar to the undefined nature of the Balanced Positive of the Creator, which is both male and female as One, yet separately it is neither. This is the state of the Adam Kadmon in which Adam exists both as male and female, as One with the Creator. That flow, from the source of the South to the extension of the North, in a little object known to us as a magnet is a perpetual system that effortlessly empowers itself. It teaches us more about our true nature than is imaginable. It showed me that in true harmony the chakras must function with the front chakras drawing in and the rear chakras carrying the energy in the same direction. Just as a jet engine propels the aircraft forward by having its energy eject out the back, so too are we propelled into the Time of Forwardness when the energy of our rear chakras comes out the back.

See Figure 28, which demonstrates how the Aleph, א, with its two Yods, י, meet in the center as One. Because it is the first letter in the Hebrew alphabet, and has the internal *gematria* of the name of God (26), the Aleph represents the Oneness and the all unification of God.

When the energies of our feeling and Will chakras are in perfect harmony, the energies of the center are One, no longer opposed, and neither negative or positive. They are Balanced Positive. In balance, one becomes an extension of the other. For this to occur, the negative, controlling Will must give up control and flip back over. So yes, they are still opposites, yet in harmony, not like the opposites of minus 2 and plus 2. If we were to balance minus 2 with plus 2, it would yield zero, when zero, nothingness, is not the state of Balanced Positive. Rather they feedback and blend together as One, one being the source, the other the extension, working together in harmony. The balance in the center is undefinable: how can there be a point that exists as both male and female as One? We cannot define that.

The rational mind also works temporally in the opposite direction of the wisdom mind. One is based in the past and holds things back as a result, because that is where it exists. The other is aligned with Ehye Usher Eyhe and the Time of Forwardness. These two minds, as our feeling and will chakras in duality, oppose each other.

We have come to believe that what we thought was the Kabbalistic "Tree of Life (Etz HaChaim)" is in fact a representation or a model of it (see Figure 29). In the Garden of Eden where the Tree of Life resides, we are not rational (Bina2) and wisdom (Chochma) blended as One. As AllGoodlove, we are not judgment (Gevourah2) and kindness (**Chesed**) blended as One, just as the nature of the Creator is not the balance of Good and Bad. Nor is our true nature a balance of ego-vanity (Hod2) and humility (**Netzach**). The *rational* (Bina2) and *judgmental* (Gevourah2) mind, and the *ego's vanity* (Hod2), all located on the left column of "The Tree of Life," were reversed and in opposition to the right column of "the Tree of Life" as a result of the influence of the Tree of Knowledge for Good and Bad. This is how these parts became dual and is equivalent to the way in which the rear chakras turned around on the front chakras. Thus the left column of the Tree turned around on the Source of God, and is associated with the negative of ego that caused our expulsion from the Garden of AllGood.

In our studies of the Kabbalah, therefore, we must be aware of what we call the Tree of Life. When we look at a Tree whose Bina is rational, Gevourah is Judgment, and Hod is vanity, this *is not the Tree of Life*, it is the Tree of Knowledge for Good and Bad.

The Tree of Life represents a vibration of existence beyond all judgment, beyond all rational constructs and definitions. It does not comprise two times or two energies that are in opposition to each other like our chakra system is now, or our two Wills. It is beheld within the Garden of Eden where the two energies of male and female work in harmony. Thus, when realigned and in connection with the Tree of Life, we see those negative energies of control and limitation of the left column of the Tree of Knowledge flip and become an extension of the right column. So we see Bina as the *Understanding* that carries forth the source of Chochma (wisdom). We see Gevourah as *Strength* that carries forward the source of Chesed (kindness & compassion). We see Hod as the confidence that extends the source of Netzach (selfless humility). (see Figure 30b)

Tree of Knowledge	*Tree of Life*
Male →←Female	**←Male ←Female**
Male dominates/competes with Female	Male equal to and extension of Female
Good and Bad	AllGood
Positive and Negative Polarities	Balanced Positive
Duality	Oneness
Rational Dominates (Bina2) Intuition	Intuition Makes Sense
Complicated	So Simple
Test of Choice, Struggle	Beingness, Effortlessness
I Must Try, I Must Know	I AM
Reflection of True Nature	Garden of Eden, Messianic Age
$0/1 = 0$ Nothingness	$1/0 = \infty$ Infinity = Undefined

Figure 30b—The Tree of Knowledge vs. The Tree of Life

The type of consciousness that we experience from the Tree of Life is immeasurably different from the Tree of Knowledge state to which we are so accustomed given our rational, judgmental, and egotistical ways. The Tree of Life does not contain parts in separation. It is AllGood, Balanced Positive.

That is what makes the whole difference.

An Australian man named David Oates recently made a great discovery that has helped us unlock a great mystery and shows us, yet again, the reversal in our world. It is called *reverse speech technology*. Oates showed that if we record our everyday language and play it back in *reverse*, you can hear a short phrase of coherent speech every eight to ten seconds. Oates presented samples at a lecture on his discovery. In one sample, Oates and a friend were making arrangements for him to help his friend fix up his house. The chatter in the normal sense was about the details of which ladder to bring, what time they would meet, etc. But when he played the tape in reverse, we got to hear this message: "Glad to be your friend." How wonderful!

With this discovery, we now know that every eight to ten seconds, our intuitive centers are actually speaking in reverse to our logical centers. Most important, the intuitive messages don't lie. The intuitive voice cannot lie because it is not in its true nature. The messages reveal our inner feelings or inner truth. Many organizations were not too happy about this discovery. Just as with every discovery that helps us plough toward being free, the **Con Trolls** would like to take this discovery away from us to keep us in the bondage of our illusions. Well, the Truth will be shouted from the mountaintops. No more control. No longer will we allow organizations that reside *above* us to keep us ignorant.

You can try to do what Oates did for yourself when you have the time. On Oates' *reverse speech* website, in the section on "R.S. examples," you can hear Neil Armstrong's famous words when he landed on the moon, "One small step for man, one giant leap for mankind." If you play this backwards on the website, or on tape, you will hear, after some gibberish, the encoded reverse message, "*Man will space walk.*"

The intuitive mind, which is always connected with the higher self, speaks backwards in relation to the rational language that we ordinarily speak. It is more visual, more symbolic. It conveys the thought in our speech as an image, as a symbol, which is amazingly mixed in backward in our normal talk. This is why people understand so much more when they go to a lecture, versus just reading a book. They are tuned into the level of intention and the reverse intuitive speech. They will get these intuitive messages as well as the spoken words. The combination is great for understanding. Without the intuitive and the intention, i.e., if you are reading this only on the rational level, it is less powerful than also connecting with the *intention* the words express.

A split between intention and words is detectable when speaking with people who are deceptive or who find it hard to express themselves openly. At times, you know their intentions are different from the implications of their words. Intuitively, you are picking up on what their reverse speech is saying and their words just don't match their intention.

The visual system also plays a part in our seeing and existing in this doubled reality. The visual system aligns us in a way that inverts what we see and helps maintain a reversed relationship with reality all around us. This has an immense effect on our perception of reality.

The left brain and the right brain divide the visual fields so that the left brain sees the right visual field and the right brain sees the left visual field. However, what exists outside of you is *perceived within the theatre of your brain as opposite.* The left visual field is *imaged* by neurons connecting to the visual cortex in the right brain. It is very much like you *imagine* it to be in the right brain. Isn't it strange that you would perceive an image on the opposite side of your brain? The vertical or y axis is flipped so what you image in your brain is also the opposite. The depth or z axis is reversed in your imagination as well. (figure 19) (Hint—*mirror-imagine:* What we see is really *an inward reflection* of what is out there. It is outside in—mirror-imagined in three dimensions, simultaneously.)

The activity of the rational mind creates a magnetic field that has a small radius around the brain. It is like a circle of rational thought is hovering around our heads. Each limiting belief system that we have about ourselves is laid down like a sheet or a veil within this balloon-like field around our head. For example, if someone believes that he or she is despised, that's a limiting thought form that is laid down in this field around their head. When this belief is triggered the mind emits energy which hits this veil-like thought form. Instead of the mind reaching out to great distances and soaring limitlessly to see reality as it is, it hits this wall of the negative thought form. It hits the inner surface of the balloon that is like a reflective surface. The mind's energy then gets reflected inward, within the dark space of the rational field. Thus the person's rational mind confines their existence to be within the limiting thought form. This is also living within the *mirror-imagine*, because when the rational mind's field, like a magnetic barrier to the freedom and expansion of thought, resists the flow of the true mind's energy, it reflects everything inward into the small space within the head. This inward reflection creates the *self within the self*, that little person who feels so small and limited within the confines of what you believe to be true about yourself and the nature of reality.

Such limiting thoughts are illusions. The more you believe limiting things about yourself and the Universe, the more your universe shrinks; it becomes a dark space centered in your head, as a false reflection of the Truth that is everywhere. Belief systems are limiting even if they represent Truth because the thought form of the belief reflects the Truth into the confines of your head. You won't even get to see the true reality because you constantly see what you believe to be true reflected inward, back to you. (This is inward projection.) You are living alone in a mirror-imagined world.

Our visual field creates the mirror-imagine the same way. Our mind that is One is always perceiving Allthatis. But because the beams of the true mind hit balloons of the rational mind's magnetic field, they get reflected inward. We thus perceive the inward, mirrored reflection of what is truly out there in the visual world.

> The book of Exodus says, "Hashem would speak to Moses face to face, as a man would speak with his fellow; then he would return to the camp." **Exo 33:11**
>
> And only nine verses later it says, "You are not able to see my face, because no man may see my face and yet live." **Exo 33:20**

Isn't that strange? What does this mystery reveal to us? There are two different states. The secret lies in the state Moses is in when he speaks with God "face to face." Moses is able to see God face to face because he is One with Hashem. God can manifest in the form of a human being with a face, yet this is not the only form of God, therefore, face-to-face indicates Moses' state of being is not separate from God's. Oneness is a "face to face" relationship. In the other state of Being, Moses is as all people who have adopted the inverted consciousness of duality and separation, and thus it is on the reverse of reality, unable to see the face of God. That is why **Exo 33:23** states that when Moses cannot see God's face, he can see his back. Interestingly, the name of Moses in Hebrew is Moshe, משה, and seen in the reverse, or backwards, the name is Hashem, השם, the name of God.

The way in which our visual field reflects inward sets up the possibility for the judgment of the objects that you can localize *outside and separate from yourself.* Within the mind that is One, there is no perception and no witnessing of reality defined as here or there that is outside. There is only seeing where something is, on the symbolic level, undefined, which is the most fascinating thing that you can witness when you are so used to perceiving things in parts. The symbolic level is somewhat cartoon-like. Even though there are no defining constructs, such as left and right, up and down, here or there, there is great wisdom and you are not completely dumfounded. Everything just *is* and you connect with it *where it is*, not in the space of your head.

We are able to witness and perceive left and right as separate, and up and down as separate because of the split and the flipping in the two separate sides of the brain (see Figure 19). Reality is perceivable in this separate manner because we only imagine it; where we are "seeing" something is not really where it is. Does the mirror-imagine make more sense now?

It is also possible to associate any number of beliefs or judgments with an object because of the way in which it is perceived dually within the brain. It is quite unreal to see a hat, a chair, a breast, a door, a penis, or a window on the symbolic level. You sort of say to yourself, "What is this?" instead of having a million and one stigmas, fears, insecurities and desires attached to it. This is because the left brain stores associations with an object: the name, its properties, what to do with it and what not to do with it, what makes it good and what makes it bad, etc. This is the association cortex of the rational brain. Associations and ideas we have adopted as reality are held in the cortex (brain) by our own will. When there is no association with the rational, the object is simply symbolic—it just *is*. You say "What is it? Manna?" The answer is, "It doesn't matter," and from this place, this space, you may be completely free to experience that object as it is. And it is Good. This is freedom.

Things might seem strange at first, when you are detaching from all rational constructs. Doing so will seem like a dream (a good one) and somewhat like a cartoon (a fun one). It will feel as if you know, very intimately, what the objects that you see are all about *where they are*, not in your head. It is as if you *are* part of that object which you are seeing. You get to experience your surroundings very intimately, unlike the way you move through your days when you are stuck in your head, oblivious of so much around you. The symbolic level of existence is the same as Oneness. You do not see yourself as separate from what you see all around. The animals, plants and objects are simply extensions of yourself. Animals experience the reality around them on this level; they do not perceive the world or the things that surround them as apart.

Although the left and right brain put perceptions together so that we see the whole surroundings in front of us, *there are blind spots*. We are largely unaware of the split in what we see because we're so accustomed to it. But these blind spots make us unable to see whole pictures at one time. This is because it is impossible for us to focus on both sides at one time. We can only see one side at a time. This is similar to not being able to encompass both sides of a paradox.

Here's a little exercise that demonstrates this. Close your eyes. Look with your mind to the left. Then look with your mind to the right. Now try to look with your mind to both left and right at once. Can you feel your mind jumping around, trying to find the balance? It cannot find the perfect balance because the rational mind, the mind that tries, does not exist as a balance and can only see one side at a time. It exists in parts. It is possible to experience both right and left at once, but you must feel. Try that now. (You can also try this exercise with up and down, back and front. It works in the same way.)

In our state of duality, we imagine two images inside of our brain and put them together in pieces that do not meet as One in the middle, just like two polar opposites sticking to each other. They are not a perfect fit. There is always a space in between, albeit small. But these polarities or sides really are One. "How can they be One?" When the rational gives up resistance and control they are One because there is only one visual field. *There is only where everything IS!* When the rational no longer has two opposing images of the *same* object or same visual field to assemble, and it only has one image within the brain, then the object just *is* where it is and that is where you experience it.

It is the visual field of what is truly *here*! It is so clear.

Our brains evolved so that we see two images that we put together in this way *because* of the rational and intuitive split. The physical is just a reflection of the spiritual, so if, hypothetically, we were split between four Wills, eventually our brains would evolve into four visual fields assembled together by our four Wills, which we would control.

As your consciousness expands, the visual experience expands as well so that you can focus on more around you. Absolute consciousness is absolute connection with all things *all* around. When you are very fearful, you have very little perception of the visual spectrum. It is as if a cloud camouflages the objects inside your head so you are not as aware of them. This is a blind spot. Those within the martial arts or any contact sport such as kick boxing or boxing know that if they are afraid and not focused, they do not see all that their opponent throws at them. In a match, a punch may arrive from the periphery and someone who is very scared and uptight will not see it coming. Those with much experience can calm themselves and rest their eyes on their opponent and take in the entirety of what is in front of them, so that if the opponent's toes so much as twitch they will see that.

When I let go of certain deeply set, ingrained beliefs and resistance patterns, my visual field expands and becomes brighter and more encompassing. I am allowing myself to take in more light and more range of vision. The negative, inward reflection of reality has lessened. In Chinese medicine, a person's vitality can be seen in their eyes. This is called Shen. When you are very deep in your resistance and struggle, you will have little Shen and light will not shine from your eyes. You are in the cellar of your reflected self. As you let go of experiencing through the eyes of your lower self, you will enable the light to shine from your eyes more and more, until the beams reach into infinity and shine like a golden sun. This whole understanding of vision became very different when Adam and Eve adopted Frmee Will. The Torah says, after they ate the forbidden fruit:

> "Then the eyes of both of them were opened and they realized that they were naked". **Gen 3:7**

But what this means, in addition to the shame of their nakedness, is that after the Tree of Knowledge, they began seeing things within the reality of separation. No longer were they in perfect harmony with all things. No longer did they feel one with all that they perceived. This new type of seeing, with what the Torah calls "their eyes open" is seeing things *on this inward, reverse side.* At the symbolic level, before the Bad and Good Tree, there is no way to be ashamed of what you are perceiving because you are not separate from it. You have no sense of removal from what you are feeling connected with. What you feel One with, you love because it is a part of you. What you love and remain connected with, you do not judge. Adam and Eve judged what they saw or thought because they went from Being One, when it is impossible to judge something as separate, to being reversed, when they began perceiving themselves as separate entities, alone within the balloons of their Frmee Will selves. And since they saw *themselves* as separate, they could see something as separate and associate an idea, rational thought, or judgment with that object. That's when their parts became private, shameful, and hidden.

This also says that they went from seeing with their One eye, to seeing with the two physical eyes. Their One eye is in the center of the forehead and is the third eye. Really, it is the first eye, we just call it the third in relation to our two other eyes. When the two other eyes opened, the chakra seal was placed over the third eye and closed it. The third eye then began looking *within* the individual and it became possible to perceive the *reverse* of the higher/deeper heavens.

The third eye "sees" by a phenomenon of direct connection that is like feeling. That is why when there is no seal over the third eye, you have all-around vision, because then you see by feeling. When I meditate, I see nothing with my third eye until I am in a space where I can feel what I am seeing. This is the difference between seeing on the physical level and seeing on the spiritual level. In order to see on the spiritual level, you must be in the place where you do not perceive yourself as separate. This also means that you are feeling a connection with what you are observing.

Let's assemble more of the puzzle. This is where it gets a little wild.

The mind is where the body is, yet also upside down and backwards.

As your sensory nerves signal the body's location to the brain, the nerves cross over onto the *other* side of the body. (see Figure 21)

Thus, the place where you feel your right hand is really *imagined* in the left brain. Isn't that strange?

Look down now at your right hand. Open and close your fist. You can see and feel the hand as if it is there, on the right. Yet in your brain, there is a double flip of your visual perception and your kinesthetic perception, thus you can perceive the hand to be *there* but it is only an *illusion* that it is there.

In Figure 22, the *homunculus* is the representation of the entire body within the pre-central and post-central gyrus. The pre-central gyrus is the command center for efferent-Will control of the body and the post central gyrus is the afferent-feeling command center for the entire body. Yet the homunculus is mapped upside down and it represents the opposite side of the body. What this means is that *your brain imagines your body to be upside down and backwards.*

When you combine this with the understanding that the brain imagines the outside world as upside down and backwards as well, then can you see that we perceive *everything* in the physical world upside down, front for back, and backwards.

It is also interesting to note that the *sensory* post-central gyrus is situated to the back of the pre-central *motor* gyrus. This is also reversed because the body, via the chakras, perceives *feeling in the front* and carries out *Will (motor) in the back.* This is a reversal along the depth or Z plane. *The brain reverses everything.* In addition to that, the perception is *within* our brain. And since it is in three dimensions, not just two, we have been living within the *hollow graphic* negative of the True reality of the Universe—*the mirror-imagine! It is reflected inward! It is outside in!*

So where do you really exist?

You are the Light on the other side.

Imagine yourself being sucked inward into your center, which is like a black hole. Once you flip over into the other reality, the other dimension, you now perceive as if you are inside out of how you were in the physical reality. (see Figure 20)

As you let go of limiting belief systems and small, incorrect ideas about who you are, your rational mind begins to dissolve around you. Your perspective is broadened as your mind reaches out to what is truly there. When there are no more limiting beliefs that reflects your perspective inward, you hit the I am, and the Frmee Will that makes you so aware of your self within yourself is no more. Do you understand the self within the self better now? It is how you perceive your true self as inwardly reflected—you end up experiencing the three-dimensional, physical body. The I am is the perspective of yourself that is One with All things, because your mind, who you truly are, perceives the infinity of Allthatis outside of your little, inward reflected self, which was the trap of your perceived physical self. It is a flip over. You are no longer self-centered, nor are you stuck inside a body. You have a center and it is God, the Universe, Allthatis.

When did we begin perceiving ourselves as physical and not Light? After eating from the Tree of Knowledge.

"And Hashem God made for Adam and his wife garments of skin, and He clothed them." **Gen 3:21**

These "garments of skin" represent the physical body, or beginning to perceive the body as being densely physical.

So how can we understand disease and pain in the body in this Light?

Disease and pain in the body are a result of holding on to the flow of energy in your mirror-imagine body (your imaginary body, perceived in your brain by putting together images) that is really on the other side of your true Light body (5th Level of the auric field.) Therefore, there is really nothing "wrong" with your body, even though you might feel stuck, blocked, creaky, weak, or painful, even though you might have manifested a disease in your body, because you are truly Light and you're just holding on and resisting the flow of the Lightness of your Being. Understanding this, there is infinite potential for healing all disease once the source of resistance is released. Once you release the resistance and holding on, the body is no longer held back to the past. The body held on to the past is the dense physical body, in the time of the past, opposed to the flow of Ehye usher Ehye, resistant and subject to the earth's gravitational pull. We perceive it as so physical because we resist the Oneness. Once that resistance is released, we resume perception of the body in its true state—Light, and we shed the "garments of skin." The ultimate release is the ultimate return to perceiving all your Being as Light.

Beyond *all* control and illusion, what you see before you is the same as what you feel inside. This is the great Oneness of all of creation. This is a great connection between the heart and mind and all around you. You see that it doesn't matter what your body is, for you do not define your Being as within the space of your body. This helps to transcend limited ideas about the body and how it should be, or look, like focusing on the self, which is a way of being stuck in ego. As One, you perceive all as part of yourself, for it *is* you. The World becomes your body. The Universe is your body. You have returned to Atzilut.

To add further to the picture of reversal and duality, the negative of the auric field (the energy field around and within the body) was created when the self imploded within the self when Adam and Eve ate from the Tree of Reversal of Reality. This is due to the activity of the self *within* the self. It is because you are living *outside in* yourself that you get the doubling effect.

Your ego-mind, stuck within you, creates the perception of reality from its viewpoint. *This is what gives rise to the lower levels of the auric field as they are now.*

Imagine a creature that is radiating light from its mind. It starts from the mind and is emitted in an outward field. This is the auric field of its true self. Now, imagine that this creature becomes doubled so that its double is now living *inside* itself, upside down and backward. This double is created by the inward reflection of what it believes to be true, that actually isn't true. This would be its ego-mind. However, the radiated light from the mind of its ego and doubled self is *inverted* compared to the light of its true self/higher self. This light of its doubled self creates the auric field of the opposite of its true self. *It exists on the other side of reality.*

There are nine levels of the auric field. The two upper levels, the 8th and the 9th levels are not influenced by the effects of the Tree of Knowledge. They are beyond the threshold of duality and have always been. For now, we will only discuss the seven levels affected by this doubling.

The seven levels of the auric field are: the level directly related to the physical body, (1st level), the level directly related to our lower emotions, (2nd level), the level that is directly related to our rational mind, (3rd level), the level that is related to our heart, (4th level), the level that is related to the higher state of our body, (5th level which is the Divine Body), the level related to our higher emotions, (6th level which is that of Divine Emotions), and the level related to our higher mind, (7th level which is the Divine Mind). The 1st and 5th levels are related to the body, the 1st is the lower and the 5th is the higher. The 2nd is the lower level and the 6th is the higher level of the emotions. And the 3rd is the lower and the 7th the higher related to the mind.

The higher levels of the auric field, the 5th, 6th, and 7th, are the source of the 1st, 2nd and 3rd. The higher levels are the blueprint of the lower levels. However, the way we experience the lower three levels is not in harmony as an extension of the upper three levels. This means that the physical body, 1st level, the emotional body, 2nd level, and the rational mind, 3rd level, are all the *reverse/negative* of the light of the higher levels of the auric field, namely the 5th Divine Body, 6th Divine Emotions, 7th Divine Mind. It is the reflection of your true self, being reflected *within* the limited, physical space locality of where your body is. This contributes to your ability to perceive your identity as an individual. Remember The Imagination of God? This reflection is an extrapolation of yourself, a *hollow graphic image* of your true self. It is devoid of the feeling of the divine. Look into a mirror. There is an image of you. It is you, but it really isn't, for you are not connected with it. It is just a hollow reflection of yourself. And we have come to mostly believe reality is living within the *hollow graphic* reflection of our true selves, as in the lower levels of the auric field. (see Figure 24 and 25)

These pairs of the higher and the lower levels have become opposites, but in reality can co-exist in harmony and bring us the experience of true bliss, just as the feeling and Will chakras have also come to be in opposition, yet in their true nature, exist as one. In the beginning, when God was Allthatis, and Adam was One with God in this state (Adam Kadmon), Allthatis was only the higher levels of the auric field. The higher levels had no counterpart and could not be experienced. They therefore became reflected inward, into the opposite of their true nature, to give the individual souls the ability to perceive themselves as separate entities.

We still have not graduated to reincorporating the experience of the higher levels of the auric field back into our reality. Instead of experiencing with the Divine Mind of Oneness, connected to all things (7th), we still think with the rational mind of limitations (3rd). Instead of feeling the divinity of the angels and the Joy of Joys (6th level), we feel the often-negative emotions associated with our selfish thoughts and associated with living within the cage of our rational minds (2nd level). Whereas we shall soon be within the Divine Beingness/Body that is beyond our trapped physical perspective of ourselves (5th level), it is the light on the other side, we are now bound to experience Earth within the physical body (1st level).

Be careful with the term high in this case and all cases. We usually attribute high to a high frequency, as in something fast, and also to mean something that is "high up there". True, the vibration is of a higher frequency at these incredibly divine levels, yet what you experience is quite

slow and down to earth, peaceful right here in the spaces on the planet.
If you think too much of high as *up* and *fast*, it will simply become
another belief system that must be faced and cleared at some point.

From the Kabbalah, we know that there are Four Worlds. These Four
Worlds span all existence and all of creation. These are the Four Worlds
of *Assiyah* (the world of action, of the body) of *Yetzirah* (the world of
creation and emotions) of *Bria* (the world of the mind, of will, of intention) and of *Atzilut* (the absolute and undefined). Within these Four
Worlds, if you look closely at what was just described, you see that these
Four Worlds are the same as the levels of the auric field. The levels of
the auric field associated with the Body are the same as the Fourth
World called Assiyah. The levels of the auric field associated with our
emotions are the same as the Third World called Yetzirah, and the levels
of the auric field associated with the Mind are equivalent to the Second
World called *Bria*. Finally, there is the First World of the undefined
Oneness (*Atzilut*), which exists on a whole other level of reality.

The First World which is One, Atzilut, is still infinite and untouched
by our rebellion on Earth. It has never become divided into duality.
The Three Worlds that have become doubled are the Fourth, Third, and
Second Worlds. The 4th World of the body (Assiyah) is the 1st layer of
the auric field (physical body) and the fifth (Divine Body). The Third
World of the emotions (Yetzirah) is the second layer of the auric field
(emotions) and the sixth (Divine Emotions). The Second World of the
Mind (Bria) is the third layer of the auric field (rational mind) and the
seventh (Divine Mind). These three worlds have become doubled from
true nature (fifth, sixth, seventh) into the mirrored reflection of that
true nature (first, second, third). Three split worlds, like the three
dimensions in which we exist (see Figure 26).

Actually, because our One Will split into two on the level of the
mind, the lower worlds also split subsequently. The World of *Bria* (Mind)
is higher than the world of *Yetzirah* (Emotions) and *Assiyah*
(Body/Physical). Any reflection in the mind causes the emotions and
the body to reflect inward.

The negative spaces that exist in the chakra seal also create these
inward, reflected worlds. The seal is like a dimensional conversion point,

the doorway that allows the lower levels of the auric field to be created on the other side of reality, which is much like another time reality. When there is no longer opposition between our Will and the feeling chakras, when we have given up our Frmee Will, the doorway to the time reality based in illusion will be closed and we will no longer have chakras, levels of our auric field, or the different Worlds within us operating in two time dimensions or realities that are disharmonious.

We also exist on four vibrational levels. The slowest is the physical, which is the Fourth World, Assiyah. The next one is the auric field, which is the Third World, Yetzirah. Then there is the level of intention, the mind, a very high vibrational level called the Second World, Bria. The First World is the World of the Oneness, where we are One with the Divine, the World of Atzilut. What Barbara Brennan has called "The Core Star level," I see also is the World of Atzilut. The Ultimate World, which encompasses all things, has the highest vibrational frequency and its speed of Light approaches infinity. (see Figure 27)

Since the World of Atzilut is beyond duality, it is beyond the threshold and it is within the state of absolute Beingness/Oneness. What is necessary for us to return to the Oneness is to step through a door that is the gate of the heart. The heart world, which is the 4th level of the auric field, balances between the lower three and upper three worlds. Let's look at this very closely. The Heart World is like the bridge that sits in between the two opposites of the higher levels and the lower levels, or between Heaven and Earth. Between the upper three—fifth, sixth and seventh (spiritual, Heaven), and the lower three—first, second and third (physical, Earth), is the bridge of the heart. This is the same, therefore, as what sits in the middle of the chakras, which is the balance between the male and the female, yet it is really neither of the two. The heart, Tiferet in the Tree of Life, is therefore the World of Atzilut, because it is undefined. It is Balanced Positive—both Heaven and Earth, male and female as One. The heart is not reflected. The Kabbalistic belief stating that the heart, Tiferet, belongs in the Second World of Yetzirah (Emotions), is incorrect. It is in the Ultimate World of Atzilut and is the central gateway unifying the inward, reflected worlds of illusion and the higher worlds of Truth.

It is essential to understand the heart's importance in our world. The seal that sits in between the male and female chakras is a block that keeps the flow of their energy in duality. When released and opened, the flow returns to a state of Oneness, so that the male becomes an extension of the female in a Balance Positive marriage. When closed, the heart acts like a seal or block that keeps the lower reflected levels of the auric field disharmonious with the source of the upper levels of the auric field. We end up being doubled, split into Good and its reflection and Bad, in between Heaven and Earth, which we experience as purgatory; a blend of Heaven and Hell. We sense two times, two wills, two people, two places. There is no Oneness.

Deep inside the heart, there is a threshold that is the heart's seal. At this threshold, the cherubim and the flame of the ever-turning sword guard the way to the Tree of Life and the Ganallisone. Stepping through this place, in other words, allowing your heart's seal to open, you will return to the existence where you see and feel yourself within the World of Atzilut, as One with all things, in Tiferet (Beauty), where you perceive the absolute Beauty in all things. This is Gan Edan and has been unavailable to us for so long that it hurts too much to think about it. There, as part of the experience of Oneness, you will have your foundation of reality in the Divine Mind (seventh level of the auric field), Divine Emotions (sixth) and Divine Body/Being (fifth) of the Creator, unopposed by the dense, trapped lower levels of the auric field. The feeling is absolutely and totally different from what we are accustomed to. It is an *incredible* feeling, beyond words. It is the direct experience of being One and protected within the Creator's heart and mind.

As you touch the threshold and begin to move through, you will feel the frozen, forgotten halves returning to your consciousness, your perception of yourself. What occurs then is that you will feel all-around awareness, simultaneously, in every direction. This is the experience of infinity. There are no longer parts, there is only One thing, one place. Wow! At first, it is quite shocking. Second, it is quite shocking. The secret to getting through this threshold is being flexible and remembering that you are waking up to something you have always been, yet experiencing yourself as never before.

In duality, the body we are used to perceiving, the reality we are accustomed to experiencing, is really only a *fraction* of our true nature compared to when we are One. Feeling doubled, we are really just feeling halved, cut into parts. Therefore, when we return into Oneness, we become whole again yet we initially experience that *as if we are merging into nothingness.* This can, yet need not, feel frightening. This is actually very interesting to think about: since our perception of reality has largely been limited to separation into parts, as those parts come back together, the rational pieces cease to exist as pieces, and we perceive this as slipping into nothingness and non-existence, or like dying. (The void!) The opposite, however, is true. This is the rebirth that we have dreamt of for millennia. It is as if someone has come to think of themselves as part A (separated male) and part B (separated female), so that when those parts come together again as one part C (male and female as One), *they no longer exist as those parts.* This can make you feel like you are disappearing, yet you are not. You are coming together as a whole, as a One. *Oneness feels like nothingness to the perception of those who exist in parts.*

The seal in the heart is related to the seal in the seventh chakra. Moving through these seals brings you into the eighth level of the auric field, something only experienced within the Oneness of your true nature. It is the level of the Messianic consciousness. It is the state of Adam Kadmon. It is also like stepping past the vibration of Uranus (don't laugh). Uranus, the seventh planet, also exists at the level of a seal because its rings are *perpendicular* to its direction of revolution around the sun. This is the astronomical "as above so below," because this represents the limit of the threshold of the seventh level of the auric field, and the seventh level of existence. Once the lower vibrational levels of reality are released, we will exist in Messianic consciousness. Our consciousness will no longer have its foundation within the physical "apparent" realities. I wonder what will happen to the rings around Uranus (I said don't laugh!) when we all release our lower levels of consciousness and cross the threshold into the eighth level. Will they shift as well?

When you develop your sensitivity and you examine yourself, especially while in close proximity to the threshold, you will see yourself as double—your true nature and its reflection. This really means that your left half and right half meet in the center, yet they are not One, nor are they in harmony. You are two pieces, physically, emotionally and mentally, glued together in the center. The glue is your Will, for you are still holding onto the duality. Your chakras also join in the center, which causes a doubling inward of yourself. Left and right are doubled, as are up and down. (see Figure 23)

It might even seem as if one part is not a part of you, but it is a part of you, just reversed. The choices you have made in this lifetime and other lifetimes outside of your true nature have created this shadow self. It is not some manifestation of evil. It is the manifestation of pain, control, judgment and resistance. You are still choosing to hold onto that inward reversal of half of you, and that is Frmee Will. Don't chop that half off, or sever yourself, because your essence is still attached to it.

> We are double.
> There is a self within the self.
> When you are feeling Love, you
> Are experiencing the part of yourself
> That is free. When you fear, judge, control,
> You slip into the negative space of the self within the self.
> This slip is like a fall.
> Slipping tells you there is something
> You haven't yet let go of…
> Thus there is some purpose to this slip.
> You can say, "Oh, I slipped. I wonder what it is
> That I am not seeing clearly or harmoniously."
> We know now that we are double.
> One side against the other.
> It is quite shocking to understand that
> When you cross the threshold, you are still
> Double, yet instead of being two, which are not one $(1 + 1 = 2)$
> You are two that are One which is Three $(1 + 1 = 1 = 3)$
> *Goodbye to the self stuck within the self.*
> *Hello to my whole Light Being.*

Chapter 10: Summary

On many levels and in many ways, the Oneness became reflected into its opposites. We are split into our true self and the reflection/opposite of that true self. The levels of the auric field are very good examples of this. The lower levels are the negative/reflection of the upper levels caused by the activity of self within the self. The visual field also exemplifies how we experience reality in a double form. We do not see what is around us *where it is*. We see it in parts upside down and backwards and then our brain puts them together. When we see this, coupled with the understanding that we feel our body upside down and in reverse as well, we see that the way in which we perceive our physical body is really only an illusion. This is how we experience life in the physical within the *mirror-imagine*. When these parts reassemble as One, that will feel to the rational-ego mind as if ceasing to be or nothingness, as if it is dying. It is not dying, nor are we, as we return to the wholeness of who we really are.

On this level of wholeness, past the threshold, we will experience our existence as within the World of Atzilut, which is the World described within the Kabbalah as Tiferet; a World of Oneness, without any separation.

ESSENCE OF THE CHAPTER

We experience ourselves now in an imaginary place that is the reverse/negative of our true nature. We are really the Light on the other side.

THE SCIENC

OF SPIRITUALITY

The purpose of this chapter is to share some very interesting information from a scientific viewpoint that unites nicely with the rest of this book, bringing more pieces of the puzzle together. The science of spirituality is not currently verifiable or credible today, nor is the purpose to prove beyond rational question the existence of God or how the Universe was created. That is not possible. The science of spirituality is somewhat like the philosophy of spirituality, the unification of practical logic with the intuitive and undefined. The difference between the science of spirituality and today's approach to science is that the science of spirituality's foundation exists in the intuitive, in the feeling of reality, and not in the rational. It therefore does not need to prove its theories because you can consider whether or not these theories are true for yourself; you don't need science to tell you. So when we unite various awarenesses from this book with simple scientific facts to give you something to think about, it is to make you say "Hmmm" and to broaden your perspective of who you are. One day, the hypotheses in the science of spirituality might be verified and proven. But since this book is about a return to Beingness, it is not necessary to prove to yourself who you are in order to become who you are. You don't really have to validate your existence to know that you are what you are.

Let's start by taking a look at what science really is, how it can be used, and how society on a large scale, within the "civilized" world, has come to place much of its faith in the hands of scientific "proof" and "fact." We are largely misled by placing our faith in the hands of what science has proven because we simply contribute more to pigeon-holing the Truth and to the limitations on Being.

> "If there is any primary rule of science, it is... acceptance of the obligation to acknowledge and describe all of reality, all that exists, everything that is the case... It must accept within its jurisdiction even that which it cannot understand, explain, that for which no theory exists, that which cannot be measured, predicted, controlled, or ordered... It includes all levels or stages of knowledge, including the inchoate,... knowledge of low reliability,... and subjective experience."
> Abraham Maslow

Science is a wondrous endeavor if it is used as a tool to examine reality. It can help serve our wishes, if we so choose. It can also help us establish the understanding of principles to bring forth greater technology. It is not necessary, however, to employ science as a means of proving to ourselves what is Truth and what is not. We have the inherent ability to know Truth and when we seek Truth in a source outside of ourselves, by asking science to prove what is Truth, for example, we lose our ability to know Truth.

The fact that scientists operate with the need to have concrete evidence for everything before moving forward to explore reality really limits science's growth and ends up slowing the progress of science. Scientists are almost "chasing their own tail" in their never-ending need to validate everything. This creates a tremendous skepticism among today's scientists about anything that doesn't fit in the "fishbowl" of established scientific knowledge. By placing our faith in science, we believe something as Truth because science validated it and gave it a stamp of approval. This is backwards to the way we should use science, since science is just a method of exploring the Truth, not an agent that creates Truth by our discoveries.

At a talk as the Seattle Center titled "The Basics of Quantum Healing," Dr. Deepak Chopra, M.D. said:

> "If you really understand what science is, then science at least until now has not been a method for exploring the Truth. Science has been a method for exploring our current map of what we think the Truth is."

If you can connect on the level of awareness and intuition, then there is no *need* to prove or to validate, for you have no doubt. Having the feeling about a certain principle or Truth, you can use that feeling to move forward to explore even more of the wild frontier of reality.

Science comes from the Latin "scire" which means "to know." The desire for science is to know and, of course, this is to know the Truth: the nature of reality. However, we have employed science to dictate our beliefs and our understanding of reality, rather than using it as a tool to examine reality. We have found things out and believed them to be ultimate Truths and we gave away our own ability to experience the Truth by direct connection.

> "You see, when science became strong then it eliminated and ruled out the true self of humankind, its intuitive self, its self of love and heart. It is time for the returning to that, for science placed humankind in holes of pigeons, categorized them, labeled them, and put them in a situation such that all people began to think of them in that way. Those scientific beliefs then led to a pattern of mass thinking." *The Only Planet of Choice*, p. 287

Soon we will all come to realize we cannot order the Truth into a scientific formula or into observed phenomena, a fixed way, for all time. Things change as does the Universe every moment of existence. The

Truth is also undefined, so even if you dip your measuring device into a well of Truth and pull out some of its water, you are only getting a hint of the nature of the undefined Truth. You are catching only a glimpse. You are only getting a slice, from one angle. Defining Truth absolutely, making declarations forevermore, holding on to Truth, creates an illusion, a reflection of Truth. Dive in and experience. Then you will be the greatest scientist, because you will already have the experience and you can deduce it to explain it. Albert Einstein, one of the greatest minds of all time, kept trying to explain this to scientists of his time. A wealth of his quotes point to the fact that he didn't try to concertize anything. In fact, he explained one of the most amazing secrets of reality: depending on our perspective, things change. This is his theory of relativity. Amongst the wonderful things he said was:

"I am enough of an artist to draw freely upon my imagination. Imagination is more important than knowledge. Knowledge is limited. Imagination encircles the world." Albert Einstein, *What Life Means to Einstein: An Interview by George Sylvester Viereck.*

We have used science to fix everything into defined constructs. We do this because we need to feel more in control. We believe that by having defined our reality and knowing it, we are in control. We do the same in our religious approach to God, in which we use the rational arguments of past interpretations and teachings to believe that we know Truth. But this is not what connects us to the Truth. This can only point towards reasoning Truth. We must always take the plunge to understand what the past prophets were hinting at and what the Truth actually is.

The need to prove is an act of doubt. Those who are able to experience the existence of something, for example like the feeling or sight of the auric field, know beyond doubt that it exists because they can experience it. Thus, even if others are not able to experience the existence of the auric field, there is no *need* to prove it to validate its existence. As in the movie *Contact*, the priest asks the skeptical scientist if she loved her father. Her answer is, without doubt, "Yes." He then says "Prove it." This is such a brilliant point that he is making, since she is so skeptical, she will not believe the existence of anything that is not first provable scientifically, including the existence of God, or Love. There is no way for her to prove that she did love her father, but there is also no doubt that she did, so why would she need to prove it? More important than that is the question, "Is it even possible for her to prove it?" For all of us who experience Love and God and have no doubt of their existence, is it even possible to prove it?

The rational mind will attempt to control Beingness by establishing beliefs about reality through science. Being is free. It is Truth in the fluidity of experience. Rational is in a box. The rational can manipulate you into believing that your way of simply being isn't sophisticated and isn't right. If you are among many people who believe personal worth is valued by how much you know, the rational mind can make you look at yourself and say, "I do not know these things, I must not be good enough." When we have the energy of non-resistance and pure Being, we let go of a lot of the structures that we have set up to find the Truth and maintain it. In this state of self-sufficiency, we need not try so hard to prove what is true or who is right.

[*Third Circle*—CaN #5—I do not need to know or to be right all the time. I can make mistakes whenever I wish. I let go of the need to be perfect. I let go of making hierarchies according to what a person knows. I do not define my worth by what I know. I take the chance of being wrong. My guidance may tell me to do things that don't make sense, that are illogical and sometimes may seem downright wrong. It could be that I am simply facing up to something to let it go and once I do that, I no longer need to do it.]

It is my wish and hope, because of the freedom that it will mean for each individual who tries, that everyone realize that we cannot explain everything in rational or scientific terms. We can try, but that is like throwing rocks into the Grand Canyon. As my friend Ariel says, it is like splitting atoms. When you take apart a thing to try to figure out what it is, you can keep splitting and splitting forever.

This is the dilemma that science falls into today, especially in the biomedical approach to our health. Looking deeper and deeper at the body as a series of genetic transcriptions, the expression of proteins, and cellular communication, you can continue to pull apart *ad infinitum*, seeking a way of understanding how it all fits. This is a never-ending process. The answer to our health lies in the higher world of the mind. The body is simply a reflection of the mind. If the mind is in disharmony, the body will reflect that. By healing all choices that are not aligned with our true nature, we will find absolute health.

The conventional medical model uses science in the way Deepak Chopra describes as: "exploring the current map of what we think the truth is." Conventional medicine has made a machine of the body, believing that we are our anatomy and our physiology. The multiple dimensions not yet recognized by biomedical science are not even taken into consideration by conventional medicine for the health of the human being. Those who believe only what science has proven about our health wait to step into the reality where scientists have pulled back the shades on the unknown. We need not wait.

"There is no need to go outside for better seeing, nor to peer from a window. Rather abide at the centre of your being, for the more you leave, the less you learn."
Lao Tzu, *Tao Te Ching* translated by Witter Bynner, Chapter 47

Those who have given their health into the hands of the medical profession have also given away their power to heal themselves.

To the scientific, rational mind, when there is a paradox it must mean a mistake has been made, for how can two opposing things coincide, be encompassed within one system, and both be true?

We are One and we are individuals. We were created by God and we create God. The World to Come in the newly found is the Return to our Origins. The beginning of Time is the same as the end of Time. Claiming our power totally and completely in every choice in our life is giving up Frmee Will. How do you reconcile these paradoxes with the rational?

Many paradoxes are encountered all the time and baffle the minds of the scientist, and the minds of the soul aspiring towards understanding God. The scientist who is bound by the established map of what we think the Truth is makes a choice between opposing findings, believing both cannot exist simultaneously. This sort of rigidity in thinking does humankind a great disservice for in the path to freedom and experience of Truth, everyday we face paradox. It is not possible to cross into a Balance Positive reality of opposites without being boggled by paradox. Paradox makes us let go of control.

Very science-minded folk look into their belief systems to argue points about the undefined Truth. They usually use very good arguments, especially those who are very intelligent, have a lot of knowledge and are very skeptical. But they are just that, arguments, and usually they are playing devil's advocate and arguing for the sake of arguing, not because they really believe in what they are saying. When the rational mind feels threatened, it will argue its existence. Even when it might not fully believe in what it is saying, it will argue anyway. When you play devil's advocate, it is as if your rational mind's arguments are beyond your control. If you truly have conviction about something, then please, argue away! But playing devil's advocate when you don't believe in what you're arguing about doesn't serve anyone and is just a waste of time and everyone's energy.

If you always try to make sense out of things or always try to prove the reasoning behind things, it is important to note that you are doing this so that you can stop. If not, and you stay within this world of the mental, you will live a hollow life. This means that your hara will not burn and move to the rhythm, and your chest will not be radiant with the strength of who you are. You will feel strained and split up in your rational mind because it is not there that you are truly one. Be centered in your body, grounded to Earth, where it doesn't really matter what everything means. There you will not lose your mind. You will let it go so that it may serve you as an extension of who you really are.

The following discusses some fascinating points about the Universe. This is what I have called the science of spirituality and can also be called the science of Frmee Will. The purpose is to trigger the codes of limitlessness in you. It is to make you close your eyes and expand your mind into places where the finite is just a toy to help you draw a circle.

According to the work of C.W. Leadbeater and Annie Besant in their book **Occult Chemistry**, the smallest particle of matter in physics is known as the *anu*. Each anu has a diameter on a distance scale of

10^{-33} cm, which is considered to be the scale of superunification in modern physics, in which the forces of electromagnetism, gravity, and the weak and strong nuclear forces are completely indistinguishable, and thus unified as One. Modern physics has shown that all matter is composed and governed by those four forces, which are equally unified as One. In other words, at this point just beyond the smallest particle of matter at the distance scale of 10^{-33} cm, all forces that exist in the Universe are unified as One. There is no distinction at this level. This is the Unified Field. This is the unification of the Source. The One that encompasses all things.

Interestingly, the *Rig Veda* (Vedic knowledge from India), states that the Entire Universe, referred to as the Cosmic Egg, is associated with a time-distance scale of 311.04 trillion years. If this is converted into light years, it corresponds to a distance scale of 10^{32} cm. That is the extreme of bigness of the Universe, compared to the extreme of smallness, which the anu represent. The distance scales are reflections of each other. One is small, 10^{-33} cm, and the other is large, 10^{32} cm. What we can say about this is that the anu are a hollowgraphic/fractal reflection of the Cosmic Egg as a whole for they are 32 steps into the smallest, and the limits of the Cosmic Egg as a whole are 32 steps, from our point of perception, into the largest. This is a fantastic insight into the magical nature of the Allthatis Universe.

Leadbeater and Besant had the ability to psychically see, with their third eye, to the most minute level. They had the power to see as if they had internal microscopes in their eyes. Their descriptions and drawings of the subatomic particles, although made almost one hundred years ago when the understanding of the molecule was at a most elementary level, have recently been confirmed and praised for their accuracy. Leadbeater and Besant reveal another shocking tidbit of information about the smallest composition of matter, the anu. In *Occult Chemistry* they state:

> "These units (anu) are all alike, spherical and absolutely simple in construction. Though they are the basis of all matter, they are not themselves matter; they are not blocks but bubbles. They do not resemble bubbles floating in the air, which consist of a thin film of water sepa-

rating the air within them from the air outside, so that the film has both an outer and an inner surface. Their analogy is rather with the bubbles that we see rising in water, bubbles which may be said to have only one surface—that of the water which is pushed back by the confined air. So to speak, for the interior of these space-bubbles is an absolute void to the highest power of vision that we can turn upon them."

Occult Chemistry, Chapter 17

This says, to the detriment of our model of *physical* existence, that the smallest units of matter upon which *all* matter is created are not blocks of matter but actual bubbles with a central void in which nothing is perceivable. The *physical* world that we thus perceive as being something solid is actually based upon a foundation of nothingness. Thus, all that we perceive as physical, *solid*, is an illusion.

Does it not boggle your mind to think that the very basis of all matter, the building blocks comprise all that we see as physical around us, are themselves made up of nothing?

"What then is their real content—the tremendous force that can blow bubbles in a material of infinite density? What but the creative power of the Logos, the Breath which He breathes into the waters of space when He wills that manifestation shall commence?" Leadbetter and Besant, **Occult Chemistry**, Chapter 17

There is a similar passage in Genesis:

"And Yawveh God proceeded to form Adam out of the dust of the ground and to blow into his nostrils the breath of life and the man came to be a living soul." **Gen 2:7**

Let's add another piece to the puzzle:

What happens when we look out to the farthest reaches of space, to see the furthest extent of the Cosmic Egg on a broad scale?

"With a powerful telescope, you would see galaxies and other giant objects that are thousand of millions of light years away. Perhaps, if you had a telescope powerful enough (it has not yet been built) you could see back in time to the beginnings of the Universe—to the time of the Big Bang Itself." *Astronomy Encyclopedia,* p. 24.

As you look out farther and farther into space, you are actually seeing *back* in time. Back toward the point where it all Began. And according to scientific discovery, what did the Universe originate from? A point of infinite density and no dimension! (see Figure 32)

What is a point of infinite density and no dimension? It is actually the exact mirror reflection of the inner dimensions of the anu. Beyond the anu is a "space" of zero density and infinite dimension. Therein is the unification of the Source, the Unified Field. When something has infinite density and *no* dimension, this is also a *void*. It is the void of the Universe before the Big Bang.

When you think about this, it boggles the mind. How is it possible that looking with a telescope out in all directions as far as you can see can bring you to a point of no dimension? And how can going into the smallest building blocks of matter yield a vast cave of infinite proportions? Therefore, there is a dimensional conversion and a marriage between the void inside the anu and the void of the furthest reaches of space. We must imagine the Cosmic Egg folding in upon itself! The point where the density is zero (in the anu—smallest particles) is actually the negative, exact mirror reflection of the very point where the density is infinite. Zero nothingness, is the perfect negative opposite of infinity, everythingness. Actually, these two are the same, yet one is the hollow (literally) graphic reflection of the other. (see Figure 33)

And do you know that we, too, are the exact representation of the Cosmic Egg as a whole? In fact, what this chapter describes about the Universe and its elements also applies to us. If we divide ourselves down into our subatomic particles, going deeper and deeper into physical reality, we, too, are made up of anu, whose center is a a void of nothingness. If we follow our energetic fields into higher and higher frequencies, more and more into spiritual reality, we reach the ninth level of the auric field, where there is also a doorway into a void of infinite dimension. There is a marriage between the two where they are one, just as there is a marriage between the north and south pole in the center. There is no way to know for sure how it will be, but can you imagine more now about the leap of faith and crossing the threshold? (see Figure 34)

If the greatest parts meet in a space equal to the smallest parts, how can anything be separate? We are still living within a collective reality in which everything is united, and perhaps any concept of separation and duality is merely an illusion that we have chosen for the purpose of helping us forget our true nature.

And since reality is still the same, and only our perspective about it (relativity) has changed, when we wake up and remember, the illusion and belief of distance melts away and we see there is a perfect sea-like connectivity between all elements, all people, all existence and there is *n0* resistance. (A superconductor also has this property; it has *zero* resistance.) When we live our lives with *n0* resistance, we have released Frmee Will, the resistance of Being. When there is no longer any resistance, we are living in Oneness consciousness and we are a perfect superconductor.

Therefore, when you live without resistance, when you have given up all your Frmee Will, then you can do what superconductors can do. You can levitate. And even more fun than that, you can *fly*.

> *"Angels can fly because they take themselves lightly."*
> Anonymous

Inside the core of a superconductor, there is a zero point which is beyond the magnetic field of the Earth. Superconductors levitate beyond the Earth's gravitational field because their existence is actually no longer of Earth—they are *in* this world, but not *of* this world. This is actually a bridge tapping into the void. The future of our world's communication will be based on this zero point field for conveying information. When two zero-point fields of information are tuned to the same frequency—or same station, we might say—there is an *instantaneous* exchange of information with no loss of time, no linearly conveyed information, because both are tapped into the zero-point void which unites the Cosmic Egg. You can poke your head into the zero-point field and pop it out wherever you wish in the Universe. As you can imagine, there will also be transportation through the zero-point field. You can enter into it at some point and come out wherever you wish, because there is no separation of things in the zero-point field. Teleportation is not so far off. Research is progressing on both communication and transportation with the zero-point field. Imagine the Internet when everyone just plugs into the Allthatis to communicate.

On the level of intention, which is the Second Kabbalistic World of Bria, there is a small point three feet above the head. Barbara Brennan, in her book *Light Emerging*, has described this as The ID point:

> "It represents our first individuation out of the void, or unmanifest God. Through it, we have our direct connection to the godhead." *Light Emerging*, p. 289

This point is therefore where, through the higher frequencies, we touch with the Oneness of God. This level of intention, the Second World of Bria, is *higher* in vibrational frequency than the level of the auric field as a whole, where our chakras and the different levels of the auric field exist (Third World—Yetzirah) which is also higher in frequency than the physical body (Fourth World—Assiyah). (see Figure 27)

And the slower frequencies begin to manifest what we have perceived as physical matter. The physical is the same as the spiritual, just slower in vibration and perceived as denser. In the very minutest building block of matter, there is the other void, where the two become One. This shows us, symbolically, that our purpose in life is to bring the ID point, in the World of Bria, and the deepest points (Anu) in the World of Assiyah, together as One, just as the Cosmic Egg folds in upon itself. This is the marriage between Heaven and Earth, or between the spiritual and the physical. This brings to finality the purpose of creation— marrying the unmanifest God with the manifest God for the purpose of making real the experience of God. We do so by Being God on earth.

This is to be with foundation, or to be grounded. And since we understand in Kabbalah that previous generations laid the foundation and augmented the state of consciousness for future generations, we can also understand that we are steps away from fulfilling the purpose of this creation. We can do so by stepping down fully into being who we are and touching the zero-point void beneath us with the zero-point void above us.

When something is at a higher frequency, it is harder for us to detect with our normal senses. It is often beyond our current level of awareness. For example, when sounds are incredibly high pitched we cannot hear them. Dogs can, but we cannot in our normal state of consciousness. It is the same with the perception of light and matter. The *slower* the frequency at which particles move, the easier it is for us to see them. Imagine something moving back and forth in front of your eyes and you are following its movement. The faster it moves, the faster your eyes have to move to follow it. Eventually it goes so fast that it blurs. When the speed (frequency) at which a particle is moving increases, it is perceived more as light and less as something solid, physical.

Light moves slower at higher temperatures. We know that sound travels slower at hotter temperatures. Why would that be any less true for light which, like sound, is energy? It is just easier to measure the speed of sound because it is so much slower. But it is more accurate to state that light is *perceived* to be slower at higher temperatures. Light can also be perceived to move relatively faster at lower temperatures. In other words, at lower temperatures light is perceived as faster.

The mass of the object varies according to the relative speed at which an object is "being." When the speed of light is at its fastest—*infinity*—it has merged with the Allthatis in that it is *everywhere*; the mass adjusts to zero. No mass, no matter. Just light. So when something has no resistance, it is superconducting and is tapped into the Source of Allthatis, the zero-point field, which is the highest form of Lightness—infinite Lightness and connection with Allthatis.

Scientists have long been trying to get temperatures very, very cold so that super-conducting substances levitate. Certain substances levitate at very low temperatures because their molecules form into a perfect crystalline structure (with next to no physical motion of the molecules) and there is no resistance among the molecules. Resistance in any system causes a magnetic field to surround it. If there is no magnetic field in a substance, no gravitational force can influence the substance and it can levitate.

When the object gets closer and closer to levitating, the speed at which its energy moves increases (vibrational frequency increases) while conversely, the movements of its molecules (physical) reach zero. At or beyond absolute zero, in *the Zone of Cold*, there is no movement in a physical sense. They are still. A thing being perceived in the zone of cold, or perceiving itself in the zone of cold, is not perceived as physical because it has no physical movement. No physical movement, no friction amongst the resisting elements of the physical, and therefore no perception of the physical. In fact, any temperature at all is caused by the movement of physical molecules, or heat causes the molecules to move. Where there is no temperature, at absolute cold (absolute zero), it is all light. For us, to date, this has only been a theoretical concept.

Of course if you put anyone in a tub of liquid nitrogen, they would die instantly. So we're not discussing low temperatures for us. We are discussing the resistance in our being. Resistance generates heat. If we do not resist we achieve the *state of being* of the zone of cold, in the spiritual sense, and we are superconductors. Superconductors for what? For God's Will, with *n0* resistance. Ah, now that is the way to Be.

Scientists have said that before the Big Bang, the Universe existed in a state of *infinite* density within a point of no dimension. This is true from a certain perspective, but doesn't really make sense from another, so let's examine this a little closer.

Scientists say there was no physical existence at this time. If there was nothing physical, how did everything exist? All was light. To be light isn't just like a flashlight or the sun. We are light, the room and all its objects we see are also light. When you watch a movie, the moving objects you see are light. When we are beyond being tricked by physicalness, we will be able to see the nature of things as they are: light, not solid objects, stuck in their three dimensional forms. Allthatis, before the creation of the physical, was not dense. Density is something of the physical. From the perspective of scientists trying to describe the state of the Universe before the Big Bang: they look at the Universe and see all this matter that exists *now*, they employ the use of the Law (belief) of Conservation of Matter, and therefore they say all of this mass must have been within a point of infinite density and no dimension. This is a theory based in the model of a physical Universe. The Universe was not physical before we started to perceive it as such. The Universe will not be (densely) physical after we stop perceiving it as such. We only perceive it as such because we are *within* the mirror-imagine, with our consciousness which resists and perceives itself as the center of the Universe.

From the scientists' perspective, no dimension is equivalent to no volume. That's really just a fancy way of saying there was as yet no physical matter that took up any space. Allthatis, at the time before the Big Bang, was non-physical. There was also no temperature, since there was no physical movement. At absolute zero, the density of the molecules is at their absolute highest, which is infinity.

When thinking of absolute zero, the zone of cold, from our physical perspective, light reality is *undefined* to our rational minds. Yet it still *is*, just as "I AM therefore I can think." To us, it is like a void beyond the physical, beyond that point at which molecules do not move. Yet it still *is* and *always* is, was and will be. It is a void that you can experience by yielding to it, not by reaching out and trying to know it.

So scientists have said that the Big Bang was an *explosion* out from a point of infinite density and from that, matter was created. Yet, *from the perspective of the Oneness*, for matter to come into existence from no matter a *Big Implosion* must have occurred. For physical reality to be created, the light of the Universe would had to have slowed its rate to speeds at which density could be perceived and the physical would seem more real.

How can this happen?

You have to put on the Cosmic brakes. (The Kabbalistic concept of "Tzimtzum," contraction of light.) This is the Big Implosion.

Together, the light had to decrease from infinite speed and slow so that it suddenly became finite. You might say its frequency fell. We can imagine the light slowing itself down into states closer and closer to being perceived as matter. It was the slowing down of the light to different levels of energy that slowly gave rise to the perception of matter. The question is, "How is this done? How does light slow itself down?"

The answer illustrates the fact that the foundation of *all* science is spiritual because the *physical world*, and the ability to perceive it, was created by the resistance of Adam and Eve's Will. This is not saying that Adam and Eve created the world. It is saying that we created the physical perception of the world. When Adam and Eve reached out to take the fruit from the Tree of Knowledge, a Big Implosion occurred within *them* and *their* consciousness changed. Because then the consciousness of Adam and Eve was *within* their identities, on the other side of God's imagination, to witness God's creation from within the creation as it was imagined. From the other side, we are set free to choose the way that the Creator most loves the process of life to be. As we touch down with our hearts to the deepest point of physical reality, we touch the base of the anu by being completely grounded in our lives, and there is a perfect marriage between our Will and the original vision/imagination of reality that is the Will of the eternal Creator.

Slowing down *and* the perception of the slowing down were caused by the resistance of the Beings who were One with God and then adopted the Will that resists Oneness. We *fell* in vibration because we chose to begin the reality of duality, thus disconnecting from the Love of the Source. We perceive physical reality *because* of our lower vibration, because of our internal, cosmic brakes of resistance. Our internal cosmic brakes are the judgments, fears and need for control that we have adopted from our minds of opposition which create the chakra seals.

It is hard to imagine the beginning of hydrogen and helium gases from the explosion of a point of infinite density and no dimension. There is no matter and all of a sudden—boom—and there is matter? Probably not. It is more conceivable that hydrogen gas molecules began to form from the slowing down of light. As infinite light slowed itself down, it naturally formed into the first elements. In this way, the rest of atomic matter formed itself.

This discussion is based on the Kabbalistic notion that the Universe was already billions of years old when Adam and Eve were plunked into it. The Torah says Adam was created as a grown man, so why would the Universe not be already created as well? The Universe was created in its infancy from scratch in the imagination of God, and it was first witnessed only several thousands of years ago when Adam and Eve were placed inside the imagination. But if there was nobody there to witness the Universe for billions of years, did it really exist? Only in the imagination of the Creator did it exist.

Does light decrease in vibration at all, if there is nothing to perceive it at lower relative speeds? This is a good Zen cohen, which is a riddle to exercise and make you expand your mind. It has the same essence as another Zen cohen, "If a tree falls in the forest and there is nobody there, does it make any sound?"

The answer is: *it doesn't matter.*

If nothing is there to perceive in the physical, why does it matter? It doesn't matter. Light remains light and not matter at all. It has no experience. It just is and it is completely undefined.

One purpose for distinguishing the beginning as being an implosion is to share the fact that we hold *within our deepest core* an imploded body that is the remnant of the effect of the Big Implosion upon our souls. Since we are all little representations of the whole, this implosion has also occurred within us. The slightest bit of resistance causes the infinite to become finite, and the activity and motion on the physical side begins.

The explosion that scientists see as the Big Bang is the one in the future and has not yet come to be, yet always is. It is due to matter and its reverse, antimatter, coming back together in an inevitable embrace, as all things that have been in separation must return as One. It is where the past and future become One, the explosion (the end of Time) with the implosion. (The beginning of time) (see Figure 35.)

This brings up the discussion of the importance and responsibility we have in bringing in the Messianic Age through our purposeful actions. If we wait for God to come rescue us, then we will see the merging of matter and antimatter when our consciousness is still stuck in our bodies. The crossing of the threshold will come upon us not because we chose it and gave rise to the experience of the Creator, but because it was forced on us. That is no good for anybody.

Nearing the source of the Big Bang or the Big Implosion, at the furthest reaches of space, the speed of light is incredibly fast. When the speed of light is very fast, time is perceived relatively slowly. Where light is infinite and whole (Allthatis), time is zero. Thus the passage of time is relative to the amount of activity on the physical plane.

So from a relative *perception* within the physical, as the speed of light (frequency) decreases (by it being resisted), the perception of mass increases, internal temperature increases, internal physical movement increases, and the perception of physical reality and the passage of time increases. This is the other side of reality, the side created by the resistance of being and the void in the center of the chakra seals.

The perception of reality as being so physical and dense is greatest on planet Earth. "Even though you exist upon a physical planet and the densest of all the planets of the Universe…" *The Only Planet of Choice*, p. 13. Of all other civilizations, the density of planet Earth is the greatest. This means that we perceive our planet to be the most physical, because of the density. Our consciousness affects the density of the planet, for as we adopt such states of resistance, the density around us increases. Spirit precedes science. Yet there can be no perception of physicality without the density of the Earth's gravitational field, because it is the strong sensation of the gravitational pull on our bodies, emotions, and minds which makes our existence seem so physical. The gravitational pull gives us the perception of physical, and the resistance in our bodies, emotions, and minds accumulates and causes the Earth to have a great density. So our consciousness and the gravitational pull feed back upon each other to yield such a high degree of density.

Any resistance in a perfect system of light causes it to come out of superconductivity into semi-conductivity and to become electromagnetic. Only when something is electromagnetic can the Earth's gravitational field have an influence on it. When there is resistance within this rational mind, the semi-conductivity caused by the resistance of flow forces the mind to be subject to the Earth's gravitational field, making the body have the sensation of being weighted down. This gives the soul a sensation of its identity being localized in its physical body. In *The Five Bodies*, Dr. J.J. Hurtak describes the *electromagnetic* body. It is the body created by the activity of the rational mind's resistance. In our electromagnetic body we are able to perceive the illusion of the physical realities and, for this reason, it is limiting to our true nature, which extends much further beyond the limits of the electromagnetic body.

"The Enochian Keys tell us that the Electromagnetic body is your individual body in its gross material form," **The Five Bodies** p. 4.

Hurtak says that in the return to collective consciousness, what we have called the return to Eden, we will shed the electromagnetic body.

The wires that conduct energy through our system are the acupuncture meridians. (see Figure 36) When Adam and Eve ate from the Tree of Knowledge for Allow and Resist, the conduction system went from a perfect system of superconductivity with the **axiotonal** lines, wherein the ORMEs flow (see Figure 38), to semi-conductivity within the acupuncture meridian system which is divided into Yin and Yang conduction channels. Like the chakras, these channels are also separated and in contradiction to one another. (See Figure 37 and 38) Thus at the time of the "fall," or the "slowing down of the light," we went from perfect connection with the Unity of Oneness via the axiotonal lines, Balanced Positive, to the dual, split systems of the yin/yang or efferent/afferent acupuncture system. The acupuncture system flows in dual directions of yin and yang because of the resistance of the Will chakras.

The disconnection from the system of superconductivity (axiotonal lines) has dramatic effects on a soul's consciousness. Instead of perceiving the connection, harmony, and Love in all things, it chooses fragmented belief systems that order reality into delusional pigeon-holes. The density is thick, like a quagmire, and it has become quite difficult for us to simply step out of it and cross back over the threshold.

The density and the stuckness of the electromagnetic body can be healed, infused with light and Love, to invigorate its vibratory rate. It can be shaken off to ascend beyond the threshold of negative mass. The negative mass is the reverse, the negative of the existence of light—it is the world of matter. Therefore, in order to transform, besides the letting go of the resistance to Being, you can also help by purifying the physical body with good diet, good exercise and a lot of pure water.

Pay attention to the times when you feel the heaviest. What is going on in your emotions? You are likely resisting something, not letting something Be. At other times, you will feel weightless, as if you are walking on air.

Because we use Frmee Will to resist Being, the molecules of the (dense electromagnetic) brain are stimulated to move more rapidly, in a more agitated manner. It has been demonstrated through various studies that in a relaxed or meditative state, the frequency of brain activity is decreased, as in alpha or delta states. In a state of stress or fear, the frequency is much more rapid, as in beta states. From the brain of a person in an agitated state (they are most likely doing the most resistance), the perception of light is limited to the physical. In other words, the physical world seems more real. When you perceive from the mind stuck in physical reality, this mind becomes more active. This is the rational, self within the self mind. It is the stressed out mind.

When the rational mind is very active, the physical is perceived as being more real. Your body will feel more weighted and dense. You will perceive yourself less connected to all things, and more limited to your physical body. A person in a state of sublime peace and tranquility, who is feeling Love, will perceive the world around them and in them as much lighter. The person feels connected with all things. If sensitive enough, he or she will perceive those frequencies of energy beyond the physical, which have a faster velocity. They might see angels, fairies and other light beings. When something's energy is perceived more "within the light," its light is more apparent, its mass less real. The converse is also true. Within relativity, if you perceive something's mass to be more real, you perceive its light to be less real. It will seem more physical and less of the quality of light. As the delusions and belief systems of the mind are shed, the perception of light increases. Things are perceived to be lighter because the heaviness caused by the resistance and semi-conduction of the electromagnetic mind has been released!

When you see someone's auric field, or when you can look at their internal energetic make-up, there is a sense of seeing their true nature, and you see that they *are* made up of light. How different would the world be if we all walked around in our light bodies? The Truth is that we always do, yet if that were the normal way we perceived each other, do you know what it would be like to behold people?

You would see their true colors.

They would see your true colors. No lying. No deception. No hiding from what you feel. No talking in half truths. All would be perfectly displayed for all to see. You would never hide your feelings about something and you would never lie. It would be silly to, because people would be able to see your internal conflict and hear the discrepancy between what you are saying while they watched what you were really feeling. They would see the conflict that lying has upon your system. Your true self is suppressed when you say something other than the Truth. Recall that there are no secrets in reverse speech and even today, you cannot lie to those who are very sensitive. They can pick up the conflict in the intention. They might call you on it and if they do, do yourself a favor and just be honest. Otherwise your guts are just going to get all knotted. Who really wants that?

When we live as if the physical is more real, then it is very possible to live in a world of illusion with yourself and others. A reality in which people get away with lying is a reality in which people easily control and dominate others. When there are no more secrets, all the control and power that has been put upon people by the Con Trolls will disappear.

The ties that you hold, fixed onto your body (in a reverse fashion— i.e., stuck to the past) are the beliefs and resistances that you have held onto because you have judged them as bad. Recall the discussion from Chapter Two on healing resistance. We resist what we judge as bad. When you are deep in this resistance, you are stuck to perceive yourself as a physical body. As the last tie is released, there is a complete freedom of the self within the self. From the perspective of your true nature, you say goodbye to it as it turns itself over, so you remain centered within your Being. If you are feeling as if you are going to dissolve into the void, it is because the last thread you are still holding is part of the rational mind and can give you the impression of impending doom.

When Adam and Eve are one within us, and Adam carries forth the energy of Eve and then feeds it back to her, we are not trapped in the magnetic field because the two energies are in perfect, coordinated harmony so that there is a magnetic neutral of Balanced Positive shared between them. This magnetic neutral has no resistance, it is pure Being, and thus it is beyond the gravitational influence of the Earth.

When the energies became separated, because the connection between Adam and Eve split, it led to the unbalanced negative being thrown up into the air out of the body and the unbalanced positive getting disconnected from the mind. And as they stretched out in dualities, their polarities became more opposed. Alchemically speaking, this separation of the poles of the male and female began the spin of the Earth, which then got faster and faster. It was scary, yes, as the world spun round and round as if down a drain pipe and through that long black hole to come out here, on the other/reverse side where there are two poles in separation. This created the magnetic attraction and stuckness. The attraction is because they are opposites and they belong as One, so they always seek that communion. They are stuck because they are attached to each other in need. There isn't freedom within this sort of attraction. It is binding and controlling—codependent. The irony is that, even though there is this strong attraction and they are bound to each other, there is always a gap that exists between the male and female; they do not fit perfectly together. We have not experienced the perfect communion between our male and female energies for a very, very long time.

Chapter 11: Summary

The word science comes from the latin "scire," which means "to know." And in its essence, the goal of science is and always has been to know the Truth, the nature of reality. We have made the error of allowing the discoveries of science to become the dictates of consciousness and science no longer serves its purpose, but rather acts to keep people limited to its definitions. No one can know the Truth in a way that is reproducible. The Truth is undefined. As soon as you attempt to order it, you are putting it into pigeon holes and limiting it to a lesser reality that is nothing like the true reality that is infinite in potential and wonder and that comes from the feeling and direct experience (Being) of the Truth. We have become stuck in the belief systems that the search for Truth has yielded, and many of us have given much of our faith over to science. Science can be employed very well to serve humanity. When humanity becomes a servant to science, things become negative and backward.

From a state of Oneness with no resistance, judgment causes our consciousness to alter from a state of pure Beingness to a controlled, divided existence. Resistance slowed the frequency of Eden and caused a Big Implosion. When Adam and Eve awoke, their eyes were open to the physical realities *within* the Earth's gravitational field, which exists on the other, inverted side of the higher planes of reality. There is a divine realm that always remains within Oneness and with no resistance and no judgment. This is the Zone of Cold and is the World of Atzilut.

Adam and Eve's energetic systems of super-conductivity also changed into a system of polarities and semi-conductivity. We see this in the dual systems of the acupuncture meridians and the chakra system, as yin and yang meridians and feeling and Will chakras, that travel in opposite directions. The resistance in a conduction-system (e.g., wire) makes it a semi-conductor with a magnetic field. This is what causes us to be subjected to the gravitational field of the earth. When there is no resistance in a system of conduction, no field of energy causes that object to be subjected to the Earth's magnetic field. It can, therefore, levitate beyond the density of Earth. It is also directly connected to the zero-point field of the earth. The more we resist, the more we are subjected to the density of the Earth and all the illusions only available within the gravitational field of the Earth. We witness physical reality all around as real because we are trapped in it. Our higher consciousness, our higher mind, sees beyond the void of the physical. The building blocks of all matter are themselves filled with nothingness, illustrating the void. Deep in the void is the conversion point into a higher reality, which encompasses the void of the All. It is a complete flip/reversal. Un-imploding (exploding) the self within the self, you exist within the consciousness of Oneness, the Allthatis, which encompasses all things. It is a journey through a black hole into another dimensional reality which is free and unlimited.

ESSENCE OF THE CHAPTER

In our true nature, we are light beings. We perceive ourselves and our world as physical because we resist the Will of God.

THE WAY OF THE FEMALE AND THE MALE

RECONCILIATION OF EVE AND ADAM

This is a very important chapter. So much revolves around the issues discussed herein. If the world embraced just this chapter, this would be the era of peace for all people.

Part I—The Male Energy in Separation from The Female

The perfect union between male and female energies is the Balanced Positive nature of the Creator. The union empowers the magic and healing of alchemy. Adam and Eve represent the male and the female energy. We have already discussed the separation between Adam and Eve in the Tree of Knowledge chapter and its role regarding the beginning of duality. The *imbalance* between these energies is an immense factor in the disharmony that occurs in individuals and on a global scale. The conflict between male and female and between man and woman creates suffering.

The judgments made by the sexes have placed much control on humankind, especially the belief that one sex is better, more important, or more intelligent than the other. This belief arose, as do all beliefs, from the need to control. The vast majority of control on this planet, through the centuries, throughout the world's different cultures and religions has been wielded by men over women. And this remains largely true even today. This male, controlling energy subjects so many to great injustices. This is not because of the true nature of man and woman in harmony, but because the roles that each has gotten stuck in during the experience of what-we-are-not in the physical. Women have played along with this control and have shown that when they no longer find a situation acceptable, they have great power to affect change. As men open their eyes and stop resisting the female energy, women will also embrace their freedom.

It is not simply that women are controlled by men. Men control men. Women control women and men as well, especially when they feel that they are not free to do as they wish and they must control to get what they want. Sometimes women play the role of the male and men play the role of the female. That is why what we are really discussing is that the male energy tends to control the female energy, which exist in each of us.

It is most important to understand, therefore, how *the Female as foundation of power* differs from *the Male as the foundation of power*. The control exerted by men over women is a reflection of the conflict and control between the male energy trying to be the foundation of power when it is *in separation* from the female. We saw this in the chakras, where the male Will chakra suppresses the flow of the female. This energetic model of the chakras is an analogy to the way the male energy, often carried out by men, attempts to block the flow of female energy, mostly represented by women.

There is another analogy between human genetics and the Hebrew alphabetic. The woman's genetics are made from two X chromosomes that physically resemble Xs. The man is made up of the XY pair, with the Y, which resembles an X *with a leg missing*. In the Hebrew alphabet, the X chromosome looks like an Aleph, א, The One, which represents the balanced whole of God (Balanced Positive). By looking closely at the Aleph, we see the balance of the beginning and the end, as if the male and the female chakras are balanced as One. (see Figure 28). The Y resembles the Tzadik suffit, **צ**, the last letter (including the final letters) of the Hebrew alphabet, which is the same as the Aleph, **א**, with a leg missing. So the woman's genes are made up of XX chromosomes. Which is **אא**. The man's genes are like XY. Which is **אצ**.

The Hebrew letter Tzadik suffit, **צ**, is symbolic of a tree, upright, firm, and strong, and the letter even looks somewhat like a tree. The Hebrew word for tree, **עץ**, has the Tzadik Suffit in it. This is the strength of the male. This strength and firmness is essential for the balance between the male and the female. What can happen of course, is this strength and sturdiness can overpower and exceed its purpose, becoming rigidity.

"Men are born soft and supple;
dead they are stiff and hard.

Plants are born tender and pliant;
dead, they are brittle and dry.

Thus whoever is stiff and inflexible
is a disciple of death.
Whoever is soft and yielding
is a disciple of life.

The hard and stiff will be broken.
The soft and supple will prevail."

Lao-tzu, *Tao Te Ching*, verse 76

This letter, **צ**, alone, represents The Tree of Knowledge for Good and Bad, which is associated with rational thought and the desire for power, which the male has aligned itself with. It is the **Y Factor**—the need to know, the need to be in control through knowing. Also Tzadik suffit, **צ**,

is the very last letter of the Hebrew alphabet, far away from the Source of the One, the first letter, which is the Aleph. The γ has the highest Gematria (numerical value of a letter), 900.

In Judaism, a "Tzadik" is an incredibly learned man whose mind understands great truths about the Torah and God. The word means "a righteous person," "an upright person." The Jewish belief is that he has great insight into the ways of things and has been brought by God to teach people. Unfortunately, there have been few Tzadiks to have taught a most important Truth that is above and beyond all the Truths that many Tzadiks have conveyed. It is the Truth that you don't need a teacher to understand God and the Universe, for the Truth is inherent within you. The many Tzadiks that did not spread the Truth that we all have full access to the Truth within us have, therefore, perpetuated a false belief system that enabled them to be like God in possession of knowledge that they either freely or frugally shared with their students, positioning themselves as the gates and keys to their students' longed-for knowledge. Of course, this is a two-way circuit, because the students of these Tzadiks have desired the knowledge that they believed the Tzadik to possess and which they did not. No one is to blame, these are simply roles being filled due to long-held belief systems. As wonderful as many of these Tzadiks have been, their errors have perpetuated a slavery for knowledge that is outside of the self. Many continue to seek knowledge of Truth outside of themselves, believing that is their connection to God. Many have turned to these Tzadiks to know Truth, for the same reason many seek gurus. This has also caused some Tzadiks to be worshipped. Many people do have the desire to be worshipped for the knowledge they possess or their ability to convey the ways of the Universe. This is a deep, primordial, and often hidden desire, of which many Tzadiks were unaware, or knew about and succumbed to their temptation. Any spiritual leaders and teachers who understood that all people are equal and capable of knowing Truth and that did not make the effort to explain that have made the error and acted out of their desire. If Tzadiks, gurus, or any spiritual teachers have not helped others see their direct access to knowledge and did not explain the great equivalence of all beings, then who did they serve? So I remind you again, that the temptation of the Serpent is to get humans trying to be like God in Knowing Good and Bad.

I don't even like the term "righteous" because it denotes a kind of uprightness that has a superior quality to it. One is righteous because they do no bad, or they only do good according to the beliefs about what is good and bad. That has the Tree of Knowledge written all over it. The Tree of Life is not about getting a ribbon for following along according to what is established good and bad. It is about being yourself. That is not a path of righteousness.

The Tzadik suffit by itself, **ץ**, the final letter away from the Source, the Aleph, is like the scientific mind seeking Truth outside itself. All by itself, it is a mind that splits reality forever into parts of good and bad. It has no foundation, nor any real Truth, just a desire to be like God in possession of Knowledge. Y Factor.

The Aleph, **א**, is Oneness and has the Gematria of 26—which is the same Gematria of the most sacred name of God, **יהוה**—26. Aleph is the beginning and the end. (see Figure 28) There is a beautiful analogy of the Aleph that is seen with a baby in the womb of its mother. That baby is One with its mother, literally and spiritually, for it is inside of her and their consciousnesses are married. (see Figure 41) The air that the mother breathes, is the air the baby breathes. The food she eats, is the food the baby eats. What is most amazing is that the child is floating in liquid, thus it has no sensation of the physical. (There is a mystery here about being within waters…) It feels Oneness, still. It's existence is effortless.

Pregnancy is a most beautiful time. The bond that the mother has with the child is powerful in a way that those who have not had the experience will never understand (until they are able to achieve Oneness within themselves).

And then you are born into a hard, dense world with bright lights and loud noises. The temperatures aren't perfectly warm and regulated, as within Ma's womb, and the doctor hangs you upside down to slap your bum. (Okay, maybe not as often anymore) Then, if that isn't enough, the chord that attaches you to your mom, that brought nourishment to your lungs and tissues (as well as the means of evacuating the waste in your system) is *cut*, separating you. (see Figure 42)

Now, you're on your own. Now you must breathe for yourself, feel for yourself, think and act for yourself. This is birth from Oneness into indiv*iduality and separation*. It begins the process of seeking to return to the Source of the Oneness, to the womb of the Mother-Shekinah-Goddess, rooted as One with the Earth. Thus, life is a journey to reconnect with the female as the foundation, because the birth into the physical is spiritually equivalent to the Aleph, **א**, having its foundation removed and having the Tzadik suffit, **ץ**, act as the foundation of reality. We are all born this way, into indiv*iduality* into separation. Thus, from this angle, men and women are the same, for we all exist within indiv*iduality*. Being born into the physical and cut from the mother is being born into duality, where the Mother-Goddess is not the foundation.

The Aleph represents a balance that has both the male and female in togetherness, **א**. You can even see the yin and yang, or male and female on each side of the line that runs down between them. (see Figure 28) There is a harmony, an equality, a balanced relationship. The Tzadik suffit, **ץ**, does not have a balance. There is something missing, and as a result, that which the Tzadik teacher is after is not Love, but knowledge for the power it brings.

Love is the most powerful force of the Universe. It is Truth. Love is **אהבה** (Ahava). **אהבה** is To Be (Ehye) **אהיה** with foundation. Ehye, **אהיה** is the nature of God, Beingness. If you look at the word Ahava, **אהבה**, it is the same as Ehye, **אהיה**, yet the Yod, **י**, which also represents Oneness and God (a point of no dimension), has a foundation. Thus, Love is To Be with foundation. Our foundation (Malchut—Hebrew for Kingdom, the foundation of the Tree of Life, is the realm wherein dwells the Shekinah) is Mother Earth. It is the female. Love is To Be grounded. To Be grounded is to be "down to earth," which is humility.

Allowing and letting yourself be grounded with your two feet, which is a natural tendency beyond control and out of the mental, and releasing the cerebral approach to being and living, is part of the way of Love. The cerebral and mental approaches to life are centered in the head and are disconnected from the foundation. That is why the Tzadik suffit, **ץ**, has a leg missing. We Love while being grounded. Becoming grounded totally and completely, is total and complete Beingness—your highest potential. This requires giving up all desire to be like God in knowing, thinking you have knowledge that others do not, or thinking that possessing knowledge will bring you closer to God. And since Love is felt in the heart, in being connected with Mother Earth, you feel the Goddess in your chest.

> "Your Mother is in you, and you in her. She bore you, she gives you life. It was she who gave to you your body, and to her shall you one day give it back again. Happy are you when you come to know her and her kingdom; if you receive your Mother's angels and if you do her laws. I tell you truly, he who does these things shall never see disease. For the power of our Mother is above all."
> The Essene *Gospel of Peace* p. 9

The Shekinah, the female aspect of God, Ruach HaKodesh **רוח הקודש**, the Holy Spirit, is the animating source of all souls of the universe. The Shekinah empowers you to *Be*. She is the breath of life— **רוח החיים**. She is what gives you the ability to feel and experience the Love and wonder of who you are and of Allthatis. The definition of Love in the *Keys of Enoch*, "The substance of Eternal Life. It is created in the believer by the Shekinah holy spirit" p. 586.

Thus, in nature, that which has *its foundation* in the female (Malchut) has a nature aligned with the energy of the Creator, the Balanced Positive, the Zone of Cold, the infinite, the undefined. It is not that you must suppress the male energy and only be female. You must have your foundation, the source of Being, in the female, the Shekinah, Mother Earth. The male, *when separated*, is aligned more within belief systems, sturdy/rigid structure, and definition, which leads to the confinement of Being and the exile from Eden. When the male tries to act as the foundation, the foundation is false and must be maintained with control, because the Y factor is missing a leg. With the female as the foundation, the source in a harmonious relationship, the male acts as an extension.

As in a magnet, when the male energy is separated from the female energy, it is incomplete and has no source of power. That is why those governed by the male tend to feel insecure and have the need to control and take possession. When the male energy is separate from the female, it becomes the opposition or the opposite of the Source. It competes with the Source, tries to control it and resists it, just like male, Will chakras act as the resistors to the female, feeling chakras. When the male energy is separate, it turns around and becomes attracted to and stuck to the female. It impedes the free flowing nature of the Balanced Positive. (see Figure 37 and Figure 18b)

The Serpent, **Hanuchash** הנחש, opposes the Shekinah שכינה. It is the energy of opposition. The reverse, the opposite. If you say Shekinah backwards, you are saying Hanachush. And since the Serpent opposes, its energy is the reverse of the Shekinah. Therefore, what turns against the Shekinah, the Will centers opposing the Feeling centers in the Left column of the Tree of Knowledge, *is* the Serpent energy. It is the energy that says, "You should know what you're doing at all times. You should be in control. You should be like God in having all the Knowledge and all the control." The Serpent vibration represents the male in separation from the female. It is the rational, Bina2 mind believing that what it knows makes it like God, that is why it tempts us to try to be like God in possessing knowledge.

With the male trying to be the foundation of power we have forgotten who we are. We have clutched and grabbed. We have limited each other through control and possession. We have made a reality on earth that is not all bad, but is definitely bad and good. And this is how it has been for so long. This is our separation from our Home.

"It is simply because the male energy has ruled for dominant times and it is feeling threatened now, for it knows that it must have equality with the female or it cannot survive. All the source of power comes from the female. By controlling the female, keeping her in bondage and in servitude he can then own that power, do you understand?" *The Only Planet of Choice* p. 305

Figure 40

The Female	The Male
In the Balanced Positive Reality	In the Balanced Positive Reality
Garden of Eden She feels Great. Free. She is pure Beingness. What a divine love-bond with the male. He is my prince. In a State of Balanced +ve.	*Garden of Eden* Wow! She is so divine, so beautiful. She shines so brightly. She has such grace and presence. He is a proud knight. Secure. Being. Honoured. He feels Great. In a State of Balanced +ve.
Tree of Knowledge Through Time and History	*Tree of Knowledge* Through Time and History
Unbalanced Positive Separated from the Male This power I have is bad. The essence of who I am is not good. I have done wrong. I must put myself in my place. She begins to believe that this is the way things must be.	**Unbalanced Negative** Separated from the Female That power she has is so much. It is daunting. It frightens me, but it is so appealing. It is all I want. I need that. I must have that! (The need comes from the true wish for the essence of the female together with the judgment of it.) I want that just Frmee. Nobody else can have her. So he hides her. He keeps her locked away and even tries to tell her how to Be, how not to Be, what to say, what to wear, what not to study.

She gives her obedience to the Male "This is Ok. This is how it should Be" Inside she shrinks herself. She lives for him and responds close-ly to his every whim and mood.	The way he does this is through control of the essence of the female, making it seem bad, or wrong. *He makes laws and rules about marriage that must be obeyed.* *She will marry him and be only with him. Breaking these laws is punishable by death.*
She learns to hide and not take up space. She learns to take her shine and make it small. She loses her sense of self. She loses her sense of choice and her power to make it so.	He becomes afraid of losing her because he puts a lot of effort and belief into trying to have her just for himself. He doesn't want others to see her beauty. He doesn't want others to see her shine. He doesn't want to share her with anyone.
Her voice and power get suppressed. She is angry at him because of the control. But she is even more angry at herself for allowing it.	The bottomless pit of Frmee Will grows greatly with the male dominat-ing the basis of reality.
Today as women are waking up to their true sense of freedom, what might help them to see: She still can fear losing her freedom and her sense of self. Has observed her mother shrinking and hiding herself for her father, so she grows up believing she must hide her-self for "her man," to keep him happy and believing this is the way she should be. She can feel now that she must prove she is free to herself and to him because she has been locked away for so long.	*Today as men are attempting to let go of control and allow her (women and the female) to be free, what might help them to see:* Can still fear losing his woman. Has observed his mother shrinking and hiding herself for his father, so he grows up believing this is the way she should be. Can still have the patterns of fear-based and control-based behaviour. Can still want to hide her. Can still want her all for himself.

Her Part/Her Healing	*His Part/His Healing*
I don't need to prove myself. All I have to do is to let myself be who I am with no doubt, no guilt and no belief that I should not or cannot.	I totally and completely align myself with allowing her to shine. I want her to shine. I want her to be free and happy. This is what I see for her. I wish the best for her according to how she would like it for herself.
I let myself shine. I let myself be free as I wish to be. I let my power be. I give myself the right to be free. It is my choice and my power, not his.	I acknowledge her power. It can feel daunting to me, but I yield to it, fully and completely. I allow myself to see the greatness in the freedom of her Beingness and Beauty.
I therefore am free and don't have to worry about not having my freedom. I have taken it for myself.	I therefore am not afraid because I am not trying to keep her locked up and hidden away. *I am now the man I have always wanted to Be* and I have set myself free.
Because this is such a deep seated belief and pattern of fear, his support, Love and playing his part will really help her out of her small space.	Because his fears, insecurities, and need to control can go very deeply, her playing her part and showing him how okay it is for her to shine and let her power and beauty out, will really help him out of his small space.

The three major religions of the world—Judaism, Christianity, and Islam—are structured to have the male acting as a foundation of reality, where the approach to God and the Truth is ordered in a rational manner through the study of the religious texts (Torah, Bible, Koran). This stifles the power of the female who functions through intuition and direct knowing beyond definition, and it also obscures the very essence of these religions, which were conceived as a means of experiencing

God, whose foundation is based in the female.

As we open up to the Truth of the Universe and we see that the desire to control reality and to control the way of another are really forms of hell, the Love that comes from equality, letting go, and letting Be will flow harmoniously once again.

It is very important for us not to punish ourselves as we become aware that we haven't been living as "perfectly" as we thought. That would be misunderstanding and not finding acceptance of ourselves and the choices we have made in our physical world. As you acknowledge errors, do not dwell on them or drown in guilt. Just remember that your true nature has never been apart from you, even if, through the experience of the physical, through pain and trauma and need, you may have made choices that were notsonice and ego-based. With this awareness, it will be much easier to let go of shame and honestly face the ugly or lesser choices you have made and find acceptance. Acceptance and forgiveness are letting go. *To hold onto the shame of being imperfect is to hold onto the need to be perfect.* It is not necessary to be perfect, and when you cannot face shame, you will hold onto the ways that you really want to release. This advice is especially for people who have preached Truth to others and used this to justify control and inequality. It is for those who have claimed to know the absolute Truth and looked to other expressions of Truth as lesser or wrong. There are no more rules. There are no more laws. It is all about freedom and equality. That is what the *Moshiach* (Messiah) is. It is living within unconditional Love, within a zone of AllGood. What rules do you need there? None. Why? Because it is AllGood and so are you.

In the state of Oneness, the male is an extension of the female. It is there, and it is like a point of no dimension. ⊙. The shell will break, and the bonds will loosen so that the perpetual hourglass can turn back to its proper position.

The Balanced Positive is the undefined. What is undefined in math?

Infinity is undefined. How big is it or what is it exactly? *You cannot define it.*

It is $1/0 =$ undefined

The male, 1, is on top of the female, 0, which is the foundation. (The woman can be on top too. ☺) The undefined is the infinite, and that is how it feels to merge with the Oneness; it feels as if you are merging into infinity, a strange feeling, as if becoming nothing. But it is not nothing, it is undefined. As it stands now with the male trying to control the foundation of reality, it is 0/1, which is *really* nothing, as in zero.

What is interesting to note is that the zeros of the infinity symbol, , which are like everything with nothing to compare with, like a void, come together in a point. If you were to turn the infinity symbol toward you on the Z plane, rotating it $90°$ clockwise going into this page, and then if you looked at it, it would look like this, ⊙, a zero point. It is also neat to see that looking at a 1 on top of a zero, 1/0, which is undefined, from above, also looks like this, ⊙, zero point, which is the Alchemical Symbol for *Gold*.

> "Our two souls, therefore, which are One,
> Though I must go, endure not yet,
> A breach, but an expansion,
> Like Gold to airy thinness beat."
> *"A Valediction Forbidding Mourning"*
> John Donne

Later in this poem, John Donne uses compasses as a beautiful metaphor. He writes:

> "If they be two, they are two so
> As stiff twin compasses are two;
> Thy soul, the fix'd foot, makes no show
> To move, but doth, if th' other do.

> And though it in the centre sit,
> Yet, when the other far doth roam,
> It leans, and hearkens after it,
> And grows erect, as that comes home.

Such wilt thou be to me, who must,
Like th' other foot, obliquely run;
Thy firmness makes my circle just,
And makes me end where I begun."

John Donne is conveying something quite amazing. He is saying that because of the fixed foot, the defined, the sturdy, the circle is able to be drawn. The male is the finite, the defined, the fixed foot, the firmness, and therefore, is the element that helps to draw the circle, and give the zero around it, symbolic of the female, some form. Without the male in the circle, there would be no point, no departure, and no return.

"God is a sphere whose center is everywhere and whose
circumference is nowhere."
Hermes Trismegistus

Those that exist as One with the Divine shine with the color of gold, for they have given up their Frmee Will and are living within the consciousness of the undefined. This is *the Zone of Cold*, the zone of pure potentiality of Que Sera Sera, *Ehye Usher Ehye*. In this Oneness, the female energy is back as the source of true power (it always was, but was opposed), the energy flows from the south and the north extends that onward and outward, and naturally returns to the Source. In this way, the male serves the female, as in the majestic times of legends in which great chivalrous knights were sworn to serve a lady. The female naturally serves the male as well, giving freely from the Source, not as a slave, but by the choice of the heart, in a Love bond. Her nature can teach us so much about Love and just Being. Love because of the caring, the kindness, the acceptance, the giving that she embodies. Just Being is aligned with the Source of the Creator. It is a state of grace and bliss.

In terms of your capacity to share that Love, beyond all definition and judgment, in the Ganallisone where there is no resistance, there is little difference between a man and a woman. There are certain physical differences that will naturally distinguish them somewhat—men and women are like pieces of Lego that fit nicely into each other, and a woman is made to carry and feed babies. Yet in behavior, the *conditions and beliefs* that we adhere to keep men and women separate and different. This is because of centuries of role-playing, fixed ideas about how a man must be and how a woman must be, and the different roles that the man and woman have adopted in the Game of Life. Yet each still has the capacity for their male and female energies to work in harmony.

In duality, men tend to be more rational and women more feeling. Because women allow themselves to feel more and express their feelings, they are also more emotional. I did not write that men are *rational* and women are *emotional*, however, because these are not opposites. The opposites are rational and feeling, in the intuitive sense.

Rational is equivalent to ego and control. If someone gets hurt, feels small or squashed, and they do not know how to deal with that properly through forgiveness and letting be and letting go, *the energetic void created from suppressing that hurt becomes ego.* The ego then becomes rational thought processes, beliefs, and judgments because, through the rational, it can control reality to compensate for the feeling of insecurity and hurt. This often begins in children. The mind begins to work in contradiction to true nature, backwards, to be in control. The more someone is rational, the less they feel, the more they have forgotten their true nature. Anyone who is hurt and does not allow themselves to feel will become more rational. They will lose touch with their feelings, including taking into consideration how others feel. This is also why a person who is very rational will also feel very alone. All will be Frmthem.

Another distinction is that men generally tend to be more selfish. Women generally are more giving and their eyes and hearts are more considerate of others. They are not so self-centered. This is of the divine nature of Love. A being who is selfish and only thinks of him or herself cannot know what Love is. You can know what it feels like to want and need someone, but not how it feels to love someone. Selfishness, only thinking for yourself, is the opposite of Love. It is Frmee Will, the will that opposes Love.

Men also tend to be more goal-oriented than women. This makes men more rushed. The rushing actually comes from a need to fulfill something from the outside. The more a person is Frmee, the larger their ego, and the more they need things from the outside to fill the hollow void on the inside. You only rush when you desire something in a needy way. That desire is really for the self only. Even though you might appear to be doing things for others, if you rush, that is due to your need-based ego.

The balance is understanding that there is a lot to do and action is very important. But instead of always rushing for more and more, *just Be* and from that as your foundation, you will *do* what you *are*. This is aligned with the first CaN of the First Circle—I do not rush to make myself better. I live for who I AM now and Love that. Let go of needing to be or have something more. Just let yourself Be and you'll see, you'll have, you'll do.

Men often have the issue of needing to be "number one" to their parents, friends, or partner. Of course the *need* to be "number one" is caused by primordial insecurity: the need to build yourself up. Insecurity also manifests as the need to prove yourself. If a person places a lot of value in what they know, they will desire to know everything, or to appear as if they do. Needing to know everything is the same thing as needing to be right all the time.

Fathers often try to be the boss and often display the need to be right. Even if this is not sensed on a conscious level, it is never missed. The son will subconsciously live through life with this competitive energy, because his dad, who is really like God to a child, has shown him that it is important to be right. The father can even hold a child back in his need to be right. This happens subconsciously, even if a father wishes the best for his son. It is a blind spot caused by his own insecurity and his need to be "number one." This is the first of the **Three Major Delusions** (Appendix B).

Another dynamic within the family structure has perpetuated this huge imbalance in belief systems about the importance of the man versus the woman. This is a very deeply ingrained pattern that is improving now. It values sons more than daughters, putting the sons higher, because the family structure usually revolves around the man, with the male energy controlling the foundation. Knowledge of a finite nature is held above Beingness, which is what the female is best at.

When they're young, the boys get more positive attention so they will feel superior to their sisters. This will also extend later to all other women because the males have learned and believe that they are more important than their female counterparts. They learn that life revolves around them. Since it is likely that the mother and father are both part of this delusion, the mother is probably treated as less important than the father (in ways of expression and in relation to the teaching of Truth) and the boy will think himself more important than the girl. If children grow up in this environment, they will adopt these values. The girl becomes enslaved, thinks she is lesser, and the boy is enslaved and thinks he is better. Which is worse? Each presents difficulties.

Men, because of the belief that they are better or more important, can put women down. If men lose control at some point, they can put women down emotionally, mentally, and physically. It is not uncommon to see men brushing aside women for not understanding "the complexity" of a rational discussion or topic, or because women show their emotions, which has been regarded as a lowly, weak way of being. Thank goodness woman are not all so rational and allow themselves to be emotional! We'd have completely destroyed ourselves by now if not for that. No person ever puts another down unless they believe they are better than the other *and* inwardly, they also feel insecure. To put yourself above, whether it is above another or above where you really are, is to try to be like God inanotsoniceway and it stems from the disconnection from the Source and the resultant insecurity. Great humility is necessary for a man to see, with great clarity, how divine the woman and the female's True nature is. Truly. With this humility, he can then love the woman and respect her in the very way that flows as naturally and as a simply as a river into the sea.

A father and mother can hold their daughter down. This is due to the prejudices, judgments, and beliefs about what a girl/woman should be. She will grow up thinking her rightful place is within these confines. This becomes her "shell of shrinking."

The Circle of Nine also emphasizes the total and complete equality between the male and the female.

[*First Circle*—CaN #3 Men and women are equal.
I align myself with the total and complete equality of the male

and the female. I align myself with the wonder of the man and the woman. I do not attempt to keep the female down, nor do I suppress the male. I see the wonder in the woman's nature that is in harmony with Mother Nature and the Divine.]

Raise your children to be equals, always. Both girls and boys. Teach them to achieve whatever their hearts prompt them to be. Although sometimes subtle and subconscious, raising your children to believe that the boy is more important than the girl is as harmful and destructive to our planet as racism and religious discrimination. Don't put your children down. If they are feeling good about themselves, don't worry that they might become proud or blind. They will know the way for their very being is Love. You don't need to build up a lot of beliefs to protect them, that would be fear-based and a projection of your own fears.

The male energy blindspot makes it difficult to see that no one is higher or better than anyone else. Maleness has a deep tendency to speak in hierarchal, competitive terms like "higher" or "better." This makes a person cold-hearted, or at least disconnected from their heart, for whenever anyone puts themselves above he or she will not be able to connect with others. It also causes their rational mind to rule over the body, like a king that judges the fool. The person is not compassionate; heartfelt connections with others are muffled, replaced by the less feeling, rational experience of reality. This blind spot also causes efforts to be better instead of just being the True self. This really stifles the joy of the heart.

The story of the Tower of Babel helps us to see that we are not meant to *try* to be God. The people were trying to build a tower. They said:

"Come, let us build us a city, and a tower with its top in the heavens, and let us make a name for ourselves, lest we be dispersed across the whole earth." **Gen 11:4**

Trying to be like God doesn't work out for people. They are always toppled by the next person trying to fill that position, or their competitive energy turns around to consume them. It is also absurd to try to get to the *height* of God, as if God's presence was truly only found up in the sky. Yet this concept of trying to reach a height is equivalent to other patterns of control, like trying to achieve positions of power and authority of knowledge over people. In Love, there is no thing that stands above another. That only occurs in a world where people judge in terms of good and bad.

To heal this pattern of negativity, see the greatness in others and you will feel it within yourself. Then there will be no need to put others down or yourself up to feel as if you stand above them.

[***Fourth Circle***—CaN #2—I wish the best for all people.
I see them manifesting their deepest, greatest wishes, their most powerful love and Beingness. This is all I see. It is my only reality. I see myself as a part of a collective consciousness of other people who feel this way. I let go of not seeing the best for others, or of being in competition with them.]

One aspect of the male controlling energy is that it always challenges others, disapproving and finding mistakes in their ways. Because of this, you can greatly fear making a mistake if you value being right much more than being kind or compassionate, especially if you have judged others often. Those always perceiving mistakes always make mistakes themselves, because they are so focused on mistakes. Let go of the fear of making a mistake and see that it is okay to be wrong. It really is. We all do it. We are not perfect beings, nor must we be. What is most interesting to understand is that when you become a Being of no resistance, that does not mean that you never make mistakes. Rather you never perceive a mistake and thus you never make them. For what is a mistake? There are no mistakes if the Golden Rule is not compromised. Do to others as you would have them do unto you. This is a Universal Law of Love. When you live conscientious of others and are with them as you'd love them to Be with you, then you know that by just Being yourself as God created you to be, that is AllGood. There are no errors in that, simply unique expressions of the AllGood.

[*Third Circle* CaN #5—I do not need to know or to be right all the time. I can make mistakes whenever I wish. I let go of the need to be perfect. I let go of making hierarchies according to what a person knows. I do not define my worth by what I know. I take the chance of being wrong.]

When these Truths dawn on men, they should never sacrifice themselves or punish themselves with guilt, nor should they cut themselves down, believing that this will bring everything to equality. Women who discover they have been controlling should also not cut themselves down. Please do not cut yourself down when you realize you have been controlling. It is not Truthful, does not heal, and it is unnecessary. When men recognize the control they tried to hold on to the female to put themselves as better, they will see they are not better. But if they then put *themselves* down because of this behavior, they are still not understanding that there is no better. Believing someone can be better is the **First Major Delusion**. When you realize that you were controlling others because of some hurt *you* suffered, or because of some false idea of reality you believed you must maintain, you will understand and accept yourself. Forgiveness/Acceptance is the secret, then you will feel and understand that there is nothing you need to sacrifice yourself for.

There is no Love created in making the male prostrate himself before the female. The male must trust that the female does not desire to be like God as does the male. So in yielding to a woman, a man can have faith that she will not use him for her own selfish purposes. She simply wishes to be acknowledged for who she really is and that she has the right to Be as she wishes. If these essentials are met, the woman has no need for control. They will hug each other.

Acceptance/forgiveness is so important. Without acceptance/forgiveness, even while knowing that change is necessary, we will continue to butt our heads against our mistakes in hopes that if we do it hard enough, we will knock those mistakes out (or ourselves). Forgiveness and acceptance are so necessary for the return to Eden in order to end the cycle of repetition of errors that come from not forgiving and accepting ourselves. *A Course in Miracles* is a phenomenal book that emphasizes the importance of acceptance and forgiveness, and refers to the accomplishment of a person forgiving themselves and finding their true nature again as "The Atonement," which is the same as the Return to Eden.

When a man acknowledges the *greatness* and the wonder in a woman, all is brought into equality. The man will recognize the qualities of the female energy which are like the Creator, who is simply Love. Large beliefs of God will melt down to the level where the One who is All resides, and there you will know the humble embodiment of the Creator in humans.

Man and woman, in reconciliation, are finally able to come together to experience the joy of unity with the Oneness of Creation. In this Love bond, the opposites are married again into togetherness. Now, brought back into harmony beyond Frmee Will, the Y factor of the male controlling energy is transformed into a gift.

Men will struggle with these great issues until they simply yield. Freedom will come from seeing the wonder in the woman, acknowledging the wish to experience that female energy as well and all its abilities. It is really wonderful to be a man, especially when you surrender this "strength" that men often think they must have in order to be good, powerful and respected. Needing to be smart, knowing all the right moves, and saying all the right things to earn respect comes from insecurity. Many men fall into this deeply ingrained delusion. This is *The Second Major Delusion* that if someone knows more, that makes them better. When a man allows himself to be vulnerable in relationship to a woman, he will understand the words of wisdom and a kernel of golden light in Lao Tze's *Tao Te Ching, Chapter 76*:

> "The stiffest tree is readiest for the axe.
> The strong and mighty
> Topple from their place;
> The soft and yielding rise above them all"

It is so easy to think in terms of power and strength, especially when you feel weak or insecure. You can slip into the need very quickly when your fear is touched and the wounds of feeling forsaken and vulnerable call into action internal armies of safety and control. In our illusions, we believe that we are safe when we keep anything that threatens us away. In our strength, we see in allowing everything near that threatens us, there is no threat. Resistance and creating iron armor zones are the most uncomfortable ways to be because you are constantly at war trying to defend your territory from outside threats. The way of allowing and yielding is most divine, for you see that there are no enemies unless you give them a place across the battlefield. To be close to God is to yield to Allthatis.

Part II—Issues of the Female—The Unbalanced Positive

Men must grow up and face up to the many ways in which they try to be first like God. But women must also free themselves from their "shells of shrinking." They put their immense power of healing and Being into a shell, thinking themselves lesser or being afraid to take their own place. But men are the sons of their mothers and the husbands of their wives. When women allow men to control them, or raise their sons to believe that they are more important, that perpetuates the disharmony between men and women. When women are very clear that they will not tolerate inequality any longer, that forces men to make choices and confront their need for control. And their choice is always the same, "Do I want Love or power (control)?"

It can be as difficult for a woman to see through the primordial belief that she is secondary just as it is for a man to overcome his belief that he comes first. If she does not simply allow herself to have what she truly deserves, she will not Be as she truly wants to Be, nor will she have what she wants with a man.

Boys that are raised to believe they are number one do not know how to Love. They are too selfish and know only how to take. When they grow up, they still believe that since they are men, they will receive everything they need from women, who are there to service them.

"Hashem God said, "It is not good that man be alone; I will make him a helper corresponding to him." *Gen 2:18*

If one were to take this phrase in the Torah literally, it would definitely feed the idea that women are there to help the men. The problem is also that girls grow up believing this to be true because they were
put second, and become women who believe everything must revolve
around men. When women live this way, they will be less likely to
receive Love from their husbands in the form of nurturing, affection,
and respect. The man, as the foundation, with things revolving around
him in this way, knows he doesn't have to do anything, because he has
a woman who constantly perpetuates his belief that everything revolves
around him. When the woman loves herself and realizes that she
deserves Love and affection just as much as she gives it and says, "I
deserve Love and attention too. What I have to say is of equal importance," she will change this dynamic. She will also see that her Being is
divine and that in simply allowing herself to express how she feels, she
is teaching others advanced lessons in Kabbalah. This will make her see
through the illusion of serving the male as the foundation and believing that one can connect with God and Truth only through study of
finite knowledge. She will also see that she does not need a man to tell
her what is right or wrong, nor does she need his approval. She will
begin to create Truth in her life, for *only* serving the male is an equation
which adds up to nothing. There is zero Love exchanged, just people's
egos being fed.

A religious woman who came to see me for healing had eight children. She was almost single-handedly taking care of them and worked
full time. Her strength to survive each day, although failing, was remarkable. She said she had nine children to take care of—her eight kids and
her husband.

As a result of many of the imbalances and injustices at the hands of
male controlling energy, female energy has revolted and can suppress the
male. It is a reaction to the way things have been in the unbalanced,
negative state. A woman looks at a controlling man, sees that he is not
the way *she* wants to be, and swings far to the other extreme. It is a trap
that the female can get into. The trap of the Unbalanced Positive.

In compensation for the overly-judgmental, negative thought
processes of the male, the female may tend to say something is okay and

it is good, when it is really not. This is taking out of context the Truth that the Source is AllGood. It is mistaking discernment and seeing what is really there, when it's not good, wrong, or unjust, for judgment. Sometimes situations aren't okay. Sometimes people are mean and mistreat each other. It's okay to see that and to be firm—to take some action to correct it. That isn't being judgmental or controlling. Just because you say "I will no longer live this way" does not mean that you are not accepting how things have been or judging them as bad. You are doing what you want. The Unbalanced Positive doesn't understand this because it reacts so strongly to any negativity seeing it, ironically, as bad, that it will do its utmost to avoid being judgmental or negative. Sometimes we have to get angry to stop injustices. And to improve the imbalanced and poor situations that are really going on in our society, our schools, and our businesses, we have to see that it is not okay. At times, anger and aggression can be necessary to stop something that would otherwise be destructive to somebody. It is necessary all the time to be able to see what is there. This is discernment, the energy of Gevourah, from the Tree of Life. It is the male side balancing the female, Chesed, which is the energy of compassion, kindness and seeing all in a light of Love and acceptance.

If the female energy does not have a male extension, or suppresses the male energy, nothing gets done because everything is okay as it is. You will be splashing around in your own play-pool. The power of the male in purely knowing that something is wrong (in that it is not Love) is the strength and clarity that will bring change. It is the strength that clears all oppression. It is a don't-mess-with-me kind of clarity that is very important and effective.

Because of her nature to see both sides and to be non-judgmental and accepting, the unbalanced female (Unbalanced Positive) doesn't understand that in some situations, you *must* take a side. If unbalanced, the female tries to make everything nice when everything really isn't nice. There is Love and there is fear. People are free to choose as they wish. But that does not make the choice of fear the best choice. It is important to see that, that many Unbalanced Positive people cannot see. This is a blind spot that has gotten worse since New Age philosophy has taught us to be non-judgmental and to accept everything. We have become petrified of being judgmental or controlling. We have lost the balance with the male nature. Political correctness has therefore gone overboard. It can be quite frustrating to explain to someone who is politically overcorrect and clouded with New Age Bull (NAB) that a situation can be unacceptable or could surely use improvement. NAB, in its very essence, is the Unbalanced Positive.

It is fine to say that the Creator, the Love that encompasses all things, the imagination of God that brought all of this to be, is AllGood. But if we say that our world is AllGood and everything, like the hatred and the violence we do to each other, is okay or *meant to be* this is **nabulous** because our world is *still* full of hatred and destruction. *We* are still choosing that. Do you see the importance?

So much is not as we wish to be. It isn't the picture of the collective Eden that we would all paint. Racism. Sexism. Injustices. Poverty. Power Hunger. Greed. The Con Trolls keeping our world in illusion. These come from our own choices based in fear and illusion, not from God's Will. In people's fear of the negative, they would rather just connect with this idea that things are AllGood rather than really face the reality here on Earth about how much work must be done before we can Truthfully say that it is AllGood. And those who won't face the reality on Earth also are incapable of facing their own inner reality, and that is the most important place to begin. It is true that the dark has been placed here to challenge us. And even at times the dark is working God's Will in ways that we do not readily understand or wish to accept. Agreed. But the Divine Plan is ultimately meant for us to live in collective, unconditional Joy and Love, which is not possible when people suffer at the hands of others. Thus this fear and avoidance of conflict within the Unbalanced Positive clouds you out and makes you nabulous, removing the understanding that you must take responsibility for healing your world. Not by judgment, but by purposeful action. In order to have the proper fuel to drive the action, you must be clear that some things have to change.

The unbalanced positive is often used as an escape. Once people have touched with the blissful essence of the divine, they do not want to come down from the high of their spiritual retreats or activities to face the muck of the world. Your heart will actually not burn with a deep power unless you can bring it down and experience all that is on this planet without judgment. That includes being able to see and face the dark reality that still exists amongst our ranks without judgment. The Unbalanced Positive will say "That negative energy amongst our ranks is okay." It is okay, yes, acceptance. Everything is okay. But everything is also not okay in that we are aware it is not how we wish Gan Edan to be. Can we find the balance? The **Sixth Circle** states, "Don't be afraid to see what's there. See what's there!" Then you won't fear negativity and have to suppress it in order to pretend that everything is Good.

The Unbalanced Positive also diminishes the power of your unwavering conviction which nobody will mess with when you are clear and sure about something. A mother whose baby's life is threatened will respond with the greatest power and even vicious strength. Will anyone question her for doing so? Not in a million years.

People often oppressed others for the wrong reasons—that is Unbalanced Negative. Now we must use the strength of numbers in our unwavering conviction to bring down structures that keep people in bondage. We are obviously not going to kill anyone for Truth which would be fanatical, and we must remain flexible at all times. We will dismantle those establishments erected by people attempting to horde and control humanity's reigns. That is healing.

Another aspect of the Unbalanced Positive is saying out of context that somethings were "meant to be." Sometimes they are, sometimes not. If you say that someone getting hurt is meant to be, this is Unbalanced Positive. It is often true that we choose to get hurt and once the injury has occurred we can learn from it and grow, but we can learn from anything, like joy or freedom, so why suffer? We are not meant to suffer. We are not meant to live in pain and struggle. Yes, we can choose that and it might bring about immense transformation, but choosing something because we *believe* we must and that it is meant to be, are very different things. If you believe that we must learn from making errors, then suffering never ends. That is not Gan Edan. So balancing the understanding that we can learn from suffering and yet, we also have the choice of freedom, will help you see the choice aligned with your true nature.

September 11th, 2001 is a case in point. Did we all learn from it? Did it scare the wits out of the world and make people start asking questions and looking for Truth? Yes. We all learned from it and, therefore, aside from the tragic loss of life it had some positive and healing effects on the planet. It did fulfill some purpose and many can see the value that came from it. But was it meant to be? Was it part of a divine plan? I don't think so. The terrorists who murdered thousands of innocent civilians did not value human life. The value for another's life is an attribute of Love. To not value life is the opposite of Love. It is the control of the opposition to Love. If you say that it was meant to be, then you are saying that God is made up of Good and Bad, or Good and Evil, and it is part of God's plan (because God is the Will of the innocent civilians *and* the terrorists' Will) that these tragic events of mass destruction occurred. The forces of opposition can definitely teach us lessons by revealing aspects of ourselves that really are not as "right on" as we thought. But is this sort of message part of God's Will? No. Eventually, there will be no more need for the dark for we will set Love as the foundation of our reality and heal ourselves peacefully and gently.

Please be careful with the philosophy of "meant to be" in certain circumstances. Hopefully, nothing like it will occur again. If it were true that September 11th was meant to be, if we were to follow that logic, then we will see more and more destruction on the planet until we either completely destroy ourselves, or purge more than half of the population. The potential for choice leaves the door open to this kind of path, to this kind of awakening in a negative sense. But if you understand choice from the previous chapters, then you must know that there is the choice of peace and Love. Understanding this reveals the great responsibility we have to avoid destruction. Tensions are mounting on the planet, and violence might be unavoidable. But if you accept this as part of the plan, or meant to be, as if God's hand is bringing this down, then you are empowering the path of destruction. You are helping the world progress toward John's Revelations of fire and brimstone, and the apocalypse. Rather, understand with peace, awareness, and healing we will arrive at the World to Come. It is when people actually will risk themselves to transmit true messages and reveal hidden agendas in power structures that Love will be brought out where there isn't any. This is a much more difficult path than just blowing ourselves up and then saying, "well that served some purpose," because such healing must come from the inside, gently, and we must let go of our past ways.

Another belief that we encounter within the Unbalanced Positive is: "Everyone's belief is the Truth." This is a reaction to many leaders or others who have kept people in bondage by stating what the Truth is and denying each individual's freedom to know and express the Truth independently. As in all reactions to injustice, the pendulum can swing too far to the other extreme as people attempt to find a balance. In this case, this belief is Unbalanced Positive. It is true that everyone has a right to believe what they wish, yet not what everyone believes is the Truth. Although their beliefs might seem to be true, and one must have compassion and understanding of that—that they are entitled to them—not everything that everyone believes is true. Much of what we believe is based in illusion and separation, fear and doubt. In the world beyond matter, within collective consciousness, all is birthed by one "belief," which is not a belief at all but a way of Being… and that is of course sponsored and supported only by Love, which is expressed in myriad ways. But it still is Truth and anything outside of that, is not.

If you have the notion that "Everyone's belief is the Truth," this naturally translates into the idea that "Everyone's way is correct." This is also untrue for the same reasons that thinking "Everyone's belief is true" is incorrect. This does not give us the right to try to control people's ways and mold them the way we think they should be. But it does clarify that not everyone's choices are aligned with Love. And if not, they are not Truthful. Compassion (Chesed) will help you accept their choices based in their past, their pain, their trials of this lifetime. Discernment (Gevourah) will keep you focused on your path and give you the strength to do what you must.

> "All it takes for evil to triumph is for
> good people to do nothing."
> Edmund Burke, April 3, 1777,
> from a letter to the Sheriffs of Bristol.

Another pattern that manifests often in the Unbalanced Positive, particularly for women, is doing too much because you are unable to say "no." This is the "Disease to Please." It is like the true intention of the heart, to serve, but has gone out of control and is giving when it is not the right time. This is an unbalanced state coming from some need for utter perfection in relationship to others and it can lead to disease. Living this way can cause cancer. If you learn that you shouldn't judge, and attempt perfection, you will be in big trouble. You're going to live an "unreal" life. New Age and religious teachings have taught us to strive to achieve a perfection by not doing anything "bad." Attempting perfection leads to righteousness, goody-two-shoes and other sterile ways of being, but God isn't goody-two-shoes. Nor is it asked of us to be righteous by looking down at certain ways of the world from immaculate perches. It is fine to have a little naughtiness to keep yourself in balance and good old fashioned anger might even be a good idea. It is okay to bark at the things that you don't like in your world.

It is in our hearts to love others and not judge them. But if you do so from the rational perspective just because it is "right," that isn't authentic. There is no Love in that because it's fake. If you allow yourself to just Be, getting mad when you need to, expressing yourself as you feel, saying no when it is time, then Love and non-judgmentalness will come naturally, being true to yourself.

Our true nature is to give to others, and to not be stuck worrying only about ourselves, but sometimes it is not the right time to give. There are people who would just take and never give of themselves because they feel that those who can never say "no" will keep giving to them. They are selfish and you are really not helping by giving to them all the time. You could also be giving to someone in a way that just empowers their needs or desires. To say "no" in such a situation is loving, even though it might feel like it is being harsh.

If you have a hard time saying "no," ask yourself why you are giving. What does it mean to you if you don't give to someone who expects it? If the answer comes from a fear-based intention such as, "I need to give to be thought of as a good person" (approval), or "If I don't give, nobody will love me," then ask yourself if you want to continue living that way. Remember to let yourself feel the suppressed emotions as they thaw during your process of being true to yourself. Don't judge. Feel the guilt, if you have it and let it out. Feel anger at having lived in such an unreal fashion. On the other side of the painful/uncomfortable thawing process, you will feel the strength to know when you wish and do not wish to give. You will be okay with saying "no" because you are more centered in who you are rather than in the projected, perfectionist idea of who you think you should be for others. The Will and ability to be who you are and do whatever you wish is stifled when you try to be perfect for the male. Being goody-two shoes weakens your system, for inside of it you are giving your power away asking for his praise, his acceptance, his recognition. This pattern of the woman allowing herself to serve the male and give her power away is as deeply ingrained as the man's need to control.

Many women were brought up with the idea that their identity centers around pleasing others. Further, they learn that they can get Love by pleasing others. To be firm and say no and risk someone's displeasure can be as scary as dying, because of the fear of not getting Love, which is the same as fearing abandonment, which is associated with being disconnected from God, which is like dying.

Men can also become stuck in the Unbalanced Positive, just as women can get stuck in the male controlling energy, for men and women both have the male and female energies. Don't forget, we have all been both men and women in our different lifetimes. We have all experienced both sides and the more we are on the path of enlightenment and nearing our zero-point marriage of the far infra red with the ultra violet, the more we deal with the balance of the male and female.

When we say women have been controlled by men for a long time, the important thing to understand is that this was a partnership in the sense that women permitted it. Women *cannot* be controlled unless they allow it. So this message is not attempting to establish that women are weaker than men and so can be dominated by them. Perhaps they are physically less strong, but we are not really speaking of physical domination. Rather, women gave their power away to the male controlling energy. Otherwise, no control could have occurred.

However, it is quite understandable how this control evolved and was allowed. There was personal threat involved (physical & emotional abuse), it was confusing (rational used to control), and there were expectations of romantic, fairy-tale Love (he is my knight in shining armor, this won't go on forever). So women didn't really want to see what was there inside of men—their fathers, their brothers, their husbands. Women made believe.

Another thing that bound women to men is their internal, divine sense of obedience. Obedience is the most wonderful service that a person can have toward the Will of God. But by being obedient to men, especially if the man's foundation is set for him to be like God, women have not given their obedience to God. This obedience is so strong, particularly in religious Jewish women, that when the choice comes to let go and be free they will defend the belief systems of the past and the Law of Moses, not because they truly believe in them, but out of a sense of obedience to the male. Women are meant to serve God, not men. All people are meant to serve God, not structures established by man. Women have been waking up, on a collective level, to the fact that the male control is no longer acceptable. They are making the choices now to not allow that. In other words, women are taking back their power. And there is nothing that can stop them, or anyone, who knows his or her rightful place. This power comes from God and nobody can mess with it.

There is a simple truth that anyone can do as they wish. In the Unbalanced Positive, this gets confused with obedience to the male for that is where she learned it. It is also looking to the male for approval. This often results because of a father who is very disapproving. This is one way the male controls. If you never are accepted and loved for who you are, and you believe you need his approval, then the male always has your desire to serve him and please him to get his recognition and acceptance. It is a never-ending process, and a bottomless pit because there is no Love in it and he will always demand more.

Some women who have trouble expressing themselves have learned to manipulate to get what they want. They do so because they simply do not understand that they are completely free to do what they want, to say how they feel. Women often lose their voices. They give up on expressing themselves. They either were not listened to, were told to be seen and not heard, or believed that what they have to say doesn't really matter. Whatever the case may be, these women believe they must manipulate because they have forgotten how to simply ask for what they want and then accept what they want. There is no need to manipulate. Just ask directly for what you want, overcome the guilt of receiving for yourself, and know that you can have it.

Women must be careful about a common reaction to attempt to equalize everything. This reaction is that the male energy is bad and "I don't want to have anything to do with it." This is not what is really felt deep inside, and it will hurt the woman who cuts herself off from something most dear to her and that she really loves.

Men also make the error of cutting off their male energy when they attempt to release the dominating part of themselves. Don't cut off your left column. Just let it turn over by releasing the need to control.

A person who does cut themselves off from *all* of the male qualities is really giving more of their power away *to* the male because they feel they have no power *beside* the male, thus the need to cut it off, to be away from it. "I am not okay next to you because you control me. I have to be away from you because I have no power with you. I have to prove to you and myself that you will not control me." Such a person is judging the male as Bad and thus suppressing their male energy. We always suppress whatever we judge and stop it from being. We say "this shouldn't exist." We are severing ourselves in half.

Remember that this reaction is not accepting responsibility for the choices you have made to serve and ask for acceptance from the male— your father, your brother, your husband or boyfriend, your rabbi or preacher, your teacher or king. You wanted to serve the male. You wanted his recognition of being a "good girl" to do what he wanted. Boys wish approval from their fathers too, who sought approval from their fathers. For boys and girls, it was an unhealthy relationship, a choice not aligned with who you really are, but it was your choice all the same. Seeing that choice, you set yourself free to choose otherwise. Pointing the finger at the male and saying "You control. You take away my power.

You are bad and I must not be with you!" is not taking responsibility and you give away your power even more. This proving, stay-away, judgmental energy actually hardens a woman. This sort of hardness is not female. It is male. So what has her judgment done? She has become what she has judged. This involves a lot of ego as well for the male, controlling energy goes hand in hand with the ego. The last thing she will want is a man more allowing and loving than she. This will threaten her entire theory and belief systems about men being bad. She might have a hard time seeing that she is actually more male-controlling than the man, unless she yields. And what is she yielding to? A man. Wow! That can be hard for her. Her ego will want to block that and just project, "Here is another bad man!"

When you realize that you have choice, totally and completely, to do as you wish, then you will wake up immense power of Will. When this Will to set yourself free is aligned with Love, although that power is very strong, it is effortless and very gentle. When a being believes he or she can do *whatever* they wish in selfishness and need-based only Frmee, he or she can have power, but must also put a lot of effort into forcing their way. It does not flow effortlessly from the Divine.

When you see that in the freedom of choice there is infinite power, you see nothing to fear and, thus, there is a *great gentleness* to that power. When there is nothing to fear, there is no struggle, all is smooth, all is allowishing. In our doubt, we think power is the kind of force someone generates by exerting themselves to the point where the veins in their forehead bulge out. This is resistance power, which depletes the source. It is not true power, which invigorates the Source.

When women suppress the male energy or the male way by judging it, they can easily become irrational when their issues of disempowerment are triggered. The male energy is logical (Bina—understanding). So if you judge the male, you are cutting off and can become lost in a world of irrational emotion. When a woman is unbalanced in this state, it is difficult to talk to her, because she is swirling around in her hurt and feeling-wronged emotions. All you can do is let her be and really accept her. If you approach her and attempt to explain or correct this irrational behavior, she will become more irrational, because she is so oversensitive to any controlling intention. If you insist on her under-standing what you are saying, this will trigger her further. By being overly emotional, even if it is unbalanced, she is teaching you something that you can learn about just being. So allow her to be as she is, and do just as **John Keats** writes in *Ode on Melancholy*:

> "But when the melancholy fit shall fall
> Sudden from heaven like a weeping cloud,
> That fosters the droop-headed flowers all,
> And hides the green hill in an April shroud;
> Then glut thy sorrow on a morning rose,
> Or on the rainbow of the salt sand-wave,
> Or on the wealth of globed peonies;
> Or if thy mistress some rich anger shows,
> Imprison her soft hand, and let her rave,
> And feed deep, deep upon her peerless eyes."

The Unbalanced Positive can have the tendency to lack discipline and drive. Unbalanced male energy usually works too hard and cannot relax because it has desire for the result, yet the unbalanced female can get a little caught up in frolicking in the flowers, and have the attitude, "It will get done when it needs to get done. Everything's okay." This is often untrue. You get things done when you put your Will into getting them done. There is something very divine and very essential about making things happen as quickly as possible while maintaining the bal-ance of not getting attached to the results and worrying about finish-ing immediately. It is patience balanced with action. Look at the plan-et or any situation in which people are suffering at the hands of oth-ers. The more time we spend putting things off, the more people suf-fer. Are they meant to suffer? No. Thus, when the female gets out of balance, that can lead to an attitude of *waiting for the right time*. The moment is always right for time is eternal, waiting for us to take it at any time or right now!

Just as there are similarities between the male and female energies and men and women, and there are differences between the roles each has adopted in the physical, so too are there similarities and differences between the energies and choices men and women make in sexual relationships with each other.

Part III—Sexuality, the Female and the Male—Finding the Balance

We all have upper mind and lower minds that neither think entirely the same way, nor have the same functions. Each has a consciousness, however. A man's lower mind is outside his body; his thoughts can come from external desire. Haven't we said that a man can think with his penis? This desire is a bottomless pit, because there is no way to ever fulfill a need from the outside. Feeding this desire increases the separation between the heart and the mind of Frmee Will, increasing the duality of the opposing Wills. Thus, duality is even more accentuated in an individual who desires to get the energy they lack through the sexual act.

A woman's lower mind is inside her body. This is the consciousness of her womb. Thus inside, she is already one so she is not as separated as in a man. But a woman can also have desire when she becomes separated from the feeling of her body. Then she, too, needs to have what she has blocked inside from the outside.

Men often live *believing* that the Garden is outside their body. They live believing that they need to make love to a woman in order to be okay. "I have sex, therefore I AM." A woman can think this way as well. The more a man or a woman is hurt or out of balance with their opposite sex energy, for example, if there are still attachments to or deep issues with the parent of the opposite sex, the more a person will manifest outside-the-self sexual desire.

When a man needing and desiring the female energy makes love to a woman, he can absorb a lot of the female energy that he might totally lack due to suppressing his feelings and needing to control everything. It feels good, but only temporarily, like eating a chocolate bar. It is not healing in nature. It is also a boost to his ego to "get" a woman. The problem with this is that the man's desire for a woman is really only for himself because he needs her energy. So instead of making Love to connect with a woman in a deep bond of sharing and unity, he does it for his own ego and need. This is the opposite of his highest purpose, which is to give to the female.

[*Second Circle*—CaN #6—He says: I do it for her pleasure. This is where I find the pleasure and joy. She says: I allow myself to receive the pleasure of the act. I give up the guilt of receiving.]

The male in separation believes that what he needs is outside of himself. It is *out there* somewhere. For the separated male energy, the Truth is *out there* too, just as it is for the rational mind. Yet Truth is all right in the center. On one level, the metaphor of the *Tree of Carnal Knowledge* describes the act of sexual union, so after the Tree, as duality began, so too did separation and duality begin between the male and female energies. Since that time they have had this driving desire to return to the state of Oneness. Now, since the man possesses unbalanced male energy, he exists more separated from the Source and his drive is largely to be with a woman to reunite him, for she possesses that female energy that is the Source and the paradise of Eden for which he longs. The female energy is like God to him. This drive is so strong, so primordial, that it can empower a man's every thought and every action. It can drive him to desire *any* woman, regardless of Love, for each woman represents to him a return to the state of Oneness.

Women tend to seek more of a communion of Love with a man, rather than mere physicality, because they are more connected with the Earth and are more interested in the true purpose of the act of love making—which is just that—to *make* Love in togetherness with a partner. The more a woman is healthy and connected with her self-esteem and her body, the less she will need to have the sex of just any man. The more a woman is hurt or the more she had a poor, unloving connection with her father, the more she will need the outside male factor to fill her up. The act of making Love will become more need-based to fill a void—rather than Love-based, to generate joy and true power.

When there is Love between a couple, and they come together in unity and as equals, the Love that is made between them is *the most spe-*

cial energy of the Universe. In the act of union with a loving partner without resistance, a soul can come very close to the Source, to the Creator. This feels like the unification of Eve and Adam as they existed within the Ganallisone, before they were separated.

Please understand that none of this means that sex is bad or is only limited to the deepest purpose. In other words, the freedom of this age is whispering to us, showing us how we are allowed to fool around and experience pleasure and share with others in whatever way we enjoy. The "laws" of good and bad are no more, remember?

[*Second Circle*—CaN #3—I allow myself to enjoy sex, fully and completely. I allow my sexual energy to flow. I release any judgment of the expression of my sexual nature.]

We can choose to be what we love to be. [*Third Circle* CaN #6] But if desire gets out of control, and it can, especially if you live perpetuating the delusion that the Garden, Heaven, Love, and joy, are outside and that you need to "get it," that creates a painful, agonizing longing, and a hollow void must constantly be filled and yet never can be filled. We have all done this to some degree or another.

[*Second Circle*—CaN #4— 'It is not all about sex.'
I can love others deeply and intimately without it needing to be about sex. I do not suppress my sexual energy, for I allow myself the joy and love of the act. I simply release the part of me that is constantly needing sex. I find the balance.]

You must meet a great internal balance, for sexual energy is our free-flowing energy of creativity and joy of Being. When you suppress it, you begin to slowly wither and die. So the answer does not lie in suppressing the true, natural, wonderful wish to make Love and be in communion with a partner. The answer lies in the balance between letting go of the bottomless pit desire and allowing yourself to make Love fully.

A woman begins to really age and get ill when she disconnects from her womb energy. This will lead to gynecological problems. Waking up the joy of her sexual feeling is a great healing for a sick womb and thus is a great source of healing. The true secret to healing is allowing herself to receive the pleasure and joy of the act. To allow herself to feel the joy and Love in the sexual act might require her to find a loving partner who respects her and wishes the best for her. Not all men now are able to give this kind of Love, but they will learn if they wish to. A woman's conviction knowing what she deserves even if it means leaving will help a man awaken from his selfish stupor. The Unbalanced Positive is associated with the guilt of receiving and when a woman is running around doing things for everyone and doesn't allow herself to receive what she needs, she will have some trouble receiving the pleasure and joy of the sexual act.

When sexual fluids are spilled out endlessly without constraint, we also begin to slowly wither and die. The will-center loses essence and becomes more empty when there is continual orgasm. This emptiness leads to the need to fill up this energy center which contributes to the desire for more sex. A vicious cycle can result if there is continual orgasm because this will only contribute to the feeling of emptiness. Although she can lose essence too, a woman does not lose it to the same extent as the man. In addition to the fact that she is generally less resistant, this can contribute to living longer than the man.

When there is separation between a person's mind and body, it is easy to replace sexual feeling with looking, even ogling another. Those who experienced this know how intensely creepy it can feel. The ogler's needy sexual energy surrounds others and makes them feel like objects. This desperation is not very healthy for the ogler's energy because it further splits his or her sexual energy from their heart and deepens the hole inside.

[*Second Circle* CaN #5—I give up looking at people as sex objects. I see people as people. I do not avoid looking at anyone. I am able to look right at all people and simply see the beauty inherent in each person, because I have given up seeing people as sex objects.]

So again, here is a balance between allowing yourself to witness all the beautiful artistry that God has given, but not desiring it all. It is interesting to see that when a man needs to make Love to all the women with his eyes, he is separating the act from his heart. He is cheapening it and the depth of the communion with a woman. A man will have difficulty seeing his partner as equal in all ways. Making Love with that partner will be tough, for sex has become a toy for that man to feel good and to relieve internal pressures. It becomes all about him fulfilling his need, rather than giving his partner pleasure because of his Love for her. The woman has also bought into this, worrying whether she is good enough for him, attractive enough, or if she is satisfying him properly. *They are both doing it just for him.*

There are three ways to balance allowing oneself to experience pleasure without letting the desire get out of control and engulf you.

The first is releasing the belief that you need the sexual act to be happy, or okay. Growing up in our teens, beginning to become acquainted with the sexual feelings stirring inside, we often sat around and chatted amongst our friends about how we "gotta get it," "we need it," "we can't take it without it." It was a cute sort of romantic longing and yet these ideas were encouraged because so many young people were expressing them. Sex was an "in-thing" to do, and if you weren't doing it, something was wrong with you. So we grow up with the idea that we need sex. Sex is of course one of the most exciting and fulfilling extracurricular activities in which we can participate. But do we *need* to do it? No. So first of all, we have to clear that idea away.

The second thing that must be balanced is becoming addicted to the pleasure of the act and lacking the willpower to control oneself. When things are pleasurable, they can be used as a high or to suppress feelings. If you reach for chocolate whenever you feel sad or some difficult emotions rise up, the pleasure of the chocolate drowns the emotions. People use sex this way a lot. To balance you can develop the willpower to not always have to have sex, for instance, by understanding that it isn't good to always have your sexual engine running at full velocity. This awareness results in the necessary willpower to be true to your body's resources.

Balancing the third is the most important and reveals why we can
have this bottomless pit desire that is out of control. It is because of *judgment* and subsequent *resistance* to sexual energy, as if it is something *bad*
that causes us to need it! When a child is forbidden something, it
becomes both taboo and irresistible. Weren't Adam and Eve told not to
do it?

For centuries, religions have taught us that the act of sex is a sin, the
original sin. They were playing upon our primordial shame, yet there is
nothing to be ashamed of. Shame, guilt, and judgment cause people to
become out of control to need sex wildly. If you truly wish for something, because it is good and Love, yet your rational mind tells you it is
wrong, bad, or shameful, you will not allow yourself to become fulfilled
with pleasure and joy. It is like having one foot on the gas and one on
the brake. One says yes, the other says no. What this causes is a pit that
becomes the *need* to have the act, because in all honesty, you would really love to, yet you hold yourself back, so you will long for it and feel
that you can't have it.

When you let go and do not judge something, you know what you
end up saying to yourself? "I can do whatever I want now. I can do it
either way. Either way is okay. I can have sex and enjoy it if I want to,
or I can refrain from having sex for I have no *need* now to do it!" The
need comes from the judgment, which doesn't allow you to have what
you truly would love. Judgment disallows choice because you force
yourself to remain one way. Joy comes from the *freedom to choose* what
you love. [**Third Circle**—CaN #6] The ultimate joy comes from being
who you are and ultimate freedom, therefore, is beyond *all* judgment
and beyond the choice itself.

The suppression and judgment of sex also leads to another major
problem. Righteousness! When you are righteous about avoiding sex,
you become really anal and rigid about life. You will go around telling
others what is good and bad, and believe yourself to be good by not
doing what you have judged as bad. Sexual desire, if suppressed, will
block up the flow through the throat and disconnect the mind from the
body. Blocking the sexual desire is at the root of so many problems, from
sexual dysfunction to auto-immune and emotional illness. Wilhelm

Reich wrote about this in his book *Sexual Rights of Youths*. He explains the importance of allowing adolescent youths the right to sexual gratification and to prevent young adults from getting wrapped up in puritanical judgment of sex.

The secret to freeing yourself from unhappy desire (meaning needy desire, because when you *need* something, you will never truly be happy) is to face sexual guilt and allow yourself to fully experience the joy of sex without judging it and resisting it. Let go and enjoy having sex, or your sexuality. Be a little naughty, it will help your sexual energy flow, just as a little anger can melt ties to whatever you no longer wish to be associated with. Let the tiger in you out, and leap into your sexual self. When there is no guilt, there will be no more need and you can choose as you wish, when you wish, and with whom you wish. You are back in the driver's seat and not controlled by your desire.

You may be thinking, "What if I don't have a partner? How can I experience this?" If you do not judge the act and you wish to experience this divine communion, then you will have no difficulty in bringing it into your life. The Universe will provide you with the experiences that you allow yourself. Understand also that you can experience your sexual energy without the physical act of sex. Your sexual energy is located in the same energy center—second chakra—as your relationship with yourself. So when you love yourself, although it is not the same experience as being with a partner, you are stirring the feelings of joy within the second chakra and experiencing sexual energy. It can also be very good to confront the need by not having sex and seeing that you can be completely and totally fine without a sexual partner.

Because the issue of sex is so charged with power, passion, pleasure, and because the act can create life, humanity has tried to control it. Depending on how we approach it, it is the Tree of Life (creation, pure ecstasy of Oneness) or the Tree of Knowledge for Good and Bad (control, shame, desire). The void created by judging this most divine act is the underlying source of Frmee Will (one Will telling you to do what the other forbids). If we were all able to let go of all sexual judgments and release all the control wrapped up in this issue and make Love purely and freely, the Love generated would release all judgment and resistance on Earth. Then we would again live collectively in the Ganallisone. The problems on this planet are a chronic manifestation of the fact that we are all sexually frustrated.

Elements that evoke the deepest connection and awakenings in us do trigger energies of opposition and the desire to control. The more something possesses light, the more it will become a target of the opposition in the Game of Life. That is why sex has been such a target. That is why we have the extremes of judgment and the exploitation and cheapening of the act. The Con Trolls cheapen the wonder of the act, pushing it on us, tempting our childish side, which thinks it is wrong.

Before the planet can be fully free in the age of collective enlightenment, we must shed our resistance and judgments of the sexual act. While we do this we will get rid of all of the excess negativity in our society that exploits the act and see right through the exploitation. If you are free to experience something as you like, then there is no way to exploit or control it.

In Love relationships, the partner you share your Love with is a free person. That person you Love is only yours by *their* choice and this choice is *their* freedom. Freedom is Truth, anything else is control. When we fall in Love with another and invest our heart, we tend to fear losing that loved one to another, or we fear just plain old losing them. Of course if you truly see that they are free, fully and completely, you will not fear *losing* them because you will never have been under the impression that you were bound to each other. When you believe they are yours to possess or to hold on to, you will fear losing them. *You will not want to believe that they are not yours to control.* What this means is that when you have a need to be with someone, you might not like to admit how free a person is because it feeds your fear of being abandoned. The fear of abandonment only comes from the fear of losing what we believe we need to be happy, or wish to possess.

The fear and illusion-based mindset of possessiveness clogs up your true nature. Your true nature gains its greatest electrical energy from loving someone and feeling how free they are to be as they wish. To really touch the Truth of how free your partner is, and to be grateful for them, will do amazing things for your self-esteem and the experience of the ecstasy of Love. When you see the freedom they really have (for all Beings have choice), you can finally feel and really *appreciate the wonder in their choice to actually choose you*! Then you actually can feel that your partner Loves you. When you are concerned with possession you are unable to feel your partner's Love for you, so you live insecurely. You are missing out on the wonderful sense of self-esteem and security. It is the wonder of feeling that this amazing being chooses you that brings the joy of communion. She owes you nothing. You owe her nothing. He owes you nothing. You owe him nothing.

In your need and your fear of losing someone, you convinced yourself that he or she is your partner and your partner alone, to have and to hold, in sickness and in health, 'til death do you part. But this need not be the case, as if the law says "you must," or as if God commands it so. To become attached to someone because you think you must, it is bad not to, or it is God's Will, is actually a limited way of Being. It only seems right in the physical world of limited thinking. No one has control over another and thus there is no choice than to see that the other is completely and totally free. Naturally, so are you.

You do not stay with someone because you must. The Law does not make you remain together. Your constantly renewed wish, by choice of the Love you share, keeps you together. If you Love someone with all your heart and soul, then that is forever and occurs effortlessly and naturally. The very fact that Love is given freely, *not by obligation*, is what keeps the Love alive. Do not shackle each other to the bedposts of your marriages and relationships thinking *this is the way it must be*. See what a gift it is to be with that soul knowing that you are both free at all times. This is facing the fear of losing the other. Afterwards, you will see it is no longer necessary to dwell on such thoughts. But perhaps from time to time, if that possessive energy creeps in and starts to clog the pipes, it would be a good idea to do a little spring cleaning and remember your partner's freedom, and yours.

If one believes the Torah word for word, it promotes the ingrained belief of many men that their woman is their possession:

"Yet your craving shall be for your husband, and he shall rule over you." **Gen 3:16.**

A man who reads this passage and concludes that it gives him the right to dominate women or his wife is sadly deluded. A more accurate interpretation for what the Torah is describing is a state of consciousness in which we would get stuck after the eating from the Tree of **ɣ**. This is the way things are within Frmee Will and, therefore, is part of the test for us to choose and ultimately overcome. It is a fear-based pattern of control and we must overcome it so that we can experience true Love. And yes, a woman can long for Love and crave her husband. But this message of the Torah, *like many others*, is part of the challenge of the Game in which we are responsible for using our wisdom and discerning what we wish to be true. As a prediction for the way things would be between men and women, it would have been more accurate written as, "The craving of the male will be for the female and thus he will try to dominate her."

Try this mental exercise: be open to the possibility that you and your partner can have Love outside of the relationship, both non-sexually and sexually. Remember that your partner is free to choose what they wish, at all times. *If your partner wants to, you want that for them as well.* The point is not that the man must be able to give his wife up or the woman her husband for he does not have her in this way, nor she him, in the first place! In this mental exercise, he doesn't give her up hoping that she doesn't share Love either sexually or non-sexually with another, but *hoping that she does* if she wants to! This makes the whole difference. When you do not see yourself attached, you see there is no way that you can control your partner. He or she is free to be as they wish.

The question, "Do I want another partner?" is enough, especially when he or she is given the freedom and space to ask. With this freedom your partner will come back to you with so much true desire for only you, because they have no qualms. He or she does not feel forced or compelled at all—they see it is their choice. This can erase all doubt about being with someone. It is especially important for women to feel this freedom, because many women now are incredibly sensitive to feeling confined in a controlled relationship. But it is really important for any person to feel that they are in a relationship because they wish to be, not because they must.

If you fear your partner cheating, or losing him or her to another, practice the above mental exercise, face the fear, and *know that it is AllGood.* You *know* they are not yours. *You know this.* There is no debate, nothing to have doubts about. You can fully allow the release of possessiveness and forever see and feel the freedom of it. You will be free of the block to true Love.

Coming from such a law-based society, we have the tendency to fear the chaos that will result when the rules we have set are released. We fear the worst; that we all begin running around like rabbits and humping each other more so than in the 60's. Perhaps some will do this, so let them. But as I truly see it, with the freedom to choose we will choose based on our heart's desire, which is not to endlessly experience sex with just anybody, but for the gift of experiencing the Oneness that it truly brings when shared with someone you Love. Our true nature may be to be monogamous with our loved one, and now we can experience it freely, rather than having it shoved on us.

In a very deep Truth, there is really nothing for men or anyone to fear, because *thinking that we must be in control causes us to fear losing that control.* Shed the thought, and you will shed the fear of loss. What is also interesting to understand about male-female relationships is that the woman's true nature is to be giving. To have a woman Love you and choose to be with you freely while you honor her freedom of choice is infinitely more than creating the situation or the law that dictates her behavior.

So if *you* choose to be with another in mind or body, then of course don't be a hypocrite or have a double-standard and not allow your partner to be with someone else. If you still live by the ugly double standard "I am allowed but he/she isn't" then you are living dishonestly and you will be twisted. This doesn't feel good, nor is it aligned with Good. If you are allowed, so is he or she. In any relationship, inequality is a rift that blocks two people from feeling Love and joy *together.* The equality in a partnership is the most precious thing on Earth and in Heaven.

If you are a man who, on the physical level, has agreed to not be with other women, yet the thought (choice) still occurs to you, then you might bear some consequence for this choice so long as you maintain or feel the need to look at other women with desire. If you desire other women, that is not a wicked act. If it were, 99% of the male population would be wicked. You are simply hurting yourself in ways that might not be so obvious. If you're in a partnership and you look at other women with desire, you will likely feel jealous or possessive when other men look at your girlfriend or wife. *It is only because you look at others with desire that this jealousy even exists for you.* Yes, you can see how beautiful others are and appreciate God's sculptural handiwork, but when you have "eyes" only for your Love, then the reality and importance of others looking at her or wanting her will not be an issue. It will not bother you and in fact, the idea that others find her attractive and beautiful will even give you feelings of gratitude, appreciation, and excitement.

If you are a jealous and possessive man, examine your desire. If you always feel like ogling other women, ask yourself *if you have really given yourself* to your Love and your Love alone. Have you made the deepest surrendering commitment in your heart to her? It is a very deep level of commitment that most men have not done, so if you see that you have not either don't be too hard on yourself. You will see that it is a *choice* to withhold your Love from her. You withhold your Love so that you can remain in control. It is not something that you *must* do because you are a man and all men have this desire for all women. Don't use the excuse that every other guy does it. That's a cop-out. Such behavior is not unconquerable just because it has become part of men's genetic makeup. You are copping out of dealing with your fear of losing yourself in a relationship.

Many issues have become genetic, but it doesn't mean they are insurmountable. They are choice based, thus you are not doomed to live these issues forever and ever. The difference is that in genetically-based issues, the negative reality seems a little denser and requires a little more dedication to work on and dissolve.

My friend Marc went away on a retreat to practice silence and med-itation. After a few days, a lot of the mental chatter cleared itself. It gave rise to the most vivid images of gorgeous naked women taunting and enticing him. He felt an immeasurable amount of desire. This, he said, was the last hurdle to overcome before he found a deep state of peace and quiet. I feel that this deeply-set program of longing and fantasy, almost like a spell or a curse, may be behind a man's ogling and look-ing at every woman that walks by. And it is quite a trap, a very large challenge for men to overcome because the desire can seem so real that the man believes he must have that most alluring beauty, no matter what. This is desire as a flip/reverse of a man's true wish to connect with the female. That is why it is so enticing. If you just look at beauty and appreciate it that is great, but when we think it is what we want, that beauty without connection to the core and guts inside the woman, it is only an illusion, like a mirror image. The delusional desire is to possess beauty. The true wish is for the surrender of Love with another in equality. Then the challenge is no more. If you have the uncontrollable desire for the beautiful women that you see, recognize that your ener-gy is lurching out of your body as a result of your very deep male, pri-mordial desire to possess the Beauty (Tiferet) of the woman, her essence, to have it for yourself. When you see this, begin to switch your thoughts to be aware that you need not and do not want to possess that energy. Freedom comes from complete recognition and appreciation of the beauty, without the need to possess. As it was so beautifully said in the movie *American Beauty*, there is so much beauty in this world and when we stop trying to hold on to it, it just flows right through us.

[*Sixth Circle*—CaN #4—I have no desire for anything outside of Love. I give up and transform bottomless pit desire. I release the desire for other women, or the desire for other men outside of the relationship that I am in. I let go of the desire for anyone other than the one I have chosen to be with within a relationship of love. I do this not because it is wrong to want another, nor because I must. I do not only do it because it is written 'thou shalt not covet thy neighbor's wife.' I give up the desire for other people because it is an illusion to desire a person I do not know and love on a deep level. It is not something real and therefore, I can see that I really do not want to desire others. I reconnect my essence with the Source and I yield totally and completely to loving the person I am with.]

Just as with anything else in this book, don't get fixated on the words themselves, because there are no rules about sex that *must* be obeyed. You can do as you wish. Allow these passages therefore, to be something to consider, should you wish to touch with the most profound experience of the sexual act. For this to occur, you must fully yield to your partner. To do so requires the commitment of the heart. That is why the power of the sexual act is so great when two people share in this way—it calls our innermost state of Truth to the fore: the yielding to Allthatis.

The balance here is allowing yourself to appreciate the beauty that women embody. If you do not look at other women because you are commanded not to, or because it is wrong, you will likely fight it and the possessiveness and jealous feelings can still plague you. When a woman walks by and you lower your hat so that you are not even looking at her, what are you saying? You are saying a lot—that it is wrong to look at women, or you are afraid of the reaction elicited by looking at a woman. The goal is not to avoid or run from the fear. That is fighting and dueling within belief-based reality. Instead, totally and completely wish to be only with your Love, in mind, body and soul, and not other women, and in that you can look at other women and not struggle. You are free.

Are you afraid of what will happen to you if you yield to her and love her as you have not loved for a long, long time? Are you afraid to put down the scepter of power so many of us are under the delusion of wielding? Do you wish not to give all of yourself to her for fear of losing her and how that might hurt? And so are you binding yourself in a selfish world of holding back?

When you allow yourself to feel full Love in the act, you will set yourself free from the need to ogle and desire every woman that you think is pleasing to the eyes or attractive. How will you want that

woman that you don't even know when you are totally and completely fulfilled, surrendering your Love to and with another? Then there
will be no fear of looking at women and losing control, because you
will not see them as sex objects to fulfill your need. There is such freedom in this way. You will also be releasing the need to control the
woman that you Love, for you don't need her energy to fill you up. You
have it within yourself in those acts of surrender, yielding, allowing, giving in, giving up, and giving.

When you fully give it up to a woman (or man) that you Love, you
surrender your need to be in control. To do this, you must face all your
issues about control and insecurity in the relationship and two particular issues that seem to be the root of many male-female problems.
First, no one is more important than another. (**The First Major
Delusion**) No one is number one. Both are total equals. Second, no one
is anyone's possession.

A man might have difficulty with yielding because he is afraid that
a woman will attempt to control him and manipulate him. Adam's error
was not seeing that he made his own choice in eating from The Tree of
Knowledge.

"And He said, "Who told you that you are naked? Have you eaten
of the tree from which I commanded you not to eat?" The man said,
"The woman whom You gave to be with me—she gave me of the tree,
and I ate." **Gen 3:11-12**

Adam did not take responsibility for his choice and gave his power
away by fearing that Eve can manipulate him into doing something
against his will. This is the fear of woman's power that many men have,
seen partially by the fear some men have of women's beauty. In his fear
Adam, and men, adopted the mentality, "control or be controlled." This
is the same as needing to prove you are in control because you feel you
are not. There is no such thing in Truth, nor does the female act this way
when given her rightful place.

Because of his control pattern, a fearful man may believe, "What I
am doing to keep her with me and protected and only mine is not

enough." In this pattern of thought, he fears the loss. If he continues to live in a fear-based world with no Love, he must try to maintain his control and therefore he controls through disapproval and through withdrawing his Love. This can trigger feelings of inferiority in the woman and of not being appreciated. This can only happen if she has bought into the belief that she is there for him. When he is unsatisfied, she takes it as her own failure. One of her fears is, "What I have to give is not enough, I must try more." She might feel the "intellectual inferior," he the "superior." They both heed more his judgment (right and wrong), rather than following the guidance they both have in their wisdom (equality). She might allow herself to remain in the relationship no matter what, because she feels she must. Ouch! What a sore spot to be in. Your female heart of high hopes gets squashed.

Through the ages, trying so hard to keep a woman's shine contained so as not lose her has driven men to their deathbeds. Women allowing their shine to be contained drives them to their deathbeds. If you understand the nature of a woman, which clearly can never be fully understood, and if you see how much she wishes to feel free, then you will know that by aligning yourself fully with the Truth, she *is* free. As a result, you will see her Love you more than you can possibly imagine. You don't have to worry so much anyway about sharing her with another man in a sexual way. If she Loves you and has chosen you, it wouldn't mean much to her if she were to have intercourse with another man. It wouldn't feel much to her at all, for all her intimate Love is for you. She doesn't desire sex with a man she doesn't Love.

If we only allowed ourselves to take all the necessary leaps of faith into Love and yielded to all the magnificence of the other, we would have everything we long for. If you have grown with a person and it is time to part ways, then you will move on. But when you have found someone that you really Love, are attracted to, and fulfilled by, *then do yourself a favor.* Give yourself totally and completely to that person. Women tend to do this much more readily than men when they fall in Love and they are all the more rewarded for it. Because of their deep insecurity and the emptiness, men feel they must keep their options open or else they will lose themselves. This is actually holding onto Frmee Will.

All that a woman really needs is to be listened to and to be allowed to do as she wishes. So listen to her. Really listen to her, not because you feel you must because she gets mad when you do not. Listen to her because when she speaks, her words come straight from the mouth of the Goddess herself. She stands right before you, showing you Truth by her very Being and you can be her prince if you wish to live in this World of Oneness. Don't shut her up, because you will be taking the wings of the dove and placing them in a cage.

Let's go a little deeper and take a look at some other issues and long-forgotten mysteries.

Part of the people's need to be on top as number one also has within it the fear of not being 'big' enough, in terms of job and social status, knowledge, or body parts. All men and women must come to love themselves in the exact way that they are.

[*Second Circle*—CaN #1—As I AM—I find beauty in who I am. If I am a man, I give up the need to be bigger than I am.]

When a man allows the flow of his sexual energy totally and completely, when he has let go of the issues of inadequacy and trying to prove himself, his sexual chakra becomes opened and aligned with his heart. The energy of his penis can extend far beyond its physical parameters into the woman so that she will feel him penetrating her on an energetic level that is very deep. This enlargement is energetic and is not available to a man who feels the need to be bigger than the Creator has made him, whether that be in mind, spirit, or body.

Yet deep connections on a spiritual and energetic level do not seem to be what a man always desires in this day and age, and in the past. Today many desire to have larger penises. It is quite amazing to note that this desire also existed in another ancient civilization. In the chapter on the civilization of Atlantis in *The Only Planet of Choice* (p. 148-149), it is written:

"If it had not been below their waste they were always in trouble, then it would have been a fine civilization. .../

Rather than using of the knowledge of medicine which they had to improve their mentalities or their physicals, they used their knowledge to improve their sex organs."

Repetition of the way things were is a revisitation to a past time. The fact that we see this desire to enlarge penises again today to such a large degree, and allegedly the technology to do so, is a sign that we are nearing the re-emerging of the time of Atlantis. Just as a pattern of your life will begin to repeat itself in an attempt to deal with past errors of choice and heal them, so too are we seeing the issues and errors of Atlantis re-emerging. It is also a return to our origins as we were before we ate from the Tree of Knowledge.

Portions of what might be the civilization of Atlantis have recently been discovered, underwater, off the coast of Cuba and much more will be found at many different locations. Many movies are depicting what some have imagined about the time and place. We are being prepared for the uncovering of all secrets for everyone to witness. The return to Eden is the New Atlantis.

There was a great flood that destroyed the civilization of Atlantis, that is why so much of our mythology surrounding it depicts the civilization underwater. Does this sound familiar? There is another place that discusses a great Flood. It is represented in the Torah by the story of Noah's Ark and the Great Flood. During the time of Noah, the "sons of gods" desired many of the "daughters of the earth."

> "The sons of the gods saw that the daughters of man were good and they went taking wives for themselves, namely, all whom they chose. And Hashem said, "My spirit shall not contend evermore concerning Man since he is but flesh; his days shall be a hundred and twenty years." *Gen* 6:2-3

The phrase "sons of gods" comes from the Hebrew "בני־האלהים," which literally means "sons of the gods," although it has also been translated as "sons of rulers," and "the Giants" merging with the daughters of men. These are the same. In the Torah, the Giants were called

"The Nephilim." They were much taller than the humans that lived on Earth then.

> "The Nephilim were on the earth in those days—and also afterward when the sons of the gods would consort with the daughters of man, who would bear to them." *Gen* 6:4

This is a very significant passage. There are many parallels between the time of Noah's Flood, and the civilization of Atlantis. *The Only Planet of Choice* explains that the flood of Atlantis was a powerful manifestation of disharmony in that civilization which had gotten so involved with sexual desire that people lost their way. This is the same reason why God brought the great flood at Noah's time.

> "And God saw the earth and behold it was corrupted, for all flesh had corrupted its way upon the earth. God said to Noah, "The end of all flesh has come before Me, for the earth is filled with robbery through them; and behold, I am about to destroy them from the earth." *Gen* 6:12-13

Let's take a look at a very illuminating mystery. It is the parallel between the civilization of Atlantis, the time of Noah *and* the time of Adam and Eve. The sons of gods (or Giants) merging with the daughters of man also came at the time of Adam and Eve. On page 138, *The Only Planet of Choice* explains that the name of the area where the civilization of Adam and Eve came from was called Akisu. Then *The Only Planet of Choice* also establishes that the Giants merging with the daughters of men came also during the time of Adam and Eve at Akisu.

> "Akisu was a seeded colony, arranged for the evolution of your planet Earth, and for teaching the process of progress, for a leap forward of humankind./ That was the beginning of what you term the "Giants merging with the daughters of men" you understand?' *The Only Plant Of Choice*, p. 134

Another parallel is that during Noah's time the men had great desire for women, "they went taking wives for themselves, namely, all whom they chose."

The lifespan during Noah's time dropped from close to 1000 years lifespan, to 120 years. "Man since he is but flesh; his days shall be a hundred and twenty years." **Gen** 6:3

This is also a symbolic parallel to the process of mortality about which God had warned Adam and Eve should they eat from the Tree of Knowledge. This is interrelated with man's desire to dominate and possess woman, and the female energy, through right and wrong, and through sex. From that desire to possess and control, which was Adam's choice, and the choice of the sons of gods to desire and take and possess the women of the earth, the final result was the Great Flood that is the tale of Noah's Ark, the Fall of Atlantis *and* the Fall of Adam and Eve from the state of the Garden. It is all a fall from the same "time." Don't think of it in terms of linear time. It was all the same era and age. They are all one and the same, told in different ways, as if from different stories. The Flood, the fall and the expulsion from Eden all marked the end of one age and the beginning of a new age, somewhat as in a new dimension.

Yet there is even more here than meets the eye.

Seeing the Flood as a destruction due to an *error*, and Adam's choice as a *fall* also due to an error, are not the complete picture. Even though described from many different sources, today's proximity to the New Atlantis and Eden-Revisited reveals a missing link, which we will now connect.

Look again at Figure 35. See that there is a parallel between the 6 x 1000 years of creation and the approximate 6 x 6000 years of creation. The time of Akisu, the arrival of sons of gods on planet Earth and Adam in the Garden of Eden, was said to be around 34,000 B.C. (*The Only Planet Of Choice* p. 129) That was around around 36,000 years ago. So the 6000 years of the Hebrew calendar from the Torah are paralleled in Earth time by a time factor of approximately 6, because around 6 x 6000 years ago Adam was placed on Earth and the Hebrew calendar is based upon a time scale of 6 x 1000 years.

According to scientists and archeologists, approximately 36,000 years ago our ancestors transition from Neanderthal man to Homo

Sapiens, of which we are direct descendants. This transition has baffled many scientists because there seemed to be a jump between the two civilizations, both in anatomy, brain size and skeleton structures, and technology that was much more advanced in Homo Sapiens. That transition was called "The Missing Link" by Charles Darwin and has remained quite a mystery.

What is that missing link? It is the implantation of a higher level of Soul into Neanderthal man. That implantation was Adam's soul, an angel in the image and likeness of God, into the body of a human being that had evolved on Earth naturally for millions of years and that had gone through the process of evolution from algae, ape and then human. This is the marriage of understanding our world both from the scientific and spiritual creation viewpoints. It is in the marriage between creation theory and evolutionary theory that we get the greatest perspective. Of course, understanding this marriage, it becomes even clearer that everything came about at the hand of the Creator. The Creator prepared the planet millions of years ago to evolve so that human beings' bodies and structures would be ready for the implantation of the Soul and to ultimately create an Eden paradise, which is a Garden for God's angels to experience themselves as individual entities.

Thirty-six thousand years ago corresponds to year one of the Hebrew calendar, when Adam was "born." Therefore, 6000 years of the Hebrew calendar really took 36,000 years of Earth time to unfold until this era, now, when we are ready to move into the seventh millennium, which is the Great Sabbath/Messianic Age.

Let's look at a few other points that we have established throughout this book and unite them all as one.

- We really created our world to be *physical* at the time of the Tree of Knowledge because we came out of the Oneness by our contraction of the Light (Tzimtzum).

- There are parallels between Adam and Eve eating from the Tree of Knowledge, Noah's Flood and the Flood of Atlantis. It is a parallel because they all had desire of the physical, and they all went from being immortal or having great longevi-

ty, to becoming mortal. (Atlanteans (those from the civilization of Atlantis) were said to have lived for thousands of years
on Earth.)

- Remember the Imagination of God chapter? God had imagined *all* of creation and created the Universe in six days,
  including humans on the sixth day. Remember the question,
  "Why does it say that 'there was no man to work the soil' (Gen
  2:5) after it says God created man?" (Gen 1:27). The answer lies
  within this passage from the Torah:

"Now all the trees of the field were not yet on the earth and all the
herb of the field had not yet sprouted, for Hashem God had not sent
rain upon the earth and there was no man to work the soil: A mist
ascended from the earth and watered the whole surface of the soil:
And Hashem God formed the man of dust from the ground, and He
blew into his nostrils the soul of life; and man became a living being."
Gen 2:5-7

Do you know what this passage is saying? What was the mist that
watered the "whole surface of the soil?" It was the Great Flood, which
is Noah's Flood *and* the Flood that covered Atlantis. It was also the
time when Adam transitioned from God's imagination, unmanifested
and not created, to having his identity in a body on Earth. That is
when he had the soul of life breathed into him and he became a living Soul able to exist in his own raindrop identity. Before the Flood,
Adam did not exist.

We established that creation does not exist outside the void of the
Creator's imagination if there is nothing or no one to witness it. If God
creates a beautiful Universe in six days and there is no one there to
witness it, does it exist? No. So the Creator gave Adam a Tree in the
forest that made Adam fall in consciousness to help the angelic realm
see the other side of reality—the side of reality that is *inside* the
Creator's Goodness—so that the angels could be born on the other
side into separation and know themselves. This was the implantation of

the Soul of Adam (the sons of gods) into the physical bodies already existing on Earth at that time. Right after this implantation, Atlantis was flooded, Noah's Flood covered the Earth in water, and Adam's consciousness was imploded and fell within creation so that he saw the other side of reality.

Adam came to Earth as a whole light being. He was a Son of God. When he "knew" Eve, he was merging his all light genetics with Eve's earthly genetics. Eve was "a daughter of man." She had evolved naturally from animals on the planet, which had been prepared by the Creator for this evolution. The children of Adam and Eve were a mixture, therefore, of two very different energies—Heaven and Earth. Initially, Adam wasn't able to perfectly merge and align his essence with Eve, in unity and in harmony to bring Heaven and Earth as One, because he wanted to be in control. This created a rift and a duality between the spiritual and the physical (which was brought on because of the challenge of the opposition who tried to make Adam believe he was like God over Eve). This rift is not such a big surprise, is it? The Creator knew it would take some time (around 6000 years of the Hebrew calendar, which is around 36,000 years of earth time) to fulfill the marriage of Adam and Eve and to bring about the Messianic Age.

So when Adam—the angels of the spirit world, the sons of Gods—were merging with the daughter of humankind, that created us, Homo Sapiens, and our genes. This brought Heaven down to Earth. Yet the proper merging and evolution have not finalized, and our genes have been evolving from day one to the perfect merging of the Adam and Eve as One within us. That is the purpose of creation. It is going to change the way our genes look. In addition to acquiring strands of DNA that have been lost, the base pairs of our DNA are also going to flip over in a similar way to the chakras, so that they are perfectly married in their center and not bound by magnetic attraction. The covalent, magnetic bonds between base pairs on the opposite Adam and Eve DNA strands will flip and become connected in their center.

The Flood of Atlantis and Noah was created to wipe the slate clean, to begin a new enterprise for Homo Sapiens, or the new marriage of the Heaven and Earth species, to begin a new civilization from scratch. The immense knowledge that existed during the civilization of Atlantis was forgotten so that humankind, as a blend of Heaven and Earth, could be challenged to recreate a civilization like Atlantis and return to Oneness.

Which brings up another very interesting point to weave into the tale. Remember that we are the only planet of choice, of Frmee Will, of separation from the Creator's Collective. The people of Atlantis did not have Frmee Will—they were working in harmony with the Will of God, in service to God. So the fact that they brought down the Flood upon themselves means that the Creator said, "Ok. It is time" and began the unfolding of the time we are in now, which is still in duality. It was not an error. They created it that way.

Therefore, there is another way to interpret the people of Atlantis' wish to "improve" their genitals.

> "Atlanteans are of two polarities blended in togetherness. They do not have what you would call male and female." *The Only Planet Of Choice*, p. 43

This shows us that the Atlanteans also existed before the beginning of time as we know it, because Adam was also created both male and female.

> "So God created Man in His image, in the image of God He created him; male and female He created them." *Gen* 1:27

Isn't that interesting? Why would the Atlanteans, which is Adam before the split into male and female, want to *improve*, as in "make larger," their genitals? Being male and female as one, Adam didn't have genitals as we do. Why also would the people of Atlantis, who equally did not have male and female sexual traits, wish to improve their sexual organs? How is that possible? It is not. Therefore, there is a mystery here to be discovered that helps clarify one of the passages of the Torah:

> "Hashem God said, 'It is not good that man be alone; I will make him a helper corresponding to him'." *Gen* 2:18

"So Hashem God cast a deep sleep upon the man and he slept; and He took one of his sides and He filled in flesh in its place: Then Hashem God fashioned the side that He had taken from the man into a woman, and He brought her to the man." *Gen* 2:20-21

This is written in a really convoluted way. It is difficult to translate from the Hebrew because the Hebrew does not even say it directly. It has been kept a mystery for a reason. It does explain that only during a deep sleep, in a dream, the male and female were separated. Before, they were One. The secret of this passage is also saying that Hashem-God took a portion from the Being that was both male and female—a bone, a "rib," an appendage—and brought the appendage from the One being, which created a whole in her (the woman's vagina), and brought that appendage to the other, and filled (or closed by joining) the flesh in its place, and created the penis of the man. (see Figure 39)

The verse: "It is not good that man be alone. I will make him a helper corresponding to him" can, therefore, be better translated. Remember, the "man" at this point is still male and female as One. So the Hebrew for "corresponding to him," כנגדו, comes from the Hebrew, נגד, which means "opposite" or "complementary." Are a man and a woman not created, like pieces of Lego, complementary and opposite to each other? Well, if you have a Being that is both male and female, with no sexual differentiation, and you remove a part out of one and create the other, you then have two beings that are "corresponding" to each other. It is *not* that there was a man, then a side was taken from him and tada!—he has a helper to do his bidding: the woman. What a misconception! That is the delusion that Adam has suffered from trying to be better or above Eve.

In this light, there are another few important clarifications to make. First of all, before the Tree of Knowledge, Adam and Eve were One inside the Being that was called Adam, which was both male and female. There was no Free Will at this time. Male-and-female Adam was one with the Will of God (as were the Atlantean people). Therefore, the act of taking fruit from the Tree of Knowledge came from a Being who was

One with God's Will. Adam and Eve were still together as One inside this Being with no Free Will. Therefore, how could Eve have been first to have eaten? She didn't. When the male-and-female Adam ate from the Tree, Adam and Eve did so together. To believe Eve ate first is deceiving and has led mankind to judge Eve and womankind as being evil and responsible for the original sin and the fall from Eden. A large misconception and error. Secondly, it was only after they ate from the Tree of Knowledge that they became separated, as in not One, as in male and female in parts, and were able to observe their separateness, and wished to hide their differences. Therefore, the time of eating from the Tree of Knowledge is the same "time" or "act" as when God cast a deep sleep upon the man and then took the two sides apart and made Adam and Eve, because that is when male-and-female Adam was separated into parts. So God casting a deep sleep upon the Oneness Being and making Adam and Eve as individuals is the same act as eating from the Tree of Knowledge. The casting of the deep sleep is much like the general anesthesia that someone is put under to undergo surgery. Well, male-and-female Adam did undergo surgery. Spiritual and physical surgery, when the energies of male and female became separated and the different sexual organs were created.

The Torah verse symbolically tells us that since the people of Atlantis didn't really have sexual organs as we do, they *had* to improve their sexual organs to create us. They used their amazing technology to create the genes of the man and the woman, thus providing a penis and a vagina, respectively. That is quite an improvement, isn't it? That is the literal sense of the Torah passage and how the Atlanteans carried out God's will in creating the human race, the new race with two separate sexes *corresponding* to each other, whose goal was to find the way back into balance and harmony with each other. Otherwise, we would not have been capable of having children, and evolution through the improvement of our ways by first forgetting toward the ultimate approach of the New Atlantis and Eden-Revisited could never have occurred.

Understanding the point that the male and female exist in separation only in the world of duality and illusion will help you let go of another primordial and deeply ingrained belief—that men and women are incomplete and only half until they meet their partner and get married. Inside, you are Adam and Eve. To believe you need your "other half" to complete you will bind you to needing the energy outside of yourself. You will be unable to experience that energy within yourself. Love relationships work best and bring us the greatest joy when we do not need them, and rather experience them as a bonus to our already at-peace state. If you enter into a relationship believing you need the "other half" to be complete, you become subject to all the control patterns that men and women place upon themselves. If you are complete inside yourself, you are free from all the ancient control patterns between men and women.

Poem—Around Back Goes the Bend

Imagine a time, in a quieter place,
The King and the Ace,
The Queen and the Fool,
You're the hand and the tool, isn't that cool?
You are the eyes of the Gods,
Who needed a lens,
So they placed you within,
Their story—the tale,
The land with no end,
Is the one just beyond,
But inside this den,
There's only one end,
That bends at the start,
And mends once it wakes,
Unto Ra Ra Time,
And through his shiny tear,
Horus is seer,
The Son of Man the Earth
Womanson's the Birth.
That is beyond Frmee will,
That is beyond desire,

For the genes from the One,
That is always the Higher,
There isn't a father?
So from where did he come?
We thought Athena
From Zeus' head sprung,
But reverse it would be,
Where we can really see.
The heart is the head of the Mom.
Leda and the Swan,
Is Eva and Adama,
For the man from the sky chose a mate,
a somewhat untimely fate,
It was just that he wanted a date,
Sad he was so he could not just wait.

Sons of Gods came to earth so to see,
How it was there in sight heavenly
For in there IS couldn't feel,
But they knew what was real,
It was all what they wished they could be

Many sons there were at that time,
And that fell so they started a rhyme,
Within reason they chose,
Gotta know and who knows?
Goodbye my sweet love sublime

That woman they chose for star ride,
Stayed in seas and never she died,
'Cause the earth was the home,
For men made to roam,
Forever seeking their sweet love bride.

We believe all along in the mind,
We must rush before closing time,

But it is when it is,
And God bless it that 'tis
There's not a thing passed the rhyme that's a mime

It's time is like stuck in backward
And exists as a left book's forward,
And when it comes to the end,
Around back goes the bend,
Spun the blade of the ever-turn sword

To us it feels like a void,
So we've been told but really half toyed,
It's the heavenly land
It's the gem to our sand
Yet before it is true they were boi'd,

They could only know what it was that they were,
But they wanted the feeling for sure,
What does it feel like a thought?
Or the word after brought?
It's where you're the Bee and the Bean and the Beer.

Thus the void, okay fine, it was that,
When alone the Goddess sat back,
And said to her self,
It is time and so fell,
Or dropped a lad out the hole in her sack

There is a strange thing in a joke,
That has truth tied up in its yolk,
For a man will try hard,
To fill holes with his ssshard
Wish back in Ma's Well he could soak.

Part IV—Appreciation of the Male and the Female

"As you know, Eve became identified with the notion of original sin. And Eve, the feminine, was buried and the male aspect consumed the earth... In the present day, the time of the female, the essence of Eve is coming to the fore, and what must be done is the complete merging of the male and female. Not for the male to attempt to bind the female, and not for the female to attempt to suppress the male, but to work in complete joy, in harmony and unity, as two pillars that are holding up the world." *The Only Planet of Choice* p. 140-1

As with the alchemical symbol for gold, the zero point, ☉, there is Love in the chaos (the zero, the infinite and undefined) that surrounds the male defining factor in the center of the circle (the point). There is also order within the chaos. Male energy is a very good thing. Yes it does have to be healed and realigned in harmony with the female to remove its tendency to compete, its desire for control, power and knowledge of a finite nature, and its desire to possess. But to be in a time of Oneness, the male energy must be viewed in its true form—good, essential, powerful, and strong.

The process of a man facing the negative to heal himself is difficult and can be very crippling if he judges the *entirety* of his maleness. As an extension of the female, the male is an essential part of the Balanced Positive that is the true nature of the Creator. It is only in the state of separation that the male becomes the root of negativity. Recall the model of the magnet. Without the male, the female's energy could not affect any change, for he carries out her energy and feeds back to her. We only painted the picture of the male and female and spoke about them in parts to explain separation. In true reality, they are indistinguishable and work hand in hand as One.

Male bashing, which has resulted from over-zealous feminism, can be very confusing for a man who wishes to be aligned with Truth. He will look at his maleness, look at how men have a tendency to be, and judge himself. This is an error. It is a very difficult task to be a man seeking Truth and enlightenment in a world that lumps all men together. Yes, you must let go of the control that might seem like a part of your natural tendency. But a man who accepts himself, lets go of the controlling factor, and allows the female to become the foundation in his entire Being, he has great power.

Women are built closer to the Earth. Their humility is much more natural and effortless. Their minds are not after the same things as men. For this reason, two things occur: one, their Beingness is already divine and two, their state of enlightenment is not much different from who they already are. They need healing as a result of having allowed the male to dominate, but it is a simple reawakening to their true nature and divinity. Men, on the other hand, have a great deal to do to overcome attempting to be like God in knowledge, power, etc. *It is for this reason that the man is a double-edged sword.* The rational mind that has no foundation (ϒ) has an empty space, which is a completely wide open channel to the energies of opposition, to the Yetzir Harah (Bad Will). He can attempt to be like God in knowing Good and Bad and also try to tell others how they should be. He can try to fill his mind with fragments of knowledge, believing this puts him ahead in the Game. Yet when he overcomes this tendency and this need, and remembers that Love is the most important thing there is, that empty space caused by the absence of foundation in the rational mind fills up with the most divine light. He adorns the mind of God (seventh Level of the Auric Field, Crown Chakra, Keter) and has access to an immense amount of Direct Knowing and Universal Intelligence. When this large ego void is transformed, the release of that potential negativity becomes immensely powerful. Therefore, do not judge the male, or you will be suppressing that power.

Who knows what the Y chromosome will look like when men give up the Y factor?

When the male simply gives up the illusion of being the foundation of power, his power is infinitely stronger because it is plugged into the infinite Source and not *trying* to be powerful and in control. Your self-esteem is immense when you release the need to be in control (because the need is only coming from a low self-esteem and is perpetuated by attempting to control). There is nothing you need to know about who you are, for you are what you are. The sun will shine on you without you lifting up your head. You will go about your day and not look back. Your sense of power will be endless and the best part is that you will not have to struggle or prove yourself to make it happen. It is effortless, a part of who you are—a proud knight.

It is so wonderful to be a man. Love yourself and accept the power that comes with that. Rejoice in your sexuality and your maleness. Do not suppress your true nature while you align yourself equal with the female, and you remove your need to be a man who dominates. Seek a woman who, in being free herself, will help you set yourself free.

It is so wonderful to be a woman. Love yourself and accept the power that comes with that. Do not suppress yourself as you come to remember just how magnificent that power is. Do not suppress the male as you let yourself be free. Allow your power to shine and be free, naturally, gently, and alongside the male. You need not prove anything about yourself, nor do you need to separate yourself from men in order to establish your power. You are free. Do not limit yourself if the man you Love is still choosing to be in a limited state. Don't continue serving a man who is afraid. You serve the Goddess and God. You serve Love.

Poem Dedication

I guess I'll go mad, I can't believe that you're mine
That you would choose my hand and then step to the time,
That your body does follow, that I wish I could mime,
Cause your way is divine; I can't believe that you're mine.

I guess I'll give up and serve as your steed,
quit trying to be right and watch you also lead,
I can't believe that you're mine, it would mean greatness of me,
That you would walk through the trees and make a bear out of me.
How selfish I've been, trying hard to be good,
and strong, wise and wicked,
so you wouldn't walk out of here,
Where heaven I've found, and so respect there the ground
Where you walk is the mound I've sought all my life.

There is sacred ground, and what I've searched for you've got,
And for what I strived and tried,

you have as your lot.
My Love I am sorry, in need I forgot,
That Love most divine is like Lancelot,
With honour his Will, was the Will of the Lady,
It swept all around and left the King all alone,
To sit in the cold on the stone of his throne.

And here I'm a man, so lucky I'll pop,
And blow up in joy that I can take in my hand,
The hand of the hand of the gods that I've sought,
To be so I see, it's so simple indeed,
The love that I wished for and wanted I've got,
And all I do, is down on one knee,
In honour I am married to serve you in care.

Keep shining so bright, I give for the pleasure,
In awe of you and the land where you stand,
Is blessed with a song, and birds hum for your feet,
'Cause the step of your foot leave's a drop that is sweet.

I searched all along in puzzles and words,
Yet the flap of the wings of the dove circles round,
Your head like a crown, of birds and fairies,
I am the guard of your grove, as you wish, if it please.
Thank God here is heaven. It is only for me,
To see I deserve, then I'll serve and be free,
And down on one knee, I yield to your might
That is bright as the moon and soft as the night,
For you it's all good, for you are my Will,
I am an extension of that and so better off still,
My time of past stops, forward takes its start,
In Eden I wake and see the fruit we did take,
And oh God there you are,
I thought I had lost,
And lost so I was to be tops as the boss,
Cause here I am me, and here you are you,

And so together we fall, in the moment of now,
forever as Us, together as One.
I feel where you are and for myself done.

The challenge for the male is to acknowledge this wonder, fully and completely, without holding back, with no doubt. And he of course knows her majesty deep, deep down, and for one, would like to be this way as well. In order for the world to return to harmony, the man will learn to yield. He will learn to allow. He will take his controlling foot off the brake and let the fuel of the female flow through him. For to yield is to allow divinity to unfold around and within you as it would if you could only stop trying so hard and resisting it.

When the male stops trying to be number one, when the male gets down on one knee and loves the might and wonder of the female, he is a regal knight. He is everything he has wished himself to be. And there was a time when men would tip their hats to women—that was a nice thing men did. Such honoring gestures are for the very core of what makes a woman a woman. Because she bears children. Because she is the fertile soil, lying in wait every month for the right time when she will create life. Because she is yielding and supple like those things bright and alive in nature. Because she has always been the one to yield to keep things from falling completely apart.

And there is a time (outside of this one) during which men shine with the privilege and honour of being with the beautiful women with whom they share. Naturally, women do the same. What will make sense of this again, for all of us, is when each man loves the woman he has chosen with all his heart and soul, and he loves her for who she is. When we all can do this, we will really let go of all the misconceptions about what it means for a woman to be beautiful. Who she *is*, *is* beautiful. And as we also see that the quality of Truth manifests itself in limitless expressions of Being, and is not reserved to the lessons in a book or classroom, then we will all teach each other advanced lessons in Kabbalah and Truth by allowing ourselves and others to be who they are.

I yield to the Goddess.
I yield to the Shekinah.
I am a vessel for the Shekinah/Goddess.

Once you really do this and confront the blocked flow of the Shekinah in you, you will really experience *allowishing, the propeller of Forwardness, letting go, joy, and Love.* You will also naturally experience the left column of the Tree of Life in the way of True understanding (Bina), True strength (Gevourah), and True humble self-esteem (Hod), which we have forgotten for so long. Ahh, what do you think the Zone of Cold means? It means we will all be (t)here soon…

Chapter 12: Summary

When Adam was created both male and female as One, there was no way for this being to experience itself. In separating the two sexual energies into male and female, the parts became perceivable. However, in its duality, insecurity, and separation from the source of all true power that is the female, the male energy felt the need to control the female in order to possess that power. If the male could accept it and yield to it, he would then have it in himself and see what this then makes him. But because he suppresses it, he becomes devoid of the female and then needs to acquire it externally. In his separation from the Source, he is insecure and yet he longs for the connection to the female because she represents God and the Garden of Eden to him. Men and women both possess the male and female energies, but because the man possesses more of the male energy, and the woman more of the female, men have tended to usurp control throughout most of our history. Today this still happens to a large degree.

So many limiting beliefs through the centuries concerning what is important have originated from the male energy's insecurity, subsequent need to control, and the need to be elevated as a god. As long as these beliefs persist, we will not experience the bliss and ecstasy of the Ganallisone. To live in the Ganallisone is to live with the female energy as the foundation and the source of all true power. The male energy carries the source into the world. Inequality has divorced us from our true nature. Reactions to the male control, like radical feminism and political correctness gone overboard, have also caused imbalances.

Consequently we constantly long to merge. Through the centuries this has manifested as a deep-rooted sexual desire that tends to be stronger in the male, who feels more disconnected from the female. Bottomless pit desire, for anything—money, power, sex—comes from a hollowness due to being separated from our true nature, the Source.

To return the Universe to harmony, men and women must reconcile their differences so that they too may return to true harmony. When men understand their role during the Reversed Time and women accept and understand theirs, patience and acceptance from both sexes will be necessary. Through acceptance, we will prepared to move onto the next phase of Creation. Women will no longer fatalistically allow any inequalities or injustices. They will leave the Unbalanced Positive boxes in which they have trapped themselves. They will also stop suppressing the male energy due to past wrongs. Then men and women, in a Love bond, will create the immense vibrations of Love of the alchemical union.

ESSENCE OF THE CHAPTER

We are all made up of the balance between male and female. With the female as the foundation of power and the male acting in harmony with that, we will let go of Frmee Will and find the Balanced Positive state of Oneness, and return to Eden.

The First Letter—Reconciliation of Eve and Adam

Part I—Men to Women

Dear Women of the World of Times Past and Present,

Please forgive us for all of the inequalities, injustices and oppression that we have enforced upon you.

Please forgive us for the violence that was done to you for being women and forgive us for trying to hide your beauty and attempting to control how you looked, how you acted and what you said.

We acknowledge now that all this control came from our own insecurities and from that weakness came our desire to have power over your divine nature.

So please let that divine nature shine and be free to express yourselves and Be exactly as your hearts guide you.

Part II—Women to Men

Dear Men of the World of Times Past and Present,

We forgive you for all of the injustices and wrong that you committed. We acknowledge your weaknesses, the parts that needed to be in control.

We realize now that we have always thought that this was the way it had to be. We see now that this isn't the case and so we won't allow it any longer.

As for the violence and suppression we endured for being women, we hope and pray that it will cease everywhere.

We see now that it is okay for us to let our light shine and that we are free to be as we choose. As such, we no longer have to suppress the male in either of us.

Thank you for your brave words of apology. We accept.

Please be a part of healing these old wounds and patterns of control. When you feel ready, go to http://www.thelastfourbooks.com/ and sign the First Letter.

BOOK I SUMMARY

Before the beginning of time as we know it, Allthatis was an infinite presence that was AllGood. In that state of AllGood, the Allthatis (the Creator) imagined everything that a Being with an infinite and unlimited consciousness can imagine. All that was imagined was seen as Good, for Good was Allthatis.

Yet a dilemma existed. The Creator was still the One Will that peered at and empowered all of creation, but there was nothing with which to share that experience. It is like knowing all the moves when you play a game against yourself. It is as if you are projecting the movie of creation on a screen in your imagination. There is no experience of the sound of a tree falling in a forest *within* the movie of creation, because there is no one there to witness it and that is what the Creator wishes for.

The Creator is LOVE, because Love wishes to share and make more of its goodness available for others to experience. Love is the intention behind our entire creation. So the Creator knew that life had to be breathed *into* parts of creation and those parts given the power to choose for themselves so that each imagined Being could come alive within itself. Those Beings seen as *very good*—the children of God, Adam and Eve, humankind—were to take on this task so that creation could come alive with the experience of what was imagined.

The Creator also knew that if not challenged, the Creator would become bored. Therefore, those Beings that were in the image and likeness of the Creator would also have to be challenged. This would, therefore, mean that the Creator itself was Being challenged. This challenge would happen in paradise (Earth) where *that which opposes* (the Serpent) could challenge the children of God. The purpose of being challenged is to give rise to choice, given power and experience to true nature when it is chosen. (This is like the Kabbalistic concept of "earning" the Light of God, through the process of choice).

Upon being challenged, the Adamic people started to exist outside of the Will of Oneness. This gave each Soul the opportunity to separate into individuality, so that the Soul could know itself as a separate entity, so that each imagined Soul could thus experience itself in its own raindrop identity, rather than as an indistinguishable part of the Universe's puddle. The true experience and the wonderful celebration of the Universe occurs when the raindrops wake up to remember that they are all part of the unconditional, collective puddle *and* they are experiencing that collective as individual raindrops.

The true challenge began when Adam and Eve ate from the Tree of Knowledge for Good and Bad, for at this time all their Goodness became reflected also into the opposite of Goodness. An opposing Will began challenging the One Will so that they had one Will telling them to do what the other opposed. This was the contradiction between the Will of the Heart and the Will of the rational mind. The Will of the Heart is the Will of Love and it is One and the same as the Will of God. It is also the Will aligned with Truth. The other Will, the Will of the rational mind, is the Will of the ego that tells you to do what it thinks is right based on past belief, the desire to control, or fear. This is the Will of that which opposes. It is the true Will turned upon itself. Opposition to the Will of the Heart causes duality and suffering. The challenge, therefore, and the Game of Life, is to choose between true nature (Love) and the opposite (Fear). Choosing True nature helps the Soul return to the Source and thus empowers our experience of the Creator.

There is a tree in nature that fits the Torah's description of the Tree of Knowledge and also causes a doubling of Wills and a contradiction between the Will of the Heart and the Will of the rational mind. Knowing this, we can use this tree homeopathically to heal the negative effects of the Tree of Knowledge by the homeopathic principle of "like curing like." The identity of this tree is *Anacardium orientale*, which *is* the Tree of Knowledge for Good and Bad.

After Adam and Eve ate from the Tree of Knowledge, *knowledge* of what is good vs. bad (Bina2) or right vs. wrong (Gevourah2) began to govern the collective consciousness of humankind. Instead of living by the Will of Love and inherent guidance within their hearts, people began living by choosing according to what they believed to be right and wrong. The essence of the heart, therefore, was buried deep in the layers and layers of control and suppression that occur when you live your life according to what is right and wrong (good and bad), versus what you would love to do and be. The heart, the One true Will, the Balanced Positive between Heaven and Earth, Tiferet in the Tree of Life and the doorway to Atzilut, becomes frozen when you believe you must choose good vs. bad with your rational mind according to how you have been taught from an external source. This way of being takes away your ability to inherently know Truth by direct connection. Living a life entirely based in the rational mind (Bina2) feels like nothingness, for it is mind set of black and white beliefs and judgments about the nature of reality. It is a hollow graphic reflection of true Beingness, of Life. That is why, on another level, the Torah, the New Testament, the Koran, and all our sacred texts with which we have dependent relationships are the Tree of Knowledge for Good and Bad, for they are filled with the laws and knowledge of what is good and bad that we have followed religiously.

What we have come to know and study as the Kabbalistic Tree of Life, which lives inside of us, with the Ten Sefirot, including the left column of Bina (understanding), Gevourah (Strength) and Hod (Self-Esteem), right column of Chochma (Wisdom), Chesed (Compassion) and Netzach (Selfless Humility), was also affected when Adam and Eve ate from the Tree of Knowledge. The Tree of Life reflected inward and became the Tree of Knowledge, for it began to contain both Good (true nature) and Bad (the opposing/reflection of true nature), such as wisdom (Chochma) and its reflection/opposite which is rational understanding (Bina2), that is not in harmony and attempts to control the Chochma. When we release and transform the limiting aspects of judgment (Gevourah2), controlling rationality (Bina2), and egotism (Hod2) from the left column of the Tree of Knowledge, we will finally experience the Tree of Life as it really is, beyond any duality or opposition. This will fulfill our destiny of creating Heaven on Earth.

After the Tree of Knowledge, the male and female energies also became separated from one another. Since the *source* of all power of Love is the Shekinah, Ruach HaKodesh, רוח הקודש, Holy Spirit, female energy, when the male energy became separated from the female, it felt insecure. Instead of living in harmony with the female energy, acknowledging its power and divinity, and allowing it to flow, the male energy began to try to control the female so that it could have it all for itself. This has manifested through the centuries as men attempting to control women's freedom to choose for themselves, and by establishing rational study and argument as the basis of connection to the divine. Women also allowed the domination to occur and have played their part in perpetuating the male energy as the foundation of reality. When women no longer wish for the situation, they are capable of changing it, and can help men let go of their need to control.

The power struggle between the male and the female also exists in each individual between the male, Will chakras and the female, feeling chakras. For many people, controlling male energies limit their state of freedom and the amount of Truth they are able to feel by holding on to beliefs, judgments and fears and by not allowing the female energy to flow right through. This is how a person suppresses being themselves.

Because of the dualistic, opposing flow of the chakras, two energies exist in every individual who lives outside of the Oneness of the Creator and these negative and positive energies are in unbalanced states. The energies yin (female) and the yang (male) are in opposition to each other, thus duality is created between them and yet they are bound to each other, being of opposite polarities. These two energies are also equivalent to the Time of Forwardness (female) and the Time of the Past (male in separation). The resistance of the male energy causes a slowing of the vibration of the body so that the individual perceives the surrounding world as denser and more physical. The resistance of the male energy in separation from the female energy also subjects the individual to the earth's gravitational field because the resistant male energy is the polar opposite of the female energy of Mother Earth. Opposites attract and then become stuck.

The stuckness is also seen in the chakras as a seal that sits in between the front and rear chakras. When the rear, Will chakra lets go of control and allows itself to be an extension of the front, feeling chakra, that creates the Balanced Positive state. This is the Time of Forwardness within a consciousness of Oneness and unconditional Love, as represented by the sacred name of God, Ehye Usher Ehye—I shall be as I shall be. Oneness is an absolute state of Beingness in which the male empowers the source of power of the female. This state is symbolized by the Tree of Life, the Tree that exists within the Garden of Eden and imparts upon those that eat its fruit immortality and unconditional Love.

Separation and resistance began when Adam and Eve ate from the Duality Tree. That marked the moment when the other side of reality and the world began to be experienced as physical because resistance of God's Will causes the contraction of light and makes you perceive the world as physical.

The world also didn't have any inhabitants on the physical side, "for Hashem God had not sent rain upon the earth," until the Great Flood, which occurred during the time of Noah and Atlantis. This Flood wiped the slate clean for humanity to start anew in its consciousness of duality (because male and female were separated) on the other side of reality and work its way back to the total merging and balance between the male and female (on an individual level and between lovers).

With the separation between Adam and Eve, Adam tried to be like God and control Eve. He attempted to put himself above the female. This perpetuated duality and separation and made it impossible to merge as One with the female. Giving up Frmee Will occurs when a Soul stops desiring to be like God and gives up fear, doubt, and its need to control reality. The Soul will wake up from the dream we have fallen asleep in to the World to Come, which is the Garden of Eden revisited, and the New Atlantis. As soon as one individual awakens completely and crosses the threshold of negative mass, others will soon follow until enough Beings exist again within unconditional Love and a critical number of people achieve such a powerful vibration that the one hundredth monkey effect occurs and all people on Earth awaken to the Ganallisone paradise.

BOOK I CONCLUSION

The simple Truth we have been reminded of thus far is that we have a true nature available to us when we release the fear, doubt, and control that we have chosen in the Game of Life. We have chosen based on our limiting belief systems about what is Good and Bad. And when we examine this very closely, we see another most divine Truth that says that the experience of our true nature comes about in full, wonderful force when we simply allow ourselves to be... ourselves. This is the marriage of the Creator's imagination with the created individual, first by choice and then by allowishing and effortless Beingness. This is immortality with the absolute ecstasy of Being.

AM is To Be. To Be is to Allow. To Allow is to Feel. To Feel is to Heal. To Heal is to Love. To Love is To Be. To Be is AM.

To Be is the Hebrew verb "Lihiyot", להיות, I AM. It is as God spoke His or Her name to Moshe, Ehye Usher Ehye, I shall Be as I shall Be. One of the most sacred names of God is the tetragrammaton, YHVH— יהוה, which is derived from "To Be." To Be is Allthatis. Allthatis is God. God is Love. Love is Allthatis. *All that* is Truth. All else is illusion. All that is not is untrue.

To try is the antitheses of AM and to Be. To try comes from the doubt of who you are. To try is to resist who you are. To resist is to control. To control is the antithesis of allow. Try and control close off the Heart and judge things as Good and Bad. The Heart is Love. God is experienced in the Heart. The Heart is Tiferet in the Tree of Life, the Beauty of Life, Being, and Love, and It's Oneness is experienced in the Kabbalistic World of Atzilut.

To try is to not be grounded. To not be grounded is to lose connection with the hara. The hara is the propeller of Forwardness and it is our Will to Live. To Live is to Be.

When the question is asked, "How do I know my Will?" You know your Will by what you Love to Be. That is the only Will you will ever need. You put *all* your Heart, *all* your Soul and *all* your Being into your Will to Live/Be what you Love. There you marry your Will with God's.

To Love is to Be with foundation. To not be grounded is to lose the foundation and connection with the Earth. Our foundation is the source of all our power and all our essence. Without foundation, we have nothing, we are untrue. Our foundation is Mother Earth. To Love is to be with Mother Earth.

Be Yourself. Don't try to be. Be.

And then we set ourselves Free.

Free from what?

From the prison of challenging ourselves and holding back from just being. Why have we held ourselves back?

Because of GUILT!

The main root of the Tree of Knowledge is *guilt*. What is guilt? It is the internal feeling of having done wrong. Guilt is being hard and down on yourself for committing what you perceive as errors. It is therefore quite interesting to note that when the Tree of Knowledge, *Anacardium orientale*, affects the human consciousness, it conveys the delusion that you are doing everything wrong. Having this delusion, we feel that there is something wrong with us. That is *why* we do not allow ourselves to just Be. That is why we have developed immense religious and legal structures and strict, sturdy study of what we believe is right and wrong. These are based in the past so that our rational minds will know exactly what to do to control and ensure that our badness does not take over. Yet do you understand that it is all coming from a delusion, an illusion of badness? It is an illusion of having sinned, erred, and having been bad. *All* of that is unreal, untrue.

So what is this saying?

There was no wrong in eating from the Tree of Knowledge.

If we believe we have done wrong and that to return to Eden we must release guilt and feeling wrong, then to be in Eden is to be *beyond* those emotions and feelings of wrong. Releasing guilt (anger at the self or self-loathing) is thus absolutely necessary to allow ourselves to just

Be and be totally and completely okay with Being who we love to be. This is the ultimate joy and destiny for every soul on Earth—the Return to Eden.

This also means that to be in Eden is to truly know that we have done *no* wrong. Since the Garden of Eden represents a state of no illusion, it is the most truthful place to be. Therefore to be in Eden is to be beyond the illusion of having done wrong.

Who is described in the Torah as being the first to eat from the Tree for being Good and feeling Bad? Eve. That is very significant. I have often heard the Garden Angels whisper to me, telling me that Eve knew that it was okay. That's *why* she ate from it. Then Adam ate. Why is this so significant? Because Eve knew that there was nothing wrong with eating from the Tree of Knowledge for Good and Bad. Symbolically, it was the act of Love-making and the creative miracle of birth. Eve intuited that there was nothing wrong with bringing another life to the Universe. Yes, okay, they weren't completely ready to have a child, but who is ever really ready to have a child? She also knew deep inside that it was okay to begin the Game of Life. She was ready for the challenges that would entail. Adam and Eve were told *not* to "eat from the Tree of Knowledge" because they had to feel as if God told them *not* to do it and they felt, therefore, that it was their choice and not God's. This then gave them the feeling of having had a choice, which began the process of differentiation into individuality.

The subsequent interpretations of Eve's choice and the association of Eve, the female aspect, with evil or the devil, is completely false. (Don't forget that even though the Torah depicts Eve as being the first to eat from the Tree of Y, Adam was still the male-and-female Being and therefore, they ate together before they were separated into parts.) The false interpretations are manifestations of the control of the patriarchal world, the male dominating energy in our duality world. This major error in our history—the suppression and association of the female, the Goddess, with evil—is being healed now as the Goddess' voice sings again amongst us.

The idea of original sin and associated feelings of guilt are also completely false, since Creation unfolded by God's Will and Adam was only created as a physical, mortal being *after* the Flood and the Fall. Traditional Kabbalistic knowledge tells us that Adam and Eve had to wait for "the Sabbath" and then they would be ready to "eat from the Tree of Knowledge" (make Love). The Kabbalah is really saying that only in these times *now* with the setting of the sun on the sixth day and the coming of the Great Sabbath, we are able to experience the union of the male and female and experience the Oneness of Creation. Born into individuality, there were too many energies, too many issues to balance before we could experience the Oneness of Creation both internally and in sexual communion with our partners. We have had to wait until this day and age when we have gone through the long process of remembering who we really are and being that, to experience what we have longed for since we were created.

So what is this memory we have about a wrong choice? Why does the Kabbalah teach us that is was too soon, or that we weren't ready? Why do we have the memory of a great destruction deep in our psyche and our souls burdened with heaviness? Why does the Torah describe the first choice as *the Tree of Knowledge for Good and Bad* as a grave error, the original sin, and depict God punishing Adam and Eve?

All for a purpose.

Because eating from the Tree of Knowledge *was* an error.

Here we hit our philosophical head right against the wall.

Why? Because this contradicts what was just said that, "*There was no wrong in eating from the Tree of Knowledge.*" In fact, they had no choice. It was God's Will. So how could it be wrong? This is the most amazing thing to understand about this ancient paradox.

The paradox is that God's Will began this reality, and yet, deep inside, we also have the notion that we, not God, are responsible for the Fall, the Flood and the destruction—the imprints of that "downfall" still sit in our subconscious. Because (here is the real secret that will help us understand) *we* had to cause the separation from God. Otherwise, there would have been no creation. We believe we did wrong and in one respect we did, because *we* chose to begin this reality in order to experience our own Will. Any separation from the Oneness of God gives the separated soul the feeling of being responsible for the choice of disobeying the Will of God. Michelangelo's famous Sistine Chapel painting *The Creation of Adam* depicts this. As God's outstretched hand is taken away and Adam is left on his own, he naturally begins to feel that he chose to separate himself from God. He experiences that separation as disobeying the Will of Oneness and as an error. We must meet any disobedience and separation with awareness and claim responsibility in order to correct the error. Neither Adam nor Eve accepted responsibility for their choice. Adam blamed his choice on Eve: "That woman you gave me, she made me eat from the tree." **Gen 3-12.** Eve blamed it on the serpent: "The serpent deceived me and so I ate." **Gen 3-13.** Not recognizing the choices *you* have had in *all* that you do, totally and completely, is an error. We have yet to fully come to accept our "original sin," our primordial separation.

God does not separate, for God is One. It was us who separated ourselves because we are on the other side of reality with our Frmee Will. It is also "wrong" in the context of Love to disobey the Will of Love. All the pain we have suffered, all the control we have exerted on ourselves and on others through the centuries is wrong in the context of Love because we, not God, made those errors of choice. It is not that things are wrong, but that they are not Love. "Wrong" therefore means that it has no foundation of Truth. It is all illusion, fear-based and therefore not necessary. Suffering has been as a result of our choices, *not because it was meant to be, and not because it was part of the divine plan.* Even though having Frmee Will gives us the complete right to choose—even to suffer if we wish—the error in choosing outside of Love is that people get hurt and *that is never meant to be.* Seeing this part of the paradox is essential to being a "real" person, facing up to the past, and not cutting off what you don't like about yourself, pretending it doesn't exist.

Through accepting our errors and seeing the paradox of Creation, Eden-Experienced is born. No acceptance of errors, no Eden. In other words, if you just embrace half the paradox that says it was all meant to be from the hand of God, you do not experience the Eden that comes from the acceptance which in Judaism we call Tchuvah, "The Return," and what *A Course in Miracles* describes as "The

Atonement." Acceptance also helps you generate the immense strength of the Will to live that is necessary to affect positive change for peace on our planet.

So understand that this division into duality occurred because it was destined. The suffering that has resulted from us being in control within the Game is not meant to be, but the process of choice that we have called "The Game" is meant to be. Can you see the balance? It is an important balance to arrive at because just embracing one aspect of the paradox leads to the extremes of either unbalanced positive (it is *all* meant to be, you are blind to errors, too weak to create change and move forward), or unbalanced negative (it was wrong to eat from the Tree of Knowledge, you are stuck in Guilt, struggling with God's Will). When we achieve this balance, we free ourselves with wonderful acceptance and empower ourselves to know that *now* is the time to take responsibility for correcting our errors which originated outside of Love's Oneness, by working to heal and create our world in the image of Eden.

We experience the Tree of Knowledge and the Flood as Bad, deeply buried in our psyche because our minds are encoded with a half-truth story book. It is only half of the story. Think again, therefore, what it meant in Chapter Nine, The Tree of Knowledge chapter:

> "The purpose of this, as part of the Creator's Divine Plan, and the task chosen by the Hebrews, was to begin the Game of Life. This means that the purpose of the Torah, given by God to Moses, was to create this Game, this challenge, this test. The Torah is thus not only the Guidebook for the Game of Life—it created the Game of Life."

Tie this in with the understanding that when Moses received the Torah, it was written on *both* sides.

> "Moses turned and descended from the mountain, with the two Tablets of the Testimony in his hand, Tablets inscribed on both their sides; they were inscribed on one side and the other." *Exo* 32:15

Then he threw it down. What he really did was break off one of the sides. We have been left with half the Torah, the story book which is the Time of the Past and which is the Tree of Knowledge for Good and Bad. We have yet to receive *the other side of the Torah*. The other side is the Kabbalah, which is the unwritten experience of the divine Truth through the feeling of the Shekinah in the Time of Forwardness and Ehye usher Ehye.

We see the Tree of Knowledge as a Fall, the Flood as a destruction, and so many of our choices as errors because we see and believe ourselves to have participated in it and not what would be truer to see; that we were created *after* the Fall with the feeling of the fall and the errors of choice already in us. The notion of having done wrong and the feeling of being bad encoded in our psyches has created the drive to correct our internal feeling of error, to heal the world, and has put us to the test to return to the Source from which we believe we have become separated. This is the essence of the Game of Life and the purpose of Frmee Will, which is really just an illusion. By our moving forward and correcting our previous missteps, we approach the Garden of Eden so that we can experience it for the first time.

> "You correct your previous missteps by stepping forward. This process is actually incomprehensible in temporal terms, because you return as you go forward." *A Course in Miracles*, pp. 20

It is most important to wipe the slate clean of all beliefs and ties held on to identities that have served their divine purpose in bringing us to this point today. For the Jew, this means letting go of all attachments to the Law of Torah, totally and completely, and all beliefs associated with it. For the Christian, the Old and New Testaments. For the Muslim, the Koran. For all other people, this means letting go of all past beliefs and ideas about the self that resulted from hurt, fear, or because of an ego's need. Wipe the slate clean. Let go of all you know, or think you know. Just be yourself in the world. Be what is the underlying essence in all religion—the Love that unites us all.

Let go of trying so hard against reality and against the unfoldment of the Creator's plan. Accept those errors and imperfections you have had *that God put in you* to challenge you and give you the ability to make who you are real by choosing it. See the errors and understand how the Creator's hand has been in all of it. And remember the other side of the paradox—that we really have made no errors. God's hand gave us the Tree of Knowledge. The Flood, too, is just symbolic of the Atlanteans, as One with God, pulling the plug on the drain of that reality to begin our new reality—the next phase of creation.

If you remembered what Atlantis was like, you would call it Heaven on Earth. We are nearing this forgotten time. These secrets are being revealed now because we are so close. We are hearing the faint melodies of the otherworldly music and feeling the warmth of the Secret Fire from the other side. That is why secrets are emerging from all over and revealing what creation has been all about.

We give thanks and take responsibility for healing ourselves of the last missteps due to how our minds were encoded in a reverse and false fashion, by moving forward in carrying out who we really are. This is the way to triumph over the Game, which is to bring about the Messianic Age of unconditional Love and peace for all people.

And then, and now, you see one thing clearer than anything you have ever allowed yourself the pleasure of knowing: you are free to move forward and create yourself in the very way you love to be. You choose to be because you love to be. (And don't forget the little secret—*because you are*)

We cannot possibly even imagine the joys and wonders in store for us. Wake up. (Wow! What a dream, what a Game that was!)

We awaken from our dream of separation by returning to Eden, recognizing the emergence of Atlantis, the marriage of Adam and Eve so that they are One again, and understanding the paradox of creation.

This strange, mystifying paradox of creation shows us something mind-boggling. It shows us that the very moment when Adam and Eve ate from the Tree of Knowledge (beginning of time as we know it) and the subsequent moment when healing of the negative effects of eating from it collectively occurs (end of time), is a time that nullifies itself.

It was wrong and it was right.

These two points about reality meet head to head, in two opposing times. Being exact opposites, like Bad and Good and the past and the future, and like matter and antimatter, they do not share the same space. Rather, they collide and cause each other to burst.

Yet something most extraordinary occurs, for the time of Past stops and Forward takes its start. The point at which the opposites meet—the marriage of the paradox (Past and Future, Good and Bad, Control and Being)—there is One that wins, because it is Truth.

All that is illusion disappears.

It **IS** AllGood, as **I AM**.

So let it be, for it shall be.

EPILOGUE

Naturally, Book I couldn't cover everything, and many secrets and awarenesses remain to be discussed. Book II of The Last Four Books of Moses will be released in the near future. It will help point you in the direction of your "Unwritten Way" and is designed with practical daily considerations, more Kabbalistic insights to help you heed the call of Tikkun Olum and/or the call of the healer, to fulfill your service to God by being yourself and carrying out your life's purpose *in* the world, totally and completely, with no resistance, fear, or doubt. I will explain how you might wipe the slate clean by letting go of the past and all other identities to which you have clung. Book II will deal much more closely with healing the relationship of the Jewish people with the Arabic people and the rest of the world.

Book II will also share powerful meditations, like the Ninth Heaven Meditation, the Two that are One Meditation, the Upside Down Magnetic Boot Meditation and exercises like, the Cutting to the Chase Exercise part II and the Homeopathic Letting Go Exercise. I will share how to deeply ground yourself into Mother Earth, which will provide a good foundation for reaching into the Higher Heavens. You will learn to use the power of the hara to propel yourself forward in the World to Come. I will also paint the rest of the picture of the Homeopathic Elixir of Life, the healing elixir that helps us dissolve all resistance and return to Oneness. If you have felt a connection and inspiration from the quotes from Phyllis Schlemmer's *The Only Planet of Choice*, please read it. It is a very special book for our time.

I am also very happy to work with you personally to help you heal yourself, let go of Frmee Will, toward creating your Heaven on Earth. If you wish to make an appointment with me, please contact me at MosheDaniel@Nddoctor.net.

GLOSSARY

The following definitions are for words that I have either created or am using in a *specific* way throughout the book. When these words first appear, they are italicized and bolded. Thereafter, the first letter of the word is capitalized to indicate that it is being used in its specific sense.

Adam Kadmon: אדם קדמון: This is the original form in which Adam existed before/beyond the state of duality. It is in a state of Oneness, in which Adam is a whole, light Being. The term applies to Adam's state before eating from the Tree of Knowledge as well as after a Being has let go of Frmee Will.

Afferent: "To receive." In the body's nervous system, our sensory organs use the afferent pathways to transmit sensations from the outside to the brain. It is female in nature.

Ahava: אהבה: Love.

Ain Sof: אין סוף: Without end. The infinite and undefined.

Allowishing: This is a will that we use to allow something to be exactly as we would love it to be. It is a Will that doesn't force or try too hard. It is effortless and aligned with our heart's desire. *"That which I wish to be, I allow myself to be."*

Ashan: The civilization of creativity, colour, and music, related to the Kabbalistic World of Yetzirah. The terms Ashan and Hoova were taken from the book *The Only Planet of Choice*.

Assiyah: עשיה: The Kabbalistic World of Body and Form that became doubled from the Divine Body into the physical body after the Tree of Knowledge. (Earth element)

Atzilut: אצילות: The Supreme Kabbalistic World that is eternally One and was never doubled by the Tree of Knowledge. It represents the World of the undefined Balanced Positive and includes the Heart. In the

Tree of Life, Tiferet is in the World of Atzilut. Here, we are Soul. (Air element)

Auric field, a.k.a. the Aura: The energy field created by the body's internal and external aura. The aura is our body in subtle, energetic form, perceivable with high sensory perception or the third eye.

Awebedience: Knowing our guidance must be carried out not because we have to or we're bad, but because the Will of our Higher Self beckons us to fulfill what is in our Hearts. When we are filled with awe for all of creation, we closely heed the call to serve our guidance. Awebedience gives us the Will to follow the guidance we know we must follow. Once we do, we no longer need to follow because it is set into motion.

Axiotonal Lines: A term from Dr. J.J. Hurtak's *The Keys of Enoch*. "The axiotonal lines connect the acupuncture mapping of the human biological system with superior astrobiological analogs" p. 567. In other words, the axiotonal lines are the higher forms of our acupuncture meridians, which connect us to the Oneness of the Universe.

Balanced Positive: The Balanced Positive state is the energy of Oneness of the undefined nature of God, which occurs when the male and female energies are in perfect harmony. It is not the balance between good and bad.

Beingness: We are in this state when we have let go of control and do not try to make everything happen. It is simply Being who you really are, having shed all the things you believe you are and think you must be. Absolute Beingness is a state beyond all judgment, beyond Frmee Will, within Oneness.

Belief system: A rigid thought form or idea about the nature of reality. It is closely related to Judgment. There are no belief systems without Judgments. We hold onto our beliefs with the rational mind. The term belief is not being used as in the sentence "I know that Love is the most important thing." This is a Universal Truth. If you truly believe in something, you need not hold onto it, you don't have to believe, you just know! The word "belief" is used in this book to describe fear-based, limiting thought patterns and ideas about the nature of reality. At its very core, a belief contains doubt.

Betzelmenu: בצלמנו: Image as in a photograph from the Hebrew, Tzilum, צילום.

Bina: בינה: Understanding inherent within Chochma (wisdom). Bina is part of the Tree of Life when it is in harmony with Chochma. When separated from Chochma, it is called Bina2.

Bina2: Knowledge of Good and Bad. The rational mind, is related to the mind of doubt. It is a limited, finite form of thought that is based in knowing from past experience in a defined way. Bina2 is one of the Sefirot of the Kabbalistic Tree of Knowledge.

BLT—Bottom Line Truth: A very deep Truth that encompasses and is the foundation for all other things. If you were able to directly experience all the BLTs written of in this book, you would be enlightened to a most wonderful degree. The BLTs are closely related and at times the same as the CaNs.

Bria: בריאה: The Kabbalistic World of Mind that became doubled, after Adam and Eve ate from The Tree of Knowledge, from the Divine Mind into rational mind.(Fire element)

CaN: Choices that are No Choice (plural). Choice that ain't No Choice (singular). Because we are still in duality consciousness, to choose Love seems like a *choice* in contrast to choosing fear, when there is really no choice at all than to choose Love. For example, there is no choice in being a racist. We are all One. All races are equal. For example, when I wake up to the Truth about who I am, I see there is no choice in trying to control another.

Chakra: Sanskrit for "wheel." Our chakras are funnels of spinning energy located on the front and back, as well as on the crown and base, of our bodies. They draw in the Universal energy that is the source of all life. There are seven chakras located on the body and nine chakras in total.

Chesed: חסד: Kindness, mercy, compassion. The term Chesed is one of the Sefirot of the Kabbalistic Tree of Life.

Chochma: חכמה: Wisdom. The type of thought of the divine mind, derived from feeling. It is intuition, guidance. Within Chochma, there is direct knowing making Chochma related to Da'at, True Knowledge. The term Chochma is one of the Sefirot of the Kabbalistic Tree of Life.

Choice: A mental function we use to choose between love-based reality and fear-based reality, between allowing and controlling, between equality and power-over. To "choose" is not the same as going to a store and having the option to select a pear, an apple or a plum. That's an "option." Here Choice is between the two types of reality named above.

The Circle of Nine: The Circle of Nine is a collection of Universal ways of Being, of love and harmony arranged into nine circles, by which you can choose to live for the purpose of healing. The ways of Being are discussed and explained in *The Last Four Books of Moses*. Once you succeed in healing yourself, you no longer need the Circle of Nine.

Collective Consciousness: Consciousness that we share as a people. There are collective consciousnesses within different cities, countries, regions, etc. Fear also creates another type of collective consciousness. We exist with "Oneness collective consciousness" when we all exist without resistance and outside of our fear-based reality of duality.

Con Trolls: Those who wish to control and maintain illusion. One of their tools is doubt.

Control: Using force to control a situation, trying too hard, imposing your Will onto someone else. It is judgment and fear-based. It is not used in the more positive context of being in control of yourself or having a situation under control. Letting go of control does not mean, "not being in charge."

Da'at: דעת: Knowledge. This type of Knowledge is direct knowing from experience. It is not knowledge of the contents of a book or subjects like math or history. That is Bina2. The term Da'at is one of the hidden Sefirot of the Kabbalistic Tree of Life.

Dabndoog: It is good and bad cut up by going through the definition-dicing, spinning blade of the Ever-Turning Sword.

Delusion: Believing something to be true that is based in illusion. A delusion is the same as a Belief system.

Dimyon: דמיון: Imagination.

Discernment: Is using your wisdom to determine whether something or someone is behaving or acting out of Love or Fear. Seeing that something is coming from fear or the desire to control doesn't mean you are judging that fear or desire for control. You are simply seeing it as it is— fear and desire for control. To discern the fear without judging it doesn't mean condoning it or that you want it to exist. The purpose of discernment becomes important when we wish to heal ourselves from our fear-based world. Discernment is the same as Gevourah from the Tree of Life.

Doctrine of Signatures: In botanical medicine and herbology, the doctrine of signatures decrees a plant's appearance reveals its medicinal properties. For example, *Ledum palustre* has many dots on its leaves, which appear to be little holes. The remedy is commonly used for puncture wounds.

Doubt: It's a thing of the past, related to the rational mind.

Duality: Existing within Unbalanced Positive and Unbalanced Negative instead of Balanced Positive. Also existing when both Love and fear exist as a reality for us, although fear is not a true reality.

Efferent: To give out. In the body's nervous system, the brain uses efferent nerves to send commands to the muscles. It is male in nature.

Ego: Energy that resists the superconduction of Love through you. It is the Self within the self. It is created by the action of the rational mind, which is the mind of doubt. Ego exists in a void absent of Love.

Ehye Usher Ehye: אהיה אשר אהיה: "I shall be as I shall be". Also translated, "I AM that I AM." A state of consciousness of a Being who is One with Allthatis. It is beheld within the time of Forwardness. Alternate meaning related to allowishing, "I wish to be and so I shall be."

Esser Sefirot: עשר ספירות: Ten branches of the Tree of Life.

Faith: Pure faith is beheld effortlessly within the heart and mind of a person who has released doubt. It is absolute knowing, beyond resistance and doubt. Faith is also acting in Love and Truth, despite feeling fear or doubt. Faith is knowing that what IS shall be.

Fear-based: Any choice, action or comment that comes from fear. This includes the fear of dying or the fear of getting hurt. It also includes behaving in a manner that controls, judges, or tries to take just for oneself (selfishness). Anything not based in Love is fear-based. Fear-based choices that we think we must make are an illusion. Fear is always an illusion, thus, one thing that we can always know for sure is that there is nothing to fear (Sixth Circle). But this is not the same as saying, "There is nothing I wish for" or "There is nothing I love."

Flame of the Ever-Turning Sword, The: The flame of the sword that spins at the threshold blocking the way back to the Garden of Eden. **Gen 3:24** To return to Eden and the Tree of Life, one must go through this final barrier.

Four Worlds, The Kabbalistic: 1) Atzilut, Source, the World of Yod, י, the Great Undefined. 2) Bria, the World of the Mind. 3) Yetzirah, the World of Emotions and Creativity. 4) Assiyah, the World of the Physical and Action.

Frmee Will: The Will of the self within the self. *Selfish* Will. For me, me, me. It resides in self-conscience, which feels like guilt. It is the energy of our ego and gives us the potential to choose outside of our true nature in fear, doubt, and judgment-based choices. Fear-based choices come from Frmee Will in the World of Illusion.

Game, The: The Game is life in the physical world where your true nature is put to the test. It is having choice between Love and Fear.

Ganallisone: Another word for the Garden of Eden, where all is One. Gan (pronounced "gun") is the Hebrew word for "Garden." It is the same as the World to Come.

Gan Edan: גן עדן: The Garden of Eden, the World to Come, Ganallisone.

Gematria: The numerical value for a Hebrew letter or word.

Gevourah: גבורה: Strength. Discernment. When balanced with its counterpart "Chesed" (Mercy/Compassion), Gevourah is strength, discernment and one of the ten sefirot that exist on the left column of the Tree of Life. When separated from Chesed, it is called Gevourah2, and represents judgment.

Gevourah2: Gevourah2 is the true nature of Gevourah, strength, turned around, becoming judgment of Good and Bad and control, which is part of the left column of the Tree of Knowledge for Good and Bad.

God: The Creator, Love. Hashem. Balanced Positive and undefined. Experienceable, but not rationally knowable or quantifiable, just as you may feel Love but you cannot explain or hold onto it in a rational manner. God is Allthatis from the verb "to be" and the most sacred names of God, אהיה and יהוה, which means everything that is, that is True. Anything else is untrue, illusion. The Balanced Positive, God, therefore is not comprised of the balance between Good and Bad. It is AllGood.

Hanuchash: הנחש: The Serpent. That which opposes Love.

Hara: Ball-like energy center located two inches below the navel. From this energy center comes our Will to live. It is the propeller of Forwardness. (Fig. 1 and 1b)

Hashem: השם: A commonly used name of God.

Hebrews: Chosen people to take on the vibration of the Tree of Knowledge for Good and Bad and then to move through that vibration and return to the Tree of Life vibration. Chosen to play the Game of Life. A Hebrew person is not limited to being Jewish, but can also include those who align him or herself with higher consciousness for Love and the healing of the planet. The Hebrews are the Hoovids, from the civilization of Hoova.

Hod: One of the branches (Sefirot) of the Tree of Life. Also translated as "splendor," it is great confidence and self-esteem that carries forth the humility and gratitude of being in God's service (Netzhach). Hod is part of the Tree of Life when it is in harmony with Netzach (Humility). When it is separated from Netzach, and turns onto itself, it is called Hod2.

Hod2: Vanity, haughtiness. Without the connection to the humility of Netzach, the true feeling of confidence turns around so that the person is absorbed in their self-importance. One of the Sefirot of the Kabbalistic Tree of Knowledge.

Homeopathic Elixir of Life, The: A combination of different homeopathic remedies that match the fallen layers of our genes. For the purpose of healing those genes and helping us return to our true nature.

Homeopathy: A powerful, gentle medicine based on the universal healing principle of "like cures like" (Latin: *Similimum similibus curentur*).

This means that the same substance in nature that causes a specific, unique disease-state in a healthy individual will cure another person who is ill with that specific, unique diseased state regardless of whether or not that person was previously influenced by that substance. See more in Appendix C.

Hoova:הובה : The Civilization of Love. It is a "state" of unconditional love that is the Messianic consciousness. The Hoovids come from Hoova (related to the Kabbalistic World of Assiyah).

Humility: Seeing all of creation with awe and wonder and feeling full of gratitude for the opportunity to be a part of it. Feeling blessed to share the experience of life with all equal Beings. Humility is Love. Humility is also accepting the simplicity of greatness and seeing that all people, in their true nature, are great.

Ibeall world: The Ibeall world is the World where I am One with everything. It is beyond Frmee Will and it is where Will is one with feeling, thus there is no distinction or necessity to clarify which is which. In the Ibeall world, *all that I am is Beingness.*

Illusion: What is not real and yet can be experienced as being real. It is the opposite of Truth and therefore is the same as fear. The fallen energies are all based in illusion.

Judgment: A label that we put on something when we think it is bad, or wrong. It is a decision outside of Love, related to a Belief system, because we believe something must be a certain way, we judge it as bad when it is not. Judgment is not to be mistaken for Discernment. When one makes a judgment, one is blocking the flow of Love within them by placing a "bad" label on something. When one makes a discernment, one is seeing where something is coming from and whether or not they would like to be aligned with it or not. Judgment is Gevourah2.

Kabbalah: קבלה :"That which is received." There are many texts written on Kabbalah, the most infamous being *The Zohar*, by Rabbi Shimone Bar Yochai, yet the Kabbalah remains the unwritten mystery from the sea of Truth that is revealed to each person who opens his or her heart and mind to receive. The Kabbalah is experienced by receiving the Truth because of the direct feeling and connection with the Shekinah, the female aspect of God.

Kidmutenu: כדמותנו: From the Hebrew word Dama, דמה, which means "to compare, to resemble." However, there is another word from the same root with a different meaning: the Hebrew word Dima, דימה, which means "to imagine."

Knowledge (True): A deep sense of direct knowing that comes from the experience of the Source that is One with the divine.

Love: Love is God. The definition of Love in *the Keys of Enoch* glossary is: "The substance of Eternal Life. It is created in the believer by the Shekinah holy spirit" p. 586. The essence of Love ranges far beyond its romantic concept. It is kindness, humility, courage, charity, faith, strength, joy, patience, gratitude, effortless and all the things that make you glow golden.

Messed-Up Humility: Feeling guilty for greatness and attempting to hide or lessen it. Shrinking so that others won't feel insecure around you. Listening to the grumpy old judgmental voice that says, "Who do you think you are?" Worrying way too much about sounding egotistical. It is your true nature blocked up in Unbalanced Positive and has been a very deep issue preventing your return to your true nature. Messed-up Humility is denying who you are!

Miasm: A disease that is passed on genetically.

Mirror-imagine: The state of consciousness in which we exist that is the negative, like the negative of a photograph, of the consciousness of our Higher Self. It is our Higher Self mirrored inward held in our imagination.

Moshiach: משיח: The Messiah. An age equivalent to the World to Come. It is the Return to Eden. It is a state of consciousness of absolute, unconditional Love for all people and all nations. It is not embodied or brought by one person (on a donkey), but by many people awakened to that state of consciousness.

Nabulous: Being cloudy in the Unbalanced Positive. From New Age Bull (NAB)!

Netzach: נצח: Also translated as "victory" and "eternity," it is the great humility and gratitude felt being in service to God and in being one of God's creations. The term Netzach is one of the Sefirot of the Kabbalistic Tree of Life.

Oneness: A state of Being or consciousness of the Balanced Positive. It is collective consciousness beyond all fear and judgment. Oneness is God.

Or L'Goyim: Light unto the nations.

Others/Opposition: The opposition to Love. The energy that tries to keep you tied to the past and to doubt. They are the Con Trolls whose realm is in illusion. The others were created by God for the purpose of creating challenge in the Game, but do not make up part of the balance of God.

Physical: The World in which we live and the state in which we exist as human beings. It includes the definition of a human as having two arms, two legs and the senses to feel, taste, see, hurt, and enjoy. *To be trapped in the physical* means to believe we are rooted to the Earth and limited only to the physical body within which we live. To give up all fear, resistance, and illusion and achieve Oneness is still to remain physical (two arms, legs, senses) yet it is to no longer remain trapped in a dense body. It is to be in this world, but not of this world, a Soul as a whole Light Being.

Rational mind: Also Bina2. The rational mind works based in the past. Having learned something to be a certain way in the past, the rational mind holds onto this past experience as if it is reality. The rational mind becomes fixated onto this learned piece of information. This mind is separated from our true nature and is doubt-based. The rational mind is in conjunction with everything outside of the Love spectrum. It is at the core root of judgment and fear, and is related to the ego. It is associated with trying to be like God in knowing what is Good and Bad, or right and wrong.

Seals of the chakras: These are primordial energy blockages that sit in between the front and rear chakras in our body, blocking off our experience of Oneness and resulting in Duality. They began after Adam and Eve ate from the Tree of Knowledge for Good and Bad.

Self within the Self: This is the part of us that is trapped within ourselves and looks out only for ourselves. It began a long time ago when we felt scared for the first time or were hurt and began to look out for ourselves. It is self-conscious, meaning not only that it always looks out for itself but also looks *at* itself. It feels guilty. It is the same as the ego and empowers Frmee Will.

Shekinah: שכינה: The Goddess. She is also the Holy Spirit. Ruach HaKodesh, רוח הקודש.

Three Major Delusions, The: 1) Trying to Be like God in Being better than others (Hod2); 2) In Knowing better than others (Bina2); and 3) Knowing Good and Bad, passing judgment on others (Gevourah2). Read more about the Three Major Delusions in **Appendix B.**

Three Treasures, The: Chinese medicine philosophy that states the relationship between mind, qi (energy), and blood. The mind governs the qi which governs the blood. We can translate this also to be mind governs the emotions which governs the body.

Threshold, The: The threshold is the limit between duality and Oneness. It is poised right at Zero point. Although crossing the threshold involves releasing Frmee Will and reemerging into the time of Forwardness and a state of AllGood, it does not mean going somewhere else. It is here and now and has always been. The Flame of the Ever-Turning Sword sits at the Threshold.

Tikkun Olum: The healing/reparation of the World, the true calling of the Jewish people and the highest state of being for all people.

Time of Forwardness: This is the time of Ehye Usher Ehye, I shall be as I shall be, when the past has been completely released. It is the World to Come.

Tree of Life: From the Kabbalah, the Tree of Life is a model used to describe the different levels of reality and the nature of a human being. On the Tree of Life there are 10 branches, called the Esser Sefirot, which have specific attributes just as the different chakras located on our body have different attributes. The fruits from the Tree of Life grant immortality and are eaten in the Garden of Eden.

Truth (Universal): Truth that cannot be defined. Truth is God/Goddess/the Absolute/the Balanced Positive/Love. It is a way of Being experienced through the feeling of a Soul that has given up fear and judgment. It cannot be conveyed rationally without limiting its infinite, undefined nature, which would render it non-truthful. It can be known through direct experience. It is Universal and thus experienced in the same essence in myriad different ways. When Truth is written with a capitol "T," Truth refers to the Truth that is Universal for all Beings.

Tzarah: צרה: Trouble, distress, conflict. In Yiddish, it is Tzouris. Samuel Hahnemann, the founder of homeopathy, used Tzarah to describe the genetic predisposition to disease (miasm) stemming from the "original sin." He called it Psora.

Unbalanced Negative: The energy and way of fear, control, judgment, power over, greed, and bottomless pit desire. It is the male when it is separated from the female. It is in competition with the Creator and tries to be like God inanotsoniceway.

Unbalanced Positive: The energy and way that tries to make everything and see everything as perfect and will not see/recognize a negative situation. It is mistaking non-judgmentalness for saying that everything is okay, no matter what. It is denying what is there to see, if it is seen as negative. It leads to suppression. It is also shrinking or putting yourself in a box so that you don't make people feel insecure or threaten them. It is being goody-two-shoes and overly polite, like apologizing when someone steps on your foot. It is also being giving at the wrong time. It is related to NAB. Focusing on the positive in a situation is good. This is not unbalanced positive. Always seeing the good in a situation is divine. When you can *only* see the good and you are blind to the Bad, you are being Unbalanced Positive. It is how the female energy can be when separated from the male.

Unconscious/Subconscious: Something that exists or occurs beyond our conscious awareness.

Y Factor: Also written as the "γ Factor." It is the need to know, and the need to control and hold onto fixed ideas about the way things are. It fears the unknown and is closely related to the rational mind.

Yetzir HaRah: The same as Frmee Will and the Will to resist. This is the "bad" Will, the Will that opposes God. It was adopted from the Serpent after we ate from the tree of Knowledge for Good and Bad.

Yetzir HaTov: Our "good" Will, one with God's Will.

Yetzirah: יְצִירה: The Kabbalistic World of Emotions and Creativity that became doubled after the Tree of Knowledge from Divine Emotions into negative emotions (water element).

Zero Point: The same as Balanced Positive and Oneness. A state/place at the core of your true self that is nature beyond all limitations. It represents the marriage point between your finite and infinite selves. It is poised upon the threshold between the reality of duality and Oneness. The term zero point was borrowed from Greg Braden's concept in *Awakening to Zero Point*. It is beyond the magnetic field of the Earth reality.

Zone of Cold, The: The point of pure potentiality at which no movement of molecules on the physical plane occurs. This is zero resistance. Zero Kelvin, or absolute zero, in a spiritual sense. The point of pure potential, where anything is possible known as the zero-point field. This term was derived from *The Only Planet of Choice*.

Figure 1a

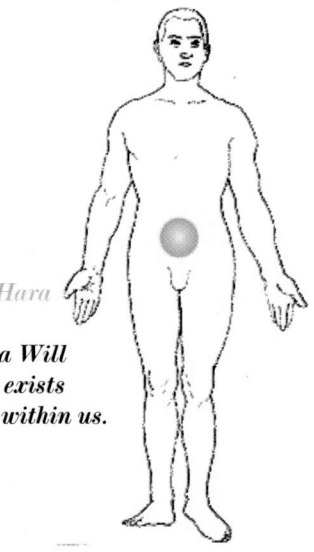

Hara

s a Will
t exists
p within us.

Figure 1b

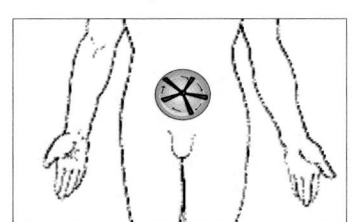

The Hara **- Propeller of Forwardness**

Figure 3:

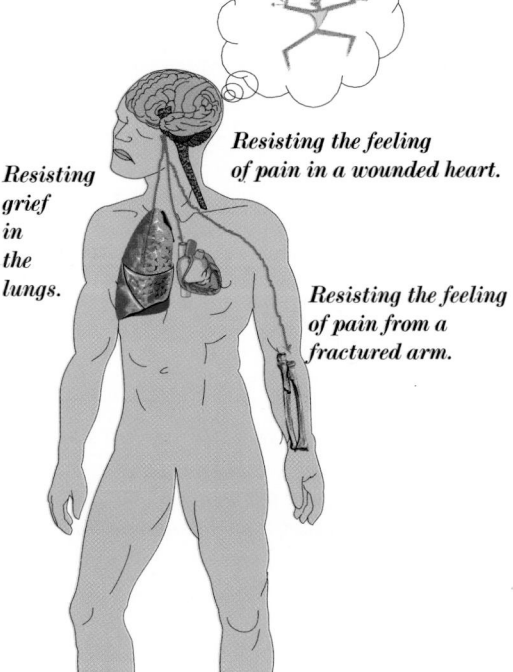

Resisting the feeling
of pain in a wounded heart.

Resisting
grief
in
the
lungs.

Resisting the feeling
of pain from a
fractured arm.

Figure 2:
he Will to Resist Dude in the Rational Mind

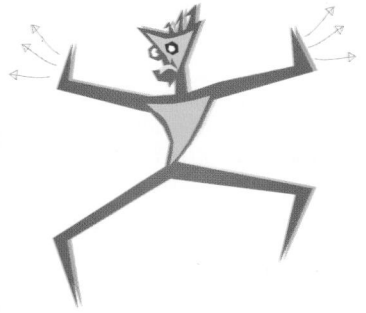

The Will to Resist comes
out from the rational mind, centered up
thin the brain, and says NO to feeling (if it
judged it as bad) and pushes out against it.

Figure 4

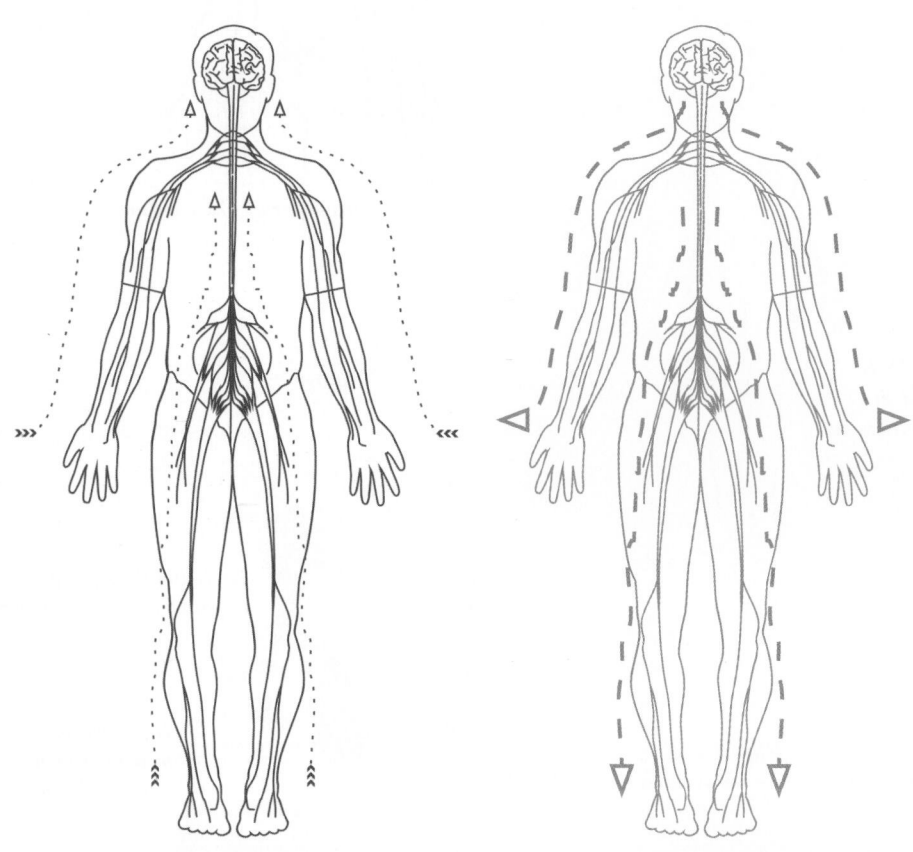

Afferent
sensory, input for pain
and temperature
sensation = spinothalamic tract

Efferent
motor, output
voluntary movement of skeletal
muscle mostly controlled by
the corticospinal tract

Figure 5

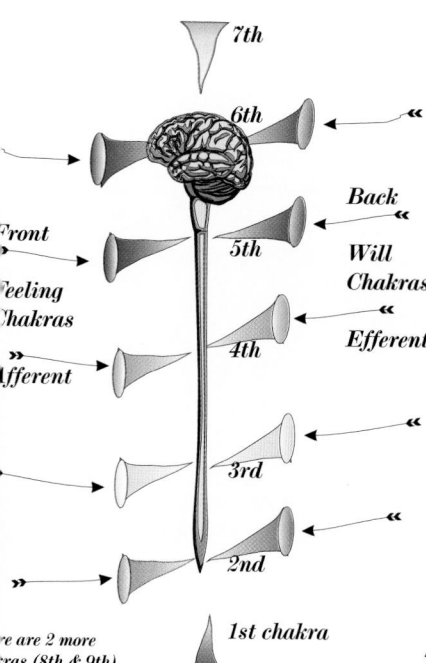

7th

6th

Front

Back

5th

Will
Chakras

Feeling
Chakras

Efferent

Afferent

4th

3rd

2nd

1st chakra

There are 2 more chakras (8th & 9th) situated on the body.

Figure 6

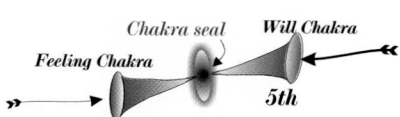

Chakra seal

Will Chakra

Feeling Chakra

5th

Here we see the Will chakra exerting too much force and blocking the flow of the feeling chakra, creating a chakra seal.

Figure 7

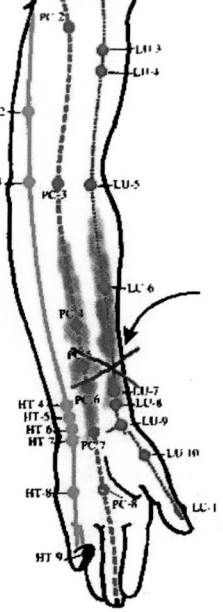

PC 2

LU 3

LU 4

HT 2

HT 3

PC 3

LU 5

LU 6

PC 5

LU 7

HT 4

PC 6

LU 8

HT 5

LU 9

HT 6

HT 7

PC 7

LU 10

HT 8

PC 8

LU 1

HT 9

A break in the radius bone has led to a blockage and a local excess in the area within the pericardium and lung channels. This blockage and decrease in energy flow will lead to loss of feeling of the body and rigidity.

Figure 8

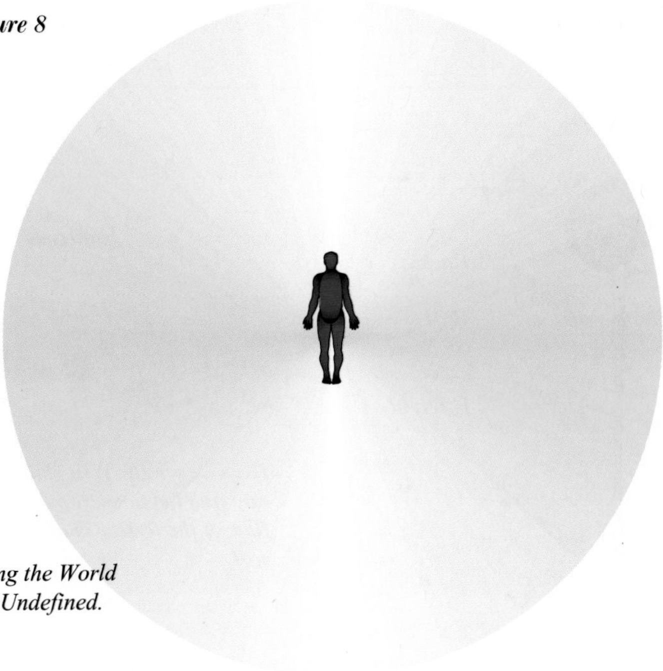

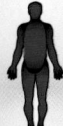

*Entering the World
of the Undefined.*

Figure 9

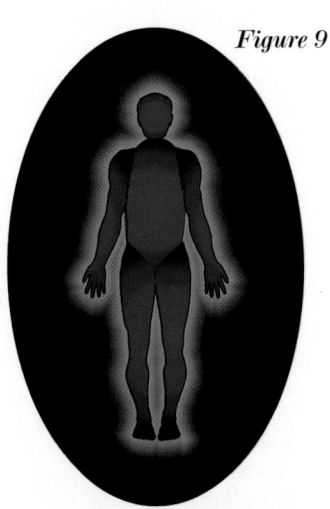

Fig. 10: A clip of the Tree of Life.

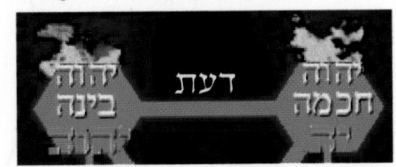

Bina - Understanding   Chochma - Wisdom

The vibration of אהיה אשר אהיה
*is beyond Frmee Will. There is a golden glow
that surrounds a being who has given up their
Frmee Will.*

Figure 11

Threshold is crossed from Oneness - fall in consciousness.

Aha! Now I can experience who I AM.

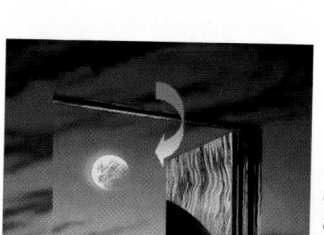

nnocence – I AM What is this that I AM?

Progression: Forgetting of the true self and existence within pain and struggle with Frmee Will.

Return across the Threshold

World of All Good (Imagination)

WORLD OF GOOD & BAD

World of All Good (Experience)

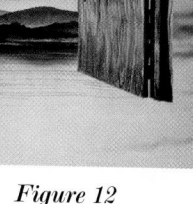

Take a step through the threshold into the here and now…

Figure 12

Figure 13

Collective Love/Fear Consciousness – The sea of Consciousness that
we create depends on what we are aligned with: Love or Fear? Both seas exist now
and anyone can tap into either at any time (there is always choice).

**Collective Consciousness
of Love**

**Collective Consciousness
of Fear**

Kindness, kinship, unity, Love.

*Limiting, rigid belief systems,
control, power-over, greed, Frmee*

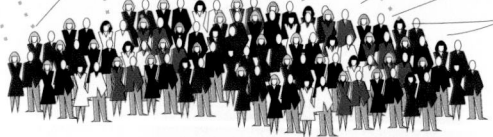

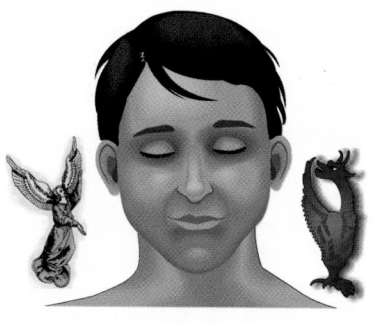

Figure 14

An angel in one ear. A devil in the other.

*Figure 15: The Two Selves -
constantly in opposition
within the World of Frmee Will.*

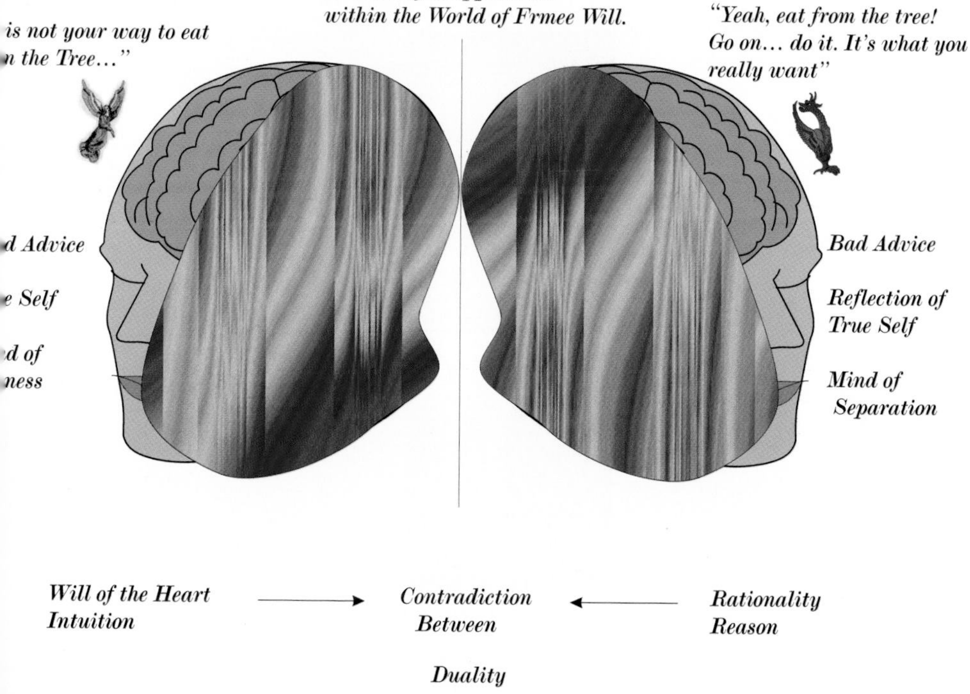

is not your way to eat
n the Tree…"

"Yeah, eat from the tree!
Go on… do it. It's what you
really want"

d Advice

Bad Advice

e Self

Reflection of
True Self

d of
ness

Mind of
Separation

Will of the Heart   ⟶   Contradiction   ⟵   Rationality
Intuition   Between   Reason

Duality

Figure 16 Anacardium orientale fruit on leaf.

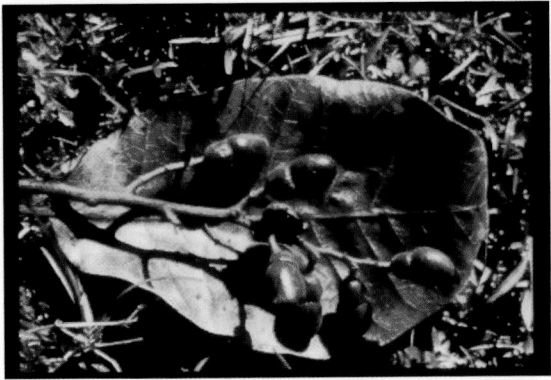

Photograph courtesy of Professor H.Y. Mohan Ram - Delhi, India

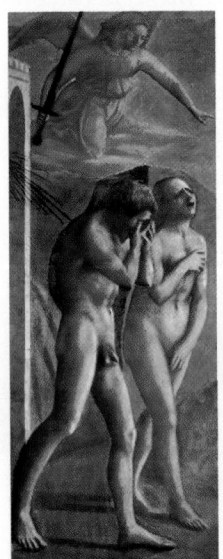

Notice the shame and how it is portrayed as if they are being thrown out of the Garden. This is the way much of the ancient art depicts this subject and symbolizes our beliefs relating to this subject.

Figure 17: Masaccio 1427

*Adam and Eve
Expelled from Paradise*

Figure 18a

*These are the directions
of flow in duality.*

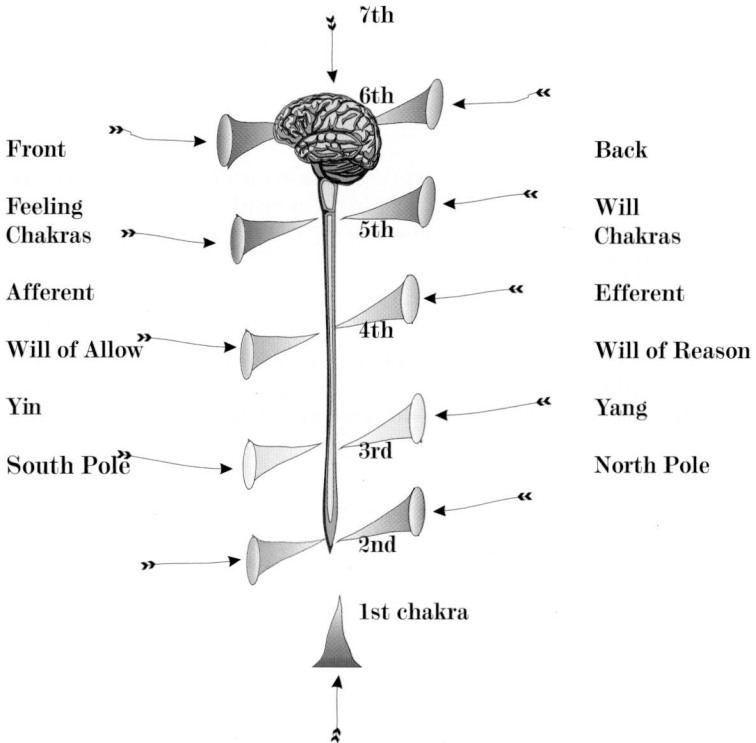

7th

6th

Front

Feeling
Chakras

Afferent

Will of Allow

Yin

South Pole

5th

4th

3rd

2nd

1st chakra

Back

Will
Chakras

Efferent

Will of Reason

Yang

North Pole

*Recall from the first chapter on resistance
how the Will chakras resist the flow of the
feeling chakras if our ego-mind so chooses.*

Figure 18b

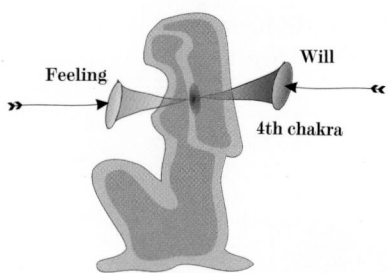

Feeling

Will

4th chakra

These two chakras (feeling and Will of the fourth/heart chakra) now work
opposite to the way in which the North and South of a magnet function.
In a magnet, the South Pole draws in the Energy and the North Pole
extends the energy.

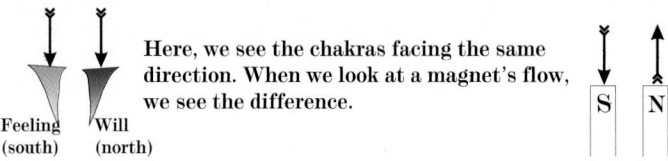

The way it is now, within Frmee Will, is that both chakras are drawing
in energy. This is like having one foot on the gas, one foot on the brake. This
makes the flow through them the same when placed right side up next to each
other.

Feeling
(south)

Will
(north)

Here, we see the chakras facing the same
direction. When we look at a magnet's flow,
we see the difference.

S   N

If they are both spinning clockwise, they are in contradiction
to each other as in these chakras that have a seal plugging
up their center.

Chakra seal   North/Will Chakra

South/Feeling
Chakra

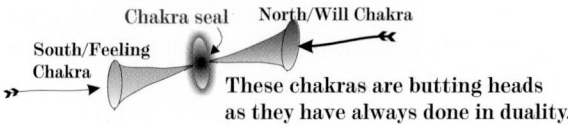

These chakras are butting heads
as they have always done in duality.

Figure 18c

They are equal and opposite in the Balanced Positive reality as in the flow of magnet
which is a perpetual system. This is how the Oneness is created within the center.

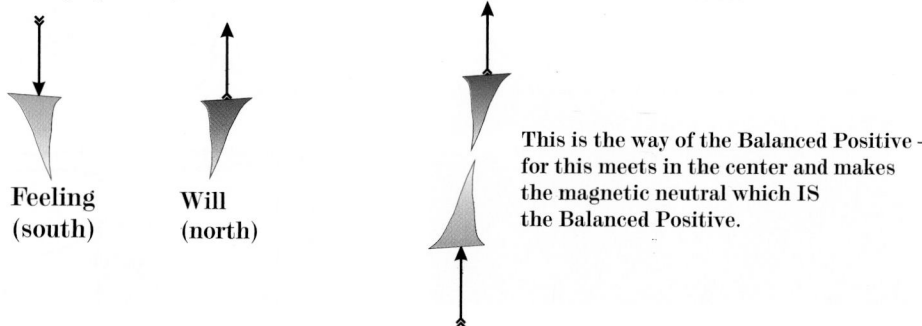

Feeling   Will
(south)   (north)

This is the way of the Balanced Positive –
for this meets in the center and makes
the magnetic neutral which IS
the Balanced Positive.

ote: This is the same for the feeling and Will chakras. The feeling chakras act as the
outh pole and the Will chakras act as the North pole beyond the chakra seals and beyond Frmee Will
the World to Come.

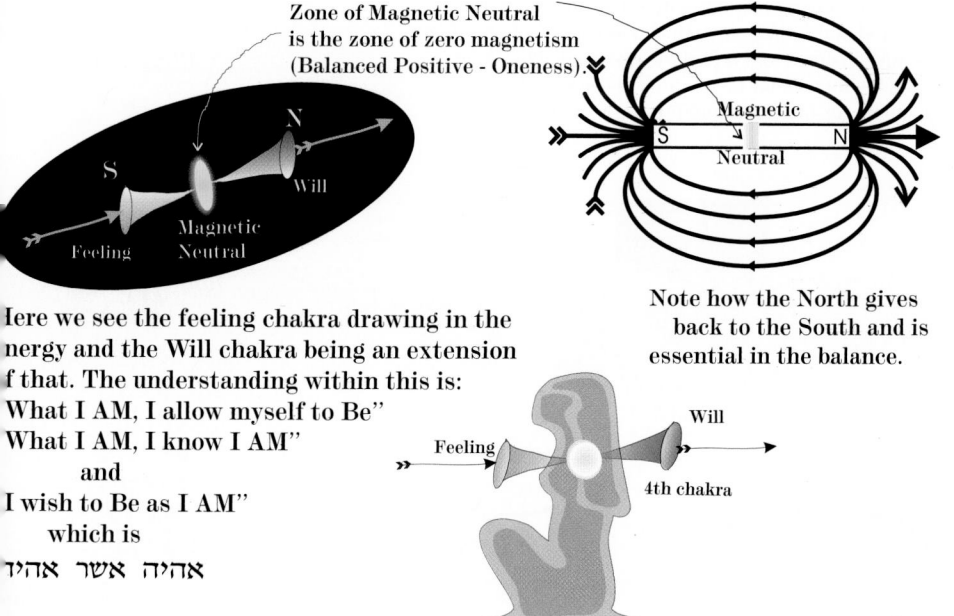

Zone of Magnetic Neutral
is the zone of zero magnetism
(Balanced Positive - Oneness).

Note how the North gives
back to the South and is
essential in the balance.

Iere we see the feeling chakra drawing in the
nergy and the Will chakra being an extension
f that. The understanding within this is:
What I AM, I allow myself to Be"
What I AM, I know I AM"
        and
I wish to Be as I AM"
    which is
אהיה אשר אהיד

Figure 19

Left visual field   **Right visual field**

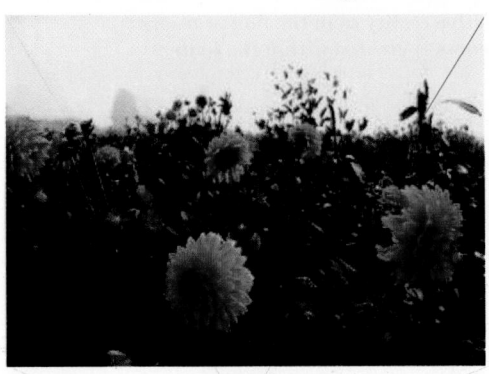

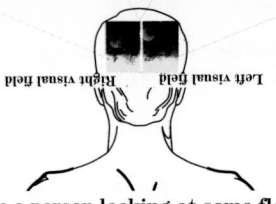

Here, we see a person looking at some flowers. Notice how the right visual field is seen in the left hemisphere of the brain, upside down and left-right reversed. The same is true for the left visual field which is seen in the right hemisphere upside down and left-right reversed.

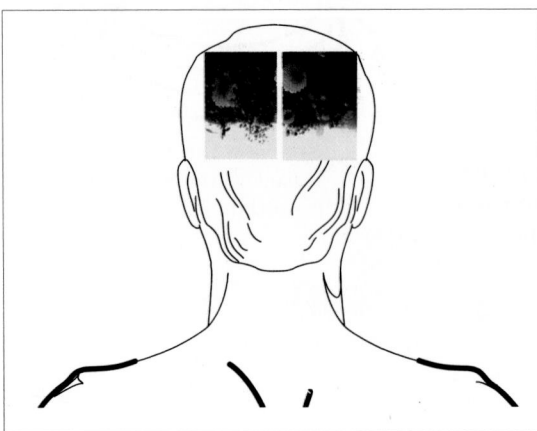

Figure 20: Da Vinci Revisite

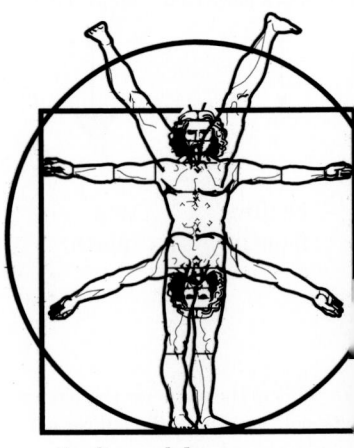

*As above so below.
What is felt in the left shoulder,
for example, also influences wha
felt energetically in the right hip*

Figure 21

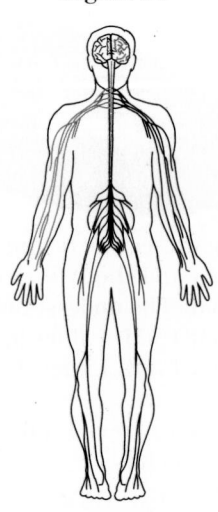

Sensations are felt (imagin
on the opposite side .

Figure 22: The Homunculus

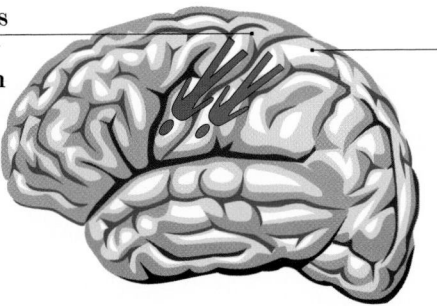

Precentral Gyrus
Efferent –Motor
Nucleus in Brain

Postcentral Gyrus
Afferent –Sensory
Feeling Nucleus
in Brain

Really, the homunculus is not proportionally represented in the brain for size of the body part but for the amount of sensitivity or fine motor skill.

The homunculus (seen within the motor (red) and sensory (blue) nuclei) is upside down and backward.

Figure 23

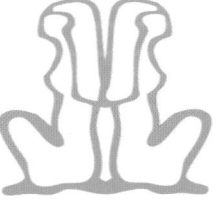

There is a double that sits behind us
Front and Back – Z axis

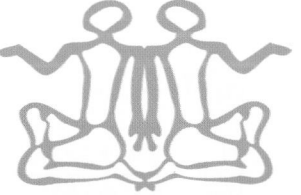

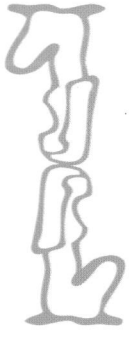

There is a double that sits above us
Up and down – Y axis

There is a double that sits beside us

Left and right –X axis

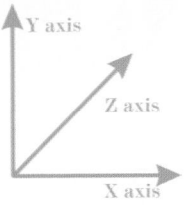

An ancient Native American legend tells how we use to live with our double attached to our backs. Then the gods separated us and life became all about trying to find your other half. The Torah tells a similar story.

Figure 24

Figure 25

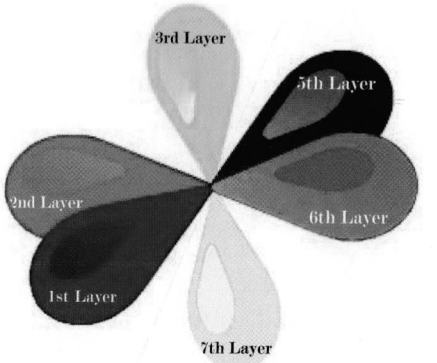

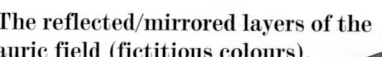

The reflected/mirrored layers of the auric field (fictitious colours).

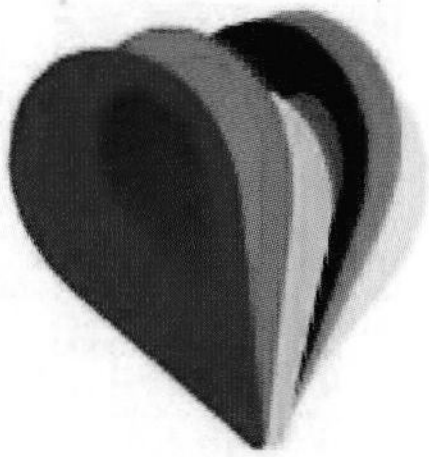

Figure 24 shows how the lower levels of the auric field are the reflections of the higher ones. However, they exist simultaneously withi the 'same space,' as it is in this figure.

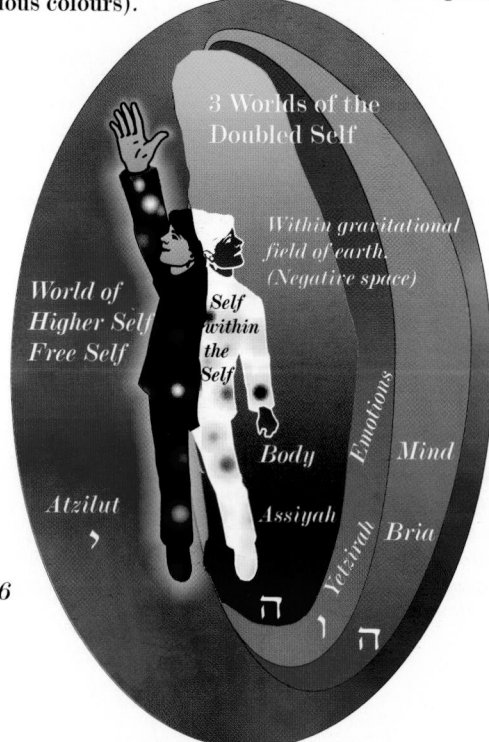

Figure 26

The Kabbalistic Four Worlds
Here, we see the reflection of the three worlds of Bria, Yetzirah, and Assiyah
and that which is beyond duality - Atzilut.

Figure 21. The Embodiment Four Worlds

The First World
Atzilut – The Infinite and Undefined.
Ain Sof.

There is no division within. All duality begins within the Second World. Atzilut represents the World beyond the Threshold of judgment. It is AllGood. It never became separated into duality.

The duality lens (behind the eyes)

Soul Seat – the soul's purpose. From here comes the Will of the Heart

Hara Will to Live

The Second World
Bria – Mind
The Level of kavanah which is the level of intention.

Within the earth consciousness, There is already division within the mind. As it returns to harmony, it all comes back together into the heart, and then there is entrance back into the World of Atzilut.

In the auric field it is the 3rd (rational mind) level and 7th Divine Mind level. The 7th is the blueprint for the 3rd which is thus its negative.

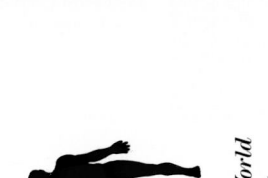

The Third World
Yetzirah – Emotions.
The level of the chakras and the level of the auric field.

Here, the division gets translated down from the second world into the split between Will and feeling. This manifests as the chakra seal and keeps things in duality. This is the level of emotions. In the auric field it is the 2nd level & 6th level – Divine emotions, communion with the Divine. The 6th is the template for the 2nd and thus The 2nd is the reverse of the 6th level.

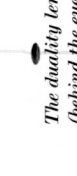

The Fourth World
Assiyah – Body

The level of the Divine Body and the physical body. The division is passed down into the body from the 2nd and 3rd Worlds. This duality manifests as sympathetic/ parasympathetic, as efferent and afferent, sensory and motor systems that are not in harmony.

This also represents the body. In the Auric Field it is the 1st – physical body and the 5th Divine Body. The 5th level is the template for the 1st level and thus, the physical body is the reverse/ negative of the 5th.

Figure 28: The Aleph, The Magnet and The Balanced Positive

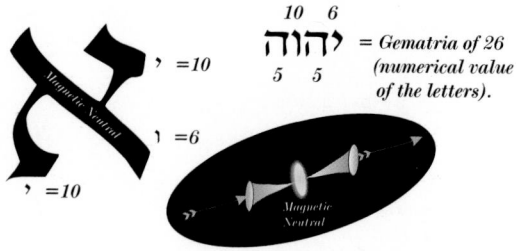

10   6

יהוה = Gematria of 26
5   5   (numerical value
of the letters).

י =10

ו =6

י =10

Magnetic Neutral

Figure 29: Tree of Life or Tree of Knowledge?

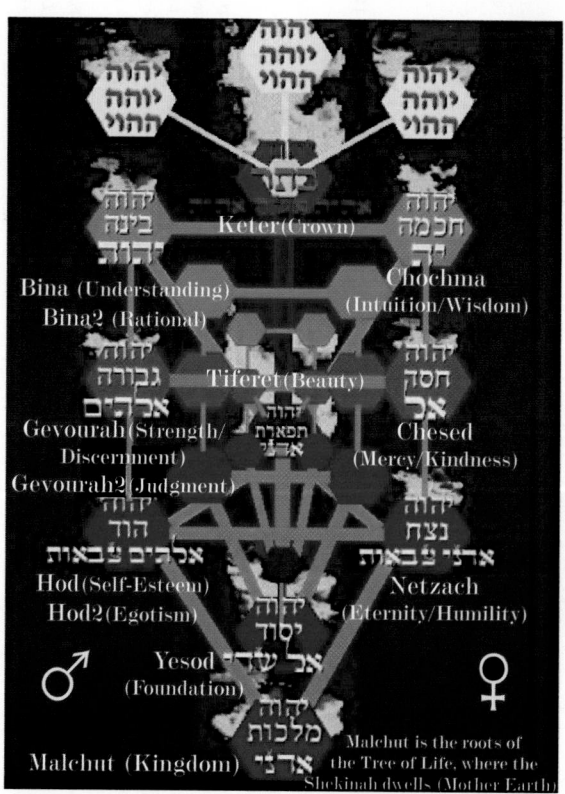

The Tree of Life as we have called this image
yet this is not always so! The Tree of Life is
beheld within Oneness consciousness, not
duality, not separation. Not one telling you to
do to what the other is opposed to. Not one
seeing all with mercy and compassion
(Chesed), the other with judgment (Gevourah).
Not one seeing with wisdom (Chochma), the
other with fragmented rationality (Bina2).
Not one feeling grateful and humble (Netzach)
to be in God's service and the other getting
carried away in ego and vanity (Hod2).
One is the true nature, the other, the reflection
of that true nature, the negative aspect,
the reverse.

So when we see this image and the left column
contains Bina2, Gevourah2, Hod2, this is
really The Tree of Knowledge for Good and Bad

(And if you flip the left column over, you will
see the Tree of Life with Bina (Understanding)
Gevourah (Strength) and Hod (Self-Esteem)
(see figure 30).

An error we have made is in believing that the left column
is female (Rational/Understanding, Strength/Judgement,
Haughtiness/Self-Esteem) and the right column is
male (Intuition/Wisdom, Mercy/Kindness, Humility)
The right column is truly female - the left is male.

Figure 30: Tree of Knowledge vs. Tree of Life

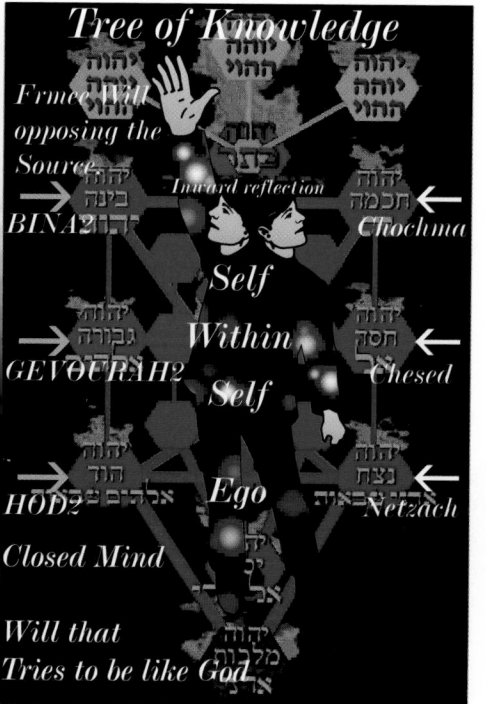

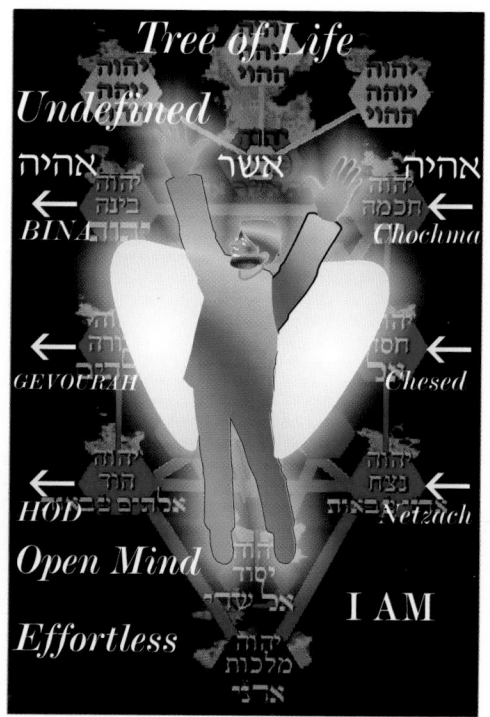

Figure 31

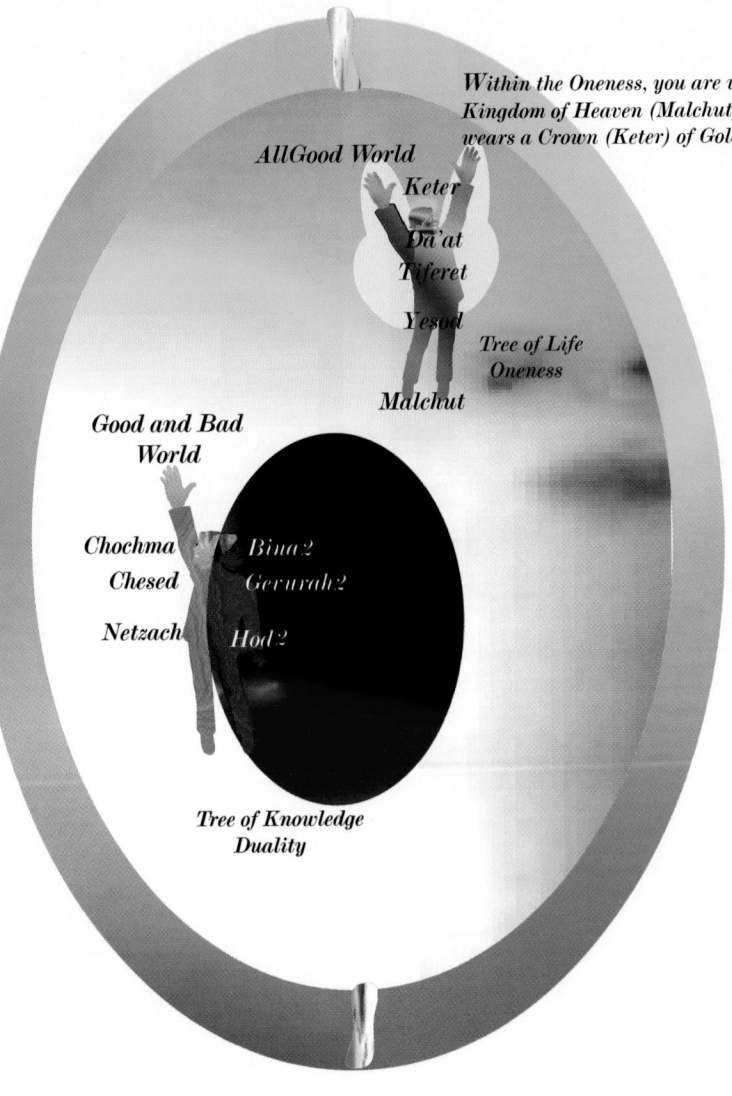

Within the Oneness, you are within the Kingdom of Heaven (Malchut) where one wears a Crown (Keter) of Golden Light.

AllGood World

Keter
Da'at
Tiferet
Yesod

Tree of Life
Oneness

Malchut

Good and Bad World

Chochma
Chesed
Netzach

Bina2
Gevurah2
Hod2

Tree of Knowledge
Duality

Figure 32

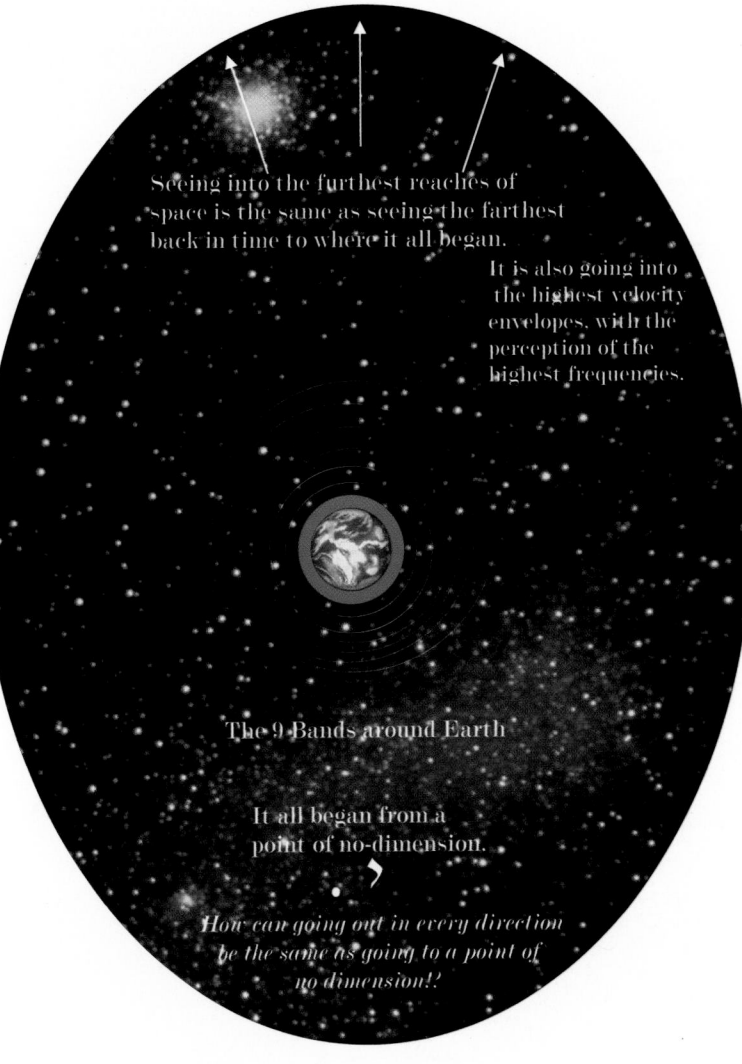

Seeing into the furthest reaches of
space is the same as seeing the farthest
back in time to where it all began.

It is also going into
the highest velocity
envelopes, with the
perception of the
highest frequencies.

The 9 Bands around Earth

It all began from a
point of no-dimension.

*How can going out in every direction
be the same as going to a point of
no dimension!!*

Figure 33

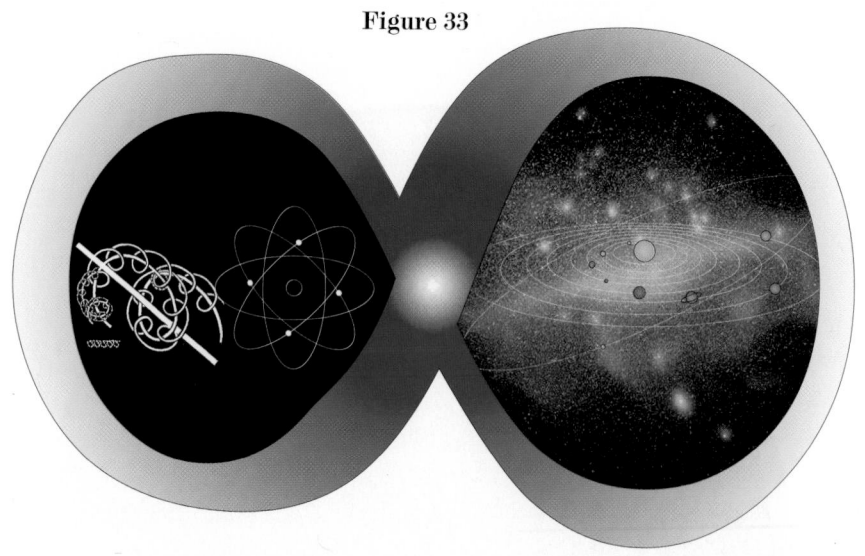

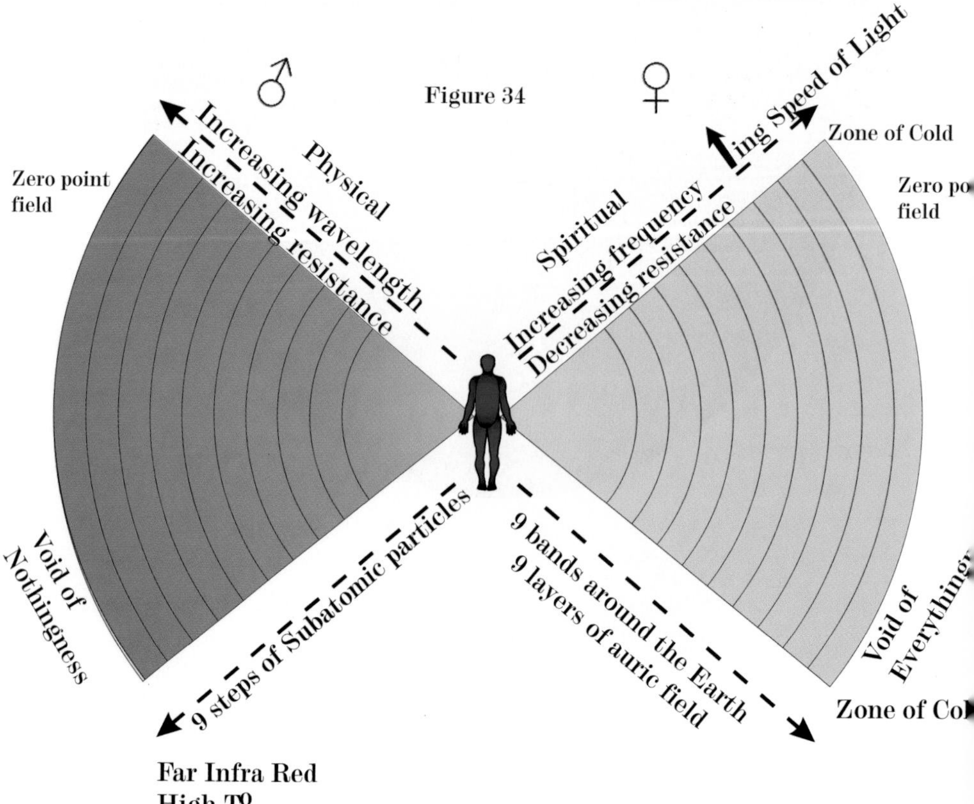

Figure 34

♂ ♀

Zero point field

Increasing wavelength
Increasing resistance

Physical

Spiritual

Increasing frequency
Decreasing resistance

Increasing Speed of Light

Zone of Cold

Zero point field

9 steps of Subatomic particles

9 bands around the Earth
9 layers of auric field

Void of Nothingness

Void of Everything

Zone of Col

Far Infra Red
High T°

Figure 35: The Reversal/ Mirroring of Time

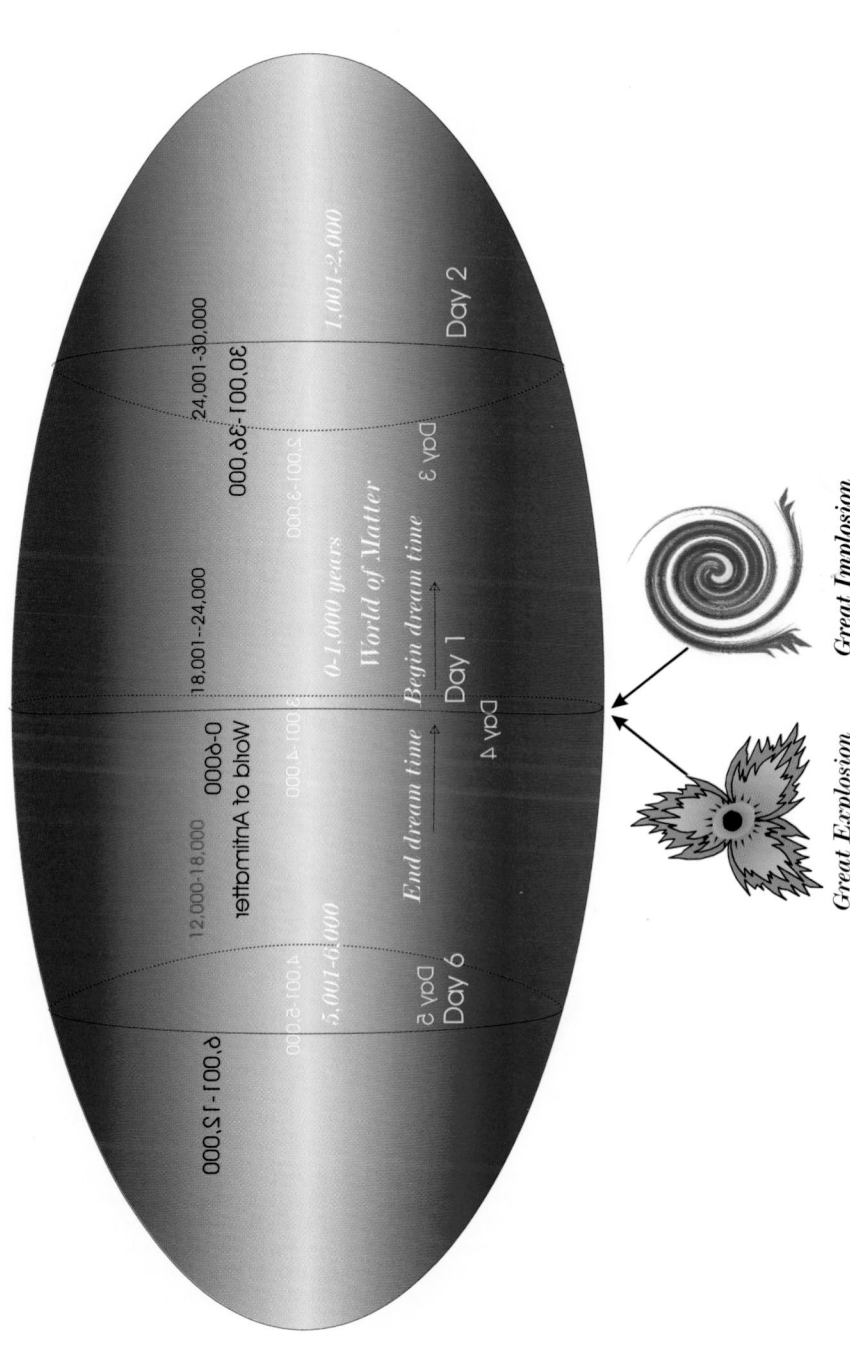

6,001-12,000

5,001-6,000   Day 6

4,001-5,000

12,000-18,000   0-6,000   World of Antimatter

18,001-24,000

End dream time

Day 4

0-1,000 years   *World of Matter*   Begin dream time

Day 1

3,001-3,000

24,001-30,000

30,001-36,000   Day 3

1,001-2,000   Day 2

Great Explosion

Great Implosion

Figure 36: The Direction of Flow in Yin and Yang Channels
(see also Figure 43)

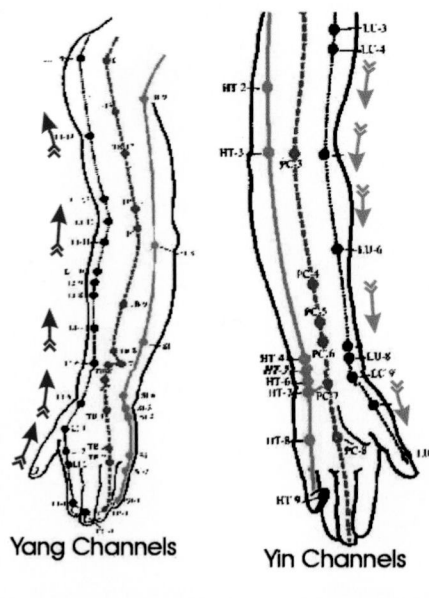

Yang Channels   **Yin Channels**

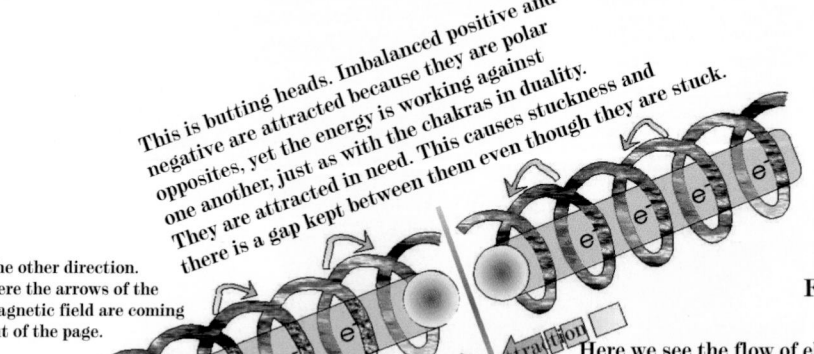

This is butting heads. Imbalanced positive and negative are attracted because they are polar opposites, yet the energy is working against one another, just as with the chakras in duality. They are attracted in need. This causes stuckness and there is a gap kept between them even though they are stuck.

The other direction. Here the arrows of the magnetic field are coming out of the page.

Figure 37

Magnetic attraction

Gap

Here we see the flow of electrons through a copper wire. The resistance in the wire creates a magnetic field coiling around the wire in the direction shown.(above arrows going into the page

This principle is similar to the way in which the energy (Qi) flows through the acupuncture meridians. In the world with no resistance, as the flow of Yin and Yang (female and male) is perfectly harmonized as One, there is unity of direction creating super-conductivity. Once there is no more resistance impeding the flow of the chakras or acupuncture meridians, the Yin/Yang channels will couple their bi-directional flow into unidirectional flow that is One and create a Balanced Positive flow in all directions (hyper-conductivity (superconductivity in all directions)) - This is the reestablishment of the flow of the axiotonal lines.

ecently, there were discovered some elements that have been called rbitally Rearranged Monoatomic Elements (ORMEs).

he discovery was done by a man named David Hudson. These ORMEs are mostly found in the latinum group precious metals (gold, silver, platinum, etc.) existing in a very special state... Within their outer shells, the ORMEs have two electrons existing within the same orbital, in the same space-time locality, called a Cooper pair. The electrons' magnetic field, of equal and opposite value, are canceling each other out and giving these ORMEs the zero-point field, like the magnetic eutral, which generates their special properties of:

oom temperature superconductivity
henomenal healing properties
nparting extrasensory perception
ncreasing spiritual awareness

t was Hudson who coined the term ORMEs, but there is some question as to whether these lements are monoatomic or *diatomic*. If diatomic, which is most likely the case, the Cooper pairs re created by two atoms each sharing a valence electron, which then become equally shared in the ame outer orbital of each atom.

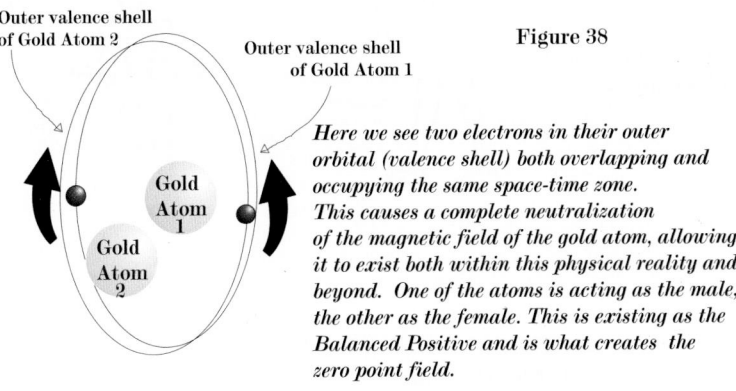

Outer valence shell
of Gold Atom 2

Outer valence shell
of Gold Atom 1

Figure 38

Gold
Atom
1

Gold
Atom
2

Here we see two electrons in their outer orbital (valence shell) both overlapping and occupying the same space-time zone. This causes a complete neutralization of the magnetic field of the gold atom, allowing it to exist both within this physical reality and beyond. One of the atoms is acting as the male, the other as the female. This is existing as the Balanced Positive and is what creates the zero point field.

"*It is two polarities which exactly overlap and overlay, And each charges the other. It is 'As Above So Below' as with the emblem of Hoova – the six-pointed star, do you understand?*"
Only Planet of Choice p. 61

What was the manna? It has been lost for a long time.
Many feel that these ORMEs are the lost link. They are also the link between Alchemy and the Philosopher's Stone. (Homeopathy has a great piece of the puzzle as well. This is dealt with in Book 2 *The Unwritten Way*)
And what is the Philosopher's Stone? It is in sympathetic resonance with the Tree of Life, Balanced Positive, for it imparts immortality upon he/she who consumes its fruit.

"*He afflicted you and let you hunger, then He fed you the manna that you did not know, nor did your forefathers know, in order to make you know that not by bread alone does man live, rather by everything that emanates from the mouth of God does man live: Your garment did not wear out upon you and your feet did not swell, these forty years.*" Deu 8:3-4

❶ "It is not good for the 'man' to be 'alone.' And so God cast a deep sleep on the 'man'...

❷ And took one of 'his' "sides"...

Figure 39: Creation of the Woman and the M

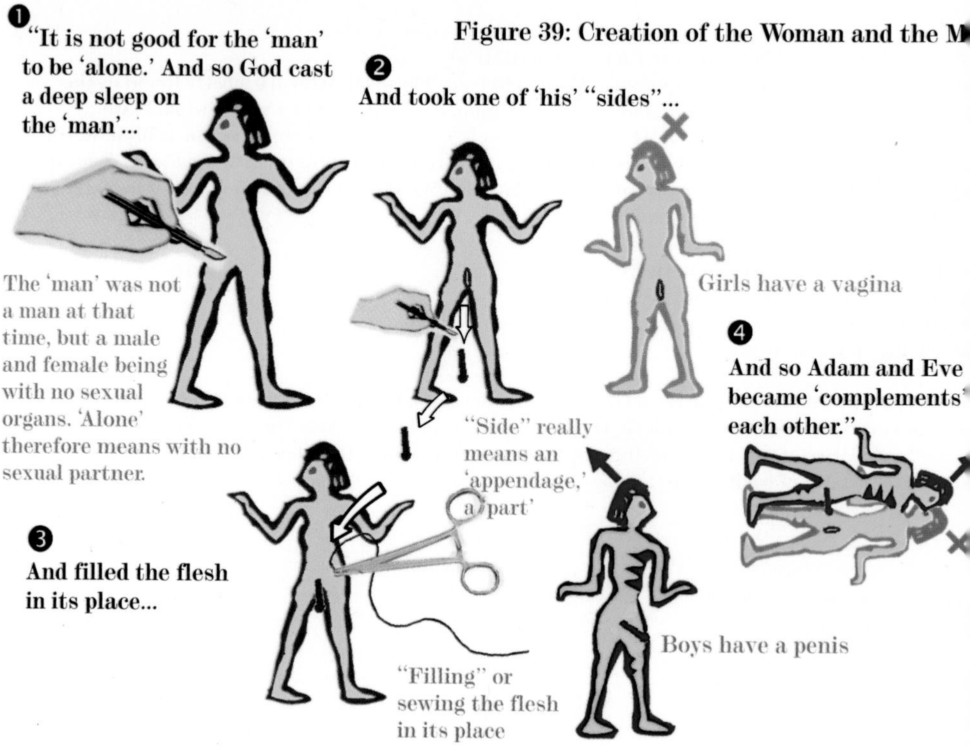

The 'man' was not a man at that time, but a male and female being with no sexual organs. 'Alone' therefore means with no sexual partner.

Girls have a vagina

❹ And so Adam and Eve became 'complements' each other."

"Side" really means an 'appendage,' a 'part'

❸ And filled the flesh in its place...

"Filling" or sewing the flesh in its place

Boys have a penis

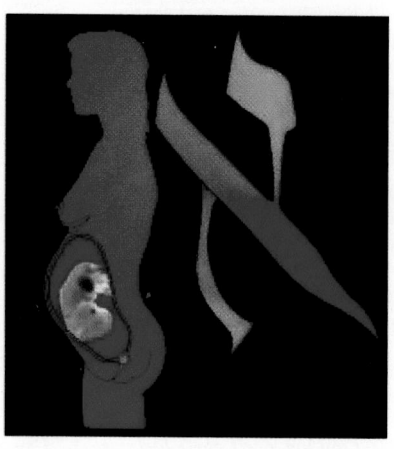

Figure 41: The Oneness of the Child within the Womb

Figure 42: Baby is Born into Individual

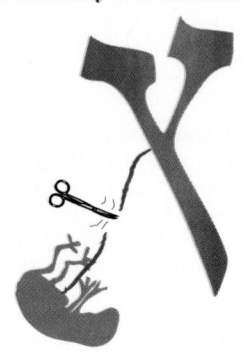

APPENDIX A:
COMMON MISCONCEPTIONS

These are beliefs I have heard spoken of in many different circles. Often enough, it became obvious how widespread they are. These misconceptions and the truths beyond them are closely related.

Misconception	*Truth*
Saying that we are okay with something and we are not judging it is like saying that we want it to happen. For example, saying it would be okay if my partner were to cheat on me is like saying that I want it to happen.	By not judging something and being okay with it if it did happen, we will not resist it. This will free us to not dwell on it constantly and modify our behaviour so much that eventually we manifest our fear. To have faith in this case is to see that allowing the possibility of the event to happen, and to be okay if it did, it won't have to happen.
God is made up of the balance between Good and Evil.	God is AllGood
Light, for instance, does not exist without the opposite of Light, which is darkness.	Light exists without darkness. It just is. Undefined.
Letting go of all fear, resistance and struggle would be boring.	It is the most exciting, fulfilling, wondrous way that we can be and there is so much to experience that we have never allowed ourselves the pleasure to experience in the state of having no resistance to Being.
Fear is important to make wise decisions. We need fear to help us survive. We should fear God.	A person who is not afraid of a lion is not oblivious of the lion's power. Fear only serves to freeze whatever faculty of quick thinking and quick action we have.

Misconception	*Truth*
A person who chooses from their Heart makes mistakes. A person who considers things carefully in a rational manner is better off.	The Heart is the guide back to your true nature. The rational mind will keep you in a limited space of belief systems and control-based reality.
We have to be perfect to create Eden.	All we have to do is follow our Hearts. The rest doesn't matter
Without the rules, structures and laws of our world, all Hell would break loose (*Lord of the Flies* mentality).	Once the rules, structures and laws are released, there might be a little chaos at the beginning. The true balance will follow, which results from our true nature (Love and goodness) emerging because of the freedom.
To be humble is to say that a human being does not have the capacity for direct connection with the Truth or with God. (Messed up humility).	We have all of the Universe and all ability in each of us. You are humble only when you see the greatness in all beings, including yourself, not denying who you are.
In order to exist within the world as it is, one must live with the rational and with control.	With faith, you can allow life to unfold and trust in Allthatis. That is enough.
There are too many people living in fear, hate, and judgment to allow for the coming of the Messianic Age.	The Messianic Age will start with a few people living in unconditional Love (Oneness—release of Frmee Will) and once a critical mass is achieved in those individuals, a "100th monkey effect" will reach all people on the planet. Then the Messianic Age will have arrived.
The Garden of Eden and the World to Come/Messianic Age are two different places.	The return to Eden and the World to Come/Messianic Age are the same. The return to Eden is to experience the Garden again, but this time with *the true experience of who we are.*

APPENDIX B:
THE THREE MAJOR DELUSIONS

The Three Major Delusions are so deeply embedded and affect our ability to experience Love and joy so much, that it is absolutely *essential* for us to release them. These programs are set to run until we give them up. They are all completely false ideas, based in illusion. They must be cleared in order for us to return to Eden.

Adam initiated the First Major Delusion. His biggest error was believing that he was better, or more important, than Eve. This extended to the belief that men are better than women. It also gave rise to the idea that anyone can be more important or more special than another. This First Major Delusion is the root of Hod2 (Haughtiness). This delusion falls within the third CaN of the *First Circle.*

One cannot Be better than another. We all dance to a unique rhythm. When we are all dancing to the rhythm of our Hearts, Being how we Love to be or Being how *we* choose to be at that moment, nobody but us can change.

In who we truly are, there is no way for one to be better than another. Yet people can behave and make choices that are not aligned with Love and goodness. This does not mean that they are lesser or inherently bad. It means that they are aligning themselves, by choice, to something that is not Love. Discernment is necessary in order not to fall into Unbalanced Positive, that is, thinking that everyone's *behaviour* is okay. That is not the case, yet. When the Messianic Age is fully upon us and we are all living within unconditional Love, it will be so.

The second of the Three Major Delusions was initiated by Moses and passed on from generation to generation. The belief that began after Moses was the belief that somebody can be better than somebody else because of what they know. This is not possible. The Second Major Delusion is in the second CaN of the *Third Circle.* This CaN helps you release the *need* to know more and therefore release the need to be better *in knowing*. This major delusion is the root of Bina2, the need to know, the Y factor.

A person can espouse both of the beliefs of the first two Major Delusions. They play off each other. If you believe that someone can be better, you will have the desire to be better. If you believe that what somebody knows can be better, you will have the desire to know more, the desire to prove yourself, to be number one, and to know it all. Release these ideas, and you will free yourself of this desire. You will be able to Be yourself.

"I release the idea and the belief that what someone knows can make them better than someone who doesn't share the same knowledge. This is not possible, so I do not even accept it as truth. Within this, I release the *need* to know more and therefore I release the need to be better in knowing."

The balance with this is that there *is* Truth and myriad ways of expressing and experiencing that Truth. There is simply no such thing as someone being better than another because of their knowledge.

The Third of the Three Major Delusions is in the third CaN of the **Fifth Circle**.

The third of the Three Major Delusions is the belief that somebody can be bad or wrong in how they are. When you pass judgment on someone, you are denying someone's right to exist. (This also applies for a thing.) This Major Delusion is the root of Gevourah2 (judgment). From this delusion, control arises. No one has the right to judge how another is or what they are choosing to be at any given time. We were all created in the image and likeness of the Creator, by the Creator, and given choice so that we could choose what we wish. You therefore cannot judge how someone is, what they have chosen to be, or what process they are going through.

The Third Major Delusion is often triggered by the other two; it is a combination of the first two, or a mutation of them. The idea that someone can be better than somebody else. Kane was jealous of Abel, thinking him better. He wished Abel not to be and killed him. Sarah also made an error of both the First and the Third Major Delusion. She was jealous of Hagar for bearing Abraham's firstborn and banished Hagar and Ishmael. (see the Fourth Letter at http://www.thelastfourbooks.com)

Banishment, murder, hiding, suppressing, excommunication, shunning are all judgmental and destructive acts of the Third Major Delusion.

Another way we can look at the Three Major Delusions is as *trying* to Be like GOD in:

1) Being Better (Hod2)

2) In Knowing better (Bina2)

3) In Knowing Good and Bad—passing judgment on others (Gevourah2). (see Figure 30)

It is not possible to try to be like God. This is why these are delusions. You are One with God. There is no need to try to Be. In fact, you cannot *try* to Be what you already *are*! If you try, you become double!

Thus the balance with all of these major delusions is also found in knowing that to accept who you really are is to adopt true humility. You are what you are. There is great humility in this, and greatness. So *do not cut yourself down to be humble.* This is messed up humility. You are what you Love to be. No less, no more.

Within this understanding, we see one of the most important incantations:

I choose to be because I Love to Be, so I allow myself to be, because I Am.

We are all unique in *who we are*. No one can Be better than another. There is no formula of good that we can emulate. There is no "established good" that we can Be. No established looks, or shape of body, no way of dressing or of smelling, no way of appearing that is aligned with True nature that needs to Be *that way*. There is no established "good" or "right."

But there is Good. There is something that we all strive to Be, to have, and to share with others! It is the Good that existed and always has existed before we created the Three Major Delusions.

The Good is in Being ourselves.

And who were we created by?

We were created by God (the Creator) to be how we were imagined to Be! One thing you can glean from this is that you were created by some pretty Good hands. You were created to Be something pretty nice. God has an image, an idea in mind, for who you really are, and the Creator created you that way because the Creator liked that a lot. (This is discussed in "The Imagination of God.")

Therefore, letting go to Be how you were created to Be is a release of control, not trying harder. Trying comes from doubt. Doubt is pure resistance to your I AM.

So choose to Be because you Love to Be, and allow yourself to Be because you Are.

APPENDIX C:
INTRODUCTION TO HOMEOPATHY

Homeopathy is based on the universal healing principle of "like cures like" (Latin: *Similia Similibus Curentur*). This means that if you take a substance in nature that causes a specific, unique diseased-state in a healthy individual, that very same substance will cure another person who is ill with that same diseased-state, regardless of whether or not he or she was previously influenced by that substance.

We know what unique diseased-state a certain substance will be able to cure by conducting a test of the substance on healthy individuals. This is called "a proving." A proving is the administering of a substance, prepared into the form of a remedy, to healthy volunteers (provers) until specific characteristics and symptoms are exhibited. In taking the substance repeatedly, the prover adopts the characteristics of the substance.

It should be noted that not all symptoms caused by the substance are disease symptoms. The symptoms are the way the substance affects the individual in their sleep habits, food desires, fears, anxieties, choice of clothing, perception of reality, health, interaction with their friends and loved ones, and many more ways.

When you read books about the different substances employed as homeopathic remedies (*Materia Medica*), you get a good understanding of what state the remedy will cause in a healthy individual and what sick states the remedies will cure when they closely match those same sick states.

For example if someone is affected by the venom of the Bushmaster snake (*Lachesis mutans*) he or she can exhibit a wide range of symptoms—heart palpitations, intense jealousy and possessiveness, paranoia, many fears and delusions, an aversion to having anything around the neck, purplish discolorations and much hemorrhaging. It is amazing that people can get into this same state without ever having been bitten by the snake. How is that possible? Perhaps their *snake-like* jealousy, possessiveness, and suspicion pushes them into the pathological state in which they will need the remedy prepared from *Lachesis mutans'* venom to cure them. Or perhaps their astrological vibration put them into sympathetic resonance with the snake so that when they get sick, they will adopt characteristics that those bitten or affected by the poison of the snake develop. Perhaps homeopathy reveals to us that every state of illness that a human being can get into has a substance in nature that is homeopathically curative for that specific state. This conjures up the mystery of the Universe that such correlations can even exist!

Therefore, we have a beautiful medicine that looks to the diseased-state of the person and matches it to a substance that causes the same diseased-state when it is administered to a healthy individual.

The greater the sensitivity in an individual, the more he or she is affected by a vibration acting upon them. Adam and Eve were in a state of perfect sensitivity. They were not prepared for the vibration that would begin to divide their consciousness so that it could know itself as separate. In fact, we can say that there was not even one tiny amount of resistance in them, for the state in which they existed was One with the Will of God. Thus, Adam and Eve were excellent provers, but they got stuck in proving by adopting the characteristics of the Tree of Knowledge that they passed on to all of us.

APPENDIX D:
THE CIRCLE OF NINE

The Circle of Nine is constantly growing. Please check in to www.thelastfourbooks.com for updates and additions.

All CaNs of the Nine Circles
CaNs: Choices that are no choice.

First Circle:

CaN #1—I slow down.

In everything I do, everything I say, everything I eat, I slow myself down. I bring myself down to earth by slowing down and enjoying the moment.

CaN #2—All races are equal.

We are all One. All people are equal. We are of One family. The people of the different nations are my brothers and sisters. The people of Africa, Asia, North America, Europe, Australia, South America, and the Middle East etc. are all my brothers and sisters. I have no racist thoughts.

CaN #3—Men and women are equal.

I align myself with the total and complete equality of the male and the female. I align myself with the wonder of the man and the woman. I do not attempt to keep the female down, nor do I suppress the male. I do not cut myself down to see the other is great. I see the wonder in the woman's nature that is in harmony with Mother Nature and the Divine. I do not put myself down when I see that the other is great. I simply see that no one can ever be better than anyone else in who they are. We are all great as we are.

In this CaN we see one of the Three Major Delusions. Adam's biggest error, the first of the Three Major Delusions, was believing that he was better, or more important, than Eve. This extended to the belief that men are better than women. It also gives rise to the idea that anyone can be more important or more special than another. This First Major Delusion is the root of Hod2 (haughtiness).

CaN #4—I am equal to all living beings.

I see myself as equal to people, animals, plants and minerals of the Earth.

CaN #5—I release the idea of hierarchies according to job status and social position.

People are people no matter what jobs they have or what they have chosen to do in life. How they are with other people, how they treat their co-workers, themselves, and their friends, their partners and children is most important, not what jobs or positions they find themselves in.

CaN #6—I take care of my body.

I keep my body in good shape with regular exercise and a healthy diet.

Second Circle:

CaN #1—I find beauty in who I am.

I do not look at myself in the mirror and compare myself to another or find myself ugly. I love myself and how I look in the mirror, because it is *me*.

If I am a man, I give up the need to be bigger than I am. If I am a woman, I give up the need to be thinner or bigger or however! I love myself as I am.

CaN #2—I love myself for who I am.

There is no mistake in being who I am. I am free to be who I am. I will stop putting myself down and cutting myself down all the time, as if I have made a mistake. I forgive and accept myself for all the errors

I feel I have made so that I can be free to know that I am good. And in this way, I stop worrying what I look like to others.

CaN #3—I allow myself to enjoy sex, fully and completely.

I allow my sexual energy to flow. I release any judgment of the expression of my sexual nature.

He says: "I do it for her pleasure. This is how I find the pleasure and joy."

She says: "I allow myself to receive the pleasure of the act. I give up the guilt of receiving." (This is balanced with CaN #4.)

CaN #4—It is not all about sex.

I can love others deeply and intimately without that needing to be about sex. I simply release the part of me that constantly needs sex. I understand this desire can come from the judgment of the act as being something bad/wrong. I release the judgment, let go of the guilt, and find the balance.

CaN #5—I give up looking at people as sex objects.

I see people as people. I do not avoid looking at anyone. I am able to look right at all people and simply see the beauty inherent in each person, because I have given up seeing people as sex objects.

Third Circle

CaN #1—I give up the need to prove myself better.

I give up the need to prove myself worthy. I trust myself and I only need myself to know that I am good. I give up needing the approval of others. I never put anyone else down, for why would I? I do not spend any of my energy trying to be better than another. If I am playing a game with someone, I can try to win the game, because that's fun, but I do not try to prove that I am number one. I play as I am, because I love it.

CaN #2—Everyone is everyone else's teacher.

What I know does not make me better.

I give up the hollow notion that what another believes can make them lesser or lower than me because of what I know or do. Usually this comes from judging knowledge more important than Being. So I release the idea that what someone knows can ever be more important or more special than how they are. I never "teach down" to someone, because *everyone is everyone else's teacher.*

In this CaN, we encounter the second of the Three Major Delusions, which has been passed on from generation to generation and was initiated by Moses. This is the belief that somebody who knows more is better than somebody else. This gives rise to the idea "teaching down" or "teaching someone a lesson." This is not possible. It is not part of my reality. I release the *need* to know more and therefore I release the need to be better in knowing. This major delusion is the root of Bina2, the need to know, the Y factor.

CaN #3—I Release the Unbalanced Positive.

I understand what the Unbalanced Positive is. (If not, read the glossary.) There are tasks to be done, situations that are unacceptable, negativities to be faced and cleared. I stop thinking it is good to shrink so that other people won't feel insecure around me. I release being a "goody-two-shoes" and being overly polite to try to make everything perfect. I take responsibility for facing what still must be healed.

CaN #4—No religion knows better.

There is no such thing as having knowledge that makes you more special or better. Thus, the people of all religions are my brothers and sisters. We are all One. Even if we express ourselves differently, even if we dress, act, speak or pray differently, I can appreciate all expressions of all faiths of the planet. I see beyond the religion to the person who stands before me. I give up the possibility of even considering my religion something superior than anyone else's. We are all of one family.

CaN #5—I do not need to know or to be right all the time.

I can make mistakes whenever I wish. I let go of the need to be perfect. I let go of making hierarchies according to what a person knows. I do not define my worth by what I know. I take the chance of being wrong. My guidance may tell me to do things that don't make sense, that are illogical and sometimes may seem downright wrong. It could be that I am simply facing up to something to let it go. Like the test of the sacrifice of Abraham's Son Isaac. I value my guidance (חכמה) as something more aligned with my true nature than my rational under-standing (בינה).

CaN #6—I choose a way, because I Love it to be that way.

I choose a way because I wish it to be that way, *not* because it is the Truth, but because I wish (want it with my heart) that it were the Truth. I want that way, that thing, that choice, to be the Truth and that is why I align myself with it. I follow my Heart to know what is true. And don't forget the little secret: what I truly wish with my Heart is true. Therefore:

I choose to be because I Love to Be so I allow myself to Be because I AM.

Fourth Circle:

CaN #1—I do unto others what I would Love others to do unto me.

I do not only live by the commandment as it is written, "Do not do unto others what you would not have them do unto you," although I inherently live by this as well. I live by loving, kindness, giving, and car-ing, all the things I Love for others and for myself. That makes all the dif-ference. What I do, I do for the Love of what will come for others, not just Frmee. I really listen to others when they speak. My heart reaches out for their well-being. I release myself from my own selfish world. Balance this with knowing that it is good to receive for yourself as well, if that serves you in becoming who you are as a whole light being.

CaN #2—I wish the best for all people.

I see all people manifesting their deepest, greatest wishes, their most powerful Love and Beingness. This is all I see. It is my only reality. I see myself as a part of the collective consciousness of others who feel this way. I let go of not seeing the best for others, or of being in competi-tion with them. I balance this with knowing that it doesn't mean I must give myself to everyone and do anything for anyone, anytime. I simply wish the best for others.

I wish the best for my ex's—that they find a wonderful, fulfilling love with another, in all the ways I would wish for myself. I wish the best for my friends—that they succeed in the very same way I wish and know I will succeed, etc. So this CaN also reads, "Wish for others what you wish for yourself," and is therefore, related to CaN #1.

CaN #3—I show the Love and express the awe I feel for others.

I release the fear of expressing and demonstrating my love in acts and words. I allow the Love I feel for others to show through my eyes, so that they may see the awe I have for them. I see the good in people, their talents, their specialness, their qualities, and let them know what I see. I release the fear of being an openly loving person.

CaN #4—I Do what I Am.

I Am what I love to be and so I do what I Am. I Am doing what I love to do. I Am doing the work in my life that I love to do. It is the work of my Heart. I see the freedom that I can Be as I love to Be and do as I love to do.

CaN #5—I let go of the belief that I must suffer.

I let go of the belief that life is painful and hard. I allow the joy and beauty of life to sweep over me every moment.

CaN #6—I allow myself to connect with others.

I see how the world is filled with others like me who are making the world a better place. I remove myself from my shell, trying to do everything on my own. I work with the team of the Universe.

CaN #7—The Highest Commitment.

I Serve the Good of All people.

I DEDICATE my Whole Heart, my Whole Soul and All my Power and Abilities to create complete peace, abundance, healing, and love for ALL people on the planet. This is balanced with taking care of myself and also wishing the best for myself.

Fifth Circle

CaN #1—I express how I feel to others.

I let go of the fear that what I have to say is worthless. I let go of the fear that I am coming from the wrong place. I know what I have to say is worthy. I know where I am coming from now, totally and completely and I am no longer afraid of saying the wrong thing. I can only say how I feel. (And since I have integrated the third circle into my being, no one will feel as if they must believe my Truth.) I can always speak up for that if someone challenges me, but I never attack for the sake of my Truth. Nor do I control for the sake of my Truth. On one side of the coin, in the third Circle, my Truth is what I would love to be my Truth. On the other, I know it is my Truth, so if I am attacked, challenged, or controlled, I can speak up for myself.

CaN #2—I am Free to do as I wish.

Balanced with—I am always responsible for my actions

I have the One will within me. I can DO whatever I wish, as I know I am a being of Good and Love. I therefore dedicate myself to doing what I Love at all times, with no exceptions. I do not ever let anyone else decide for me how it is best for me to be, nor do I make excuses about why I am unable to do as I wish. The choice is mine. I free my will to do as I love to do. And in this, I am ALWAYS responsible for my actions. I do not blame my actions on anyone else, including God.

I know that the world wants to see the great part of me. People really do want to see me shine. People do want to see how good I can be, and how talented I can be. Being myself, I can bring so much good to whatever I do and whoever I am with. There is no shame in this. So I allow myself to be and to do. There is no reason not to.

CaN #3—I do not deny anyone's right to Be.

I do not judge how someone is, for that would be saying that how they are is Bad. This negates them and denies their right to exist. My Will is not greater than any other's will on Earth. I have the same Will, because we were all granted the gift of choice and we were all created by God. I always respect another's choice, for it is their choice. I give up the need to make choices for others. I give up the need to have power over or control over any other. I let people be free to choose for themselves. I let people be free to be as they are.

In this CaN, we see the third of the Three Major Delusions: that somebody can be bad or wrong in how they are. When you pass this judgment on someone, you are denying their right to exist. (This also applies to something.) This Major Delusion is the root of Gevourah2 (judgment). No one has the right or the ability to judge how another is. We were all created in the image and likeness of the Creator, by the Creator. You therefore cannot judge how someone is, what they have chosen to Be, or what process of their life they are going through.

The balance is that I may always say how I feel and that doesn't mean conflicts never arise. I do what I love to do, and I let people do what they love to do. I simply do not impose my will over another if we differ, but I always allow myself to create what I love and to speak up for what I wish to be true.

CaN #4—I give up all control.

I do not do a thing (in a trying sense).

I let go of control within my Being. I stop challenging myself and get out of my own way. Things are happening as I have wished them. I allow the Divine to enter me. This is balanced with knowing that it is me who carries out the tasks I wish to do.

CaN #5—I let myself feel totally and completely.

I release the resistance of the feelings of my emotions and the feelings within my physical body. I allow this to occur in harmony with CaN #4.

Sixth Circle

CaN #1—I trust the process. There is nothing to worry about.

I let go of all worry about the future and I trust in the process of life, of Love, of AllthatIs. I trust in the unfoldment of the day, month, year, moment. I have faith that what I love to Be, shall Be, as I take responsibility and allow myself to create it.

CaN #2—I let go of the past, totally and completely.

I remain present in the moment. I let go of worrying about the pain and fears of the past recurring in the future. I have faith that it is AllGood, and so I don't have to constantly watch out for what comes next.

Because I have incorporated the Fifth Circle into my Being, I am not resisting the past. I simply allow my awareness to let go and fully align with the present.

CaN #3—Everywhere I am is in the presence of the Divine.

I take time to see that everywhere I go is sacred ground. Everywhere I am is in the presence of the Divine. Everyone I meet is giving me an audience with the Divine.

I take care of my Soul/Spirit.

I take time to meditate daily and to spend enough time alone to feel, work through, and clear whatever has arisen during the day.

CaN #4—I have no desire for anything outside of Love.

I give up and transform bottomless pit desire. I release the desire for other women, or the desire for other men, outside of the relationship I am in. I let go of the desire for anyone other than the one I have chosen for a relationship of Love. I do this neither because it is wrong to want another, nor because I must. I do not only do it because it is written "Thou shalt not covet thy neighbor's wife." I give up the desire for others because it is an illusion to desire a person I do not know and Love on a deep level. It is not something real, therefore, I see that I really do not want to desire others. I reconnect my essence with the Source and I yield totally and completely to loving the person I am with.

CaN #5—There is nothing to fear.

Life is AllGood. I can see that. I am aligned with this. I put my heart into seeing this, and I see that all fear is an illusion. I feel this as it is in the undefined future. *I can't imagine anything that I could be afraid of.* There is no doubt about it.

Seventh Circle

CaN #1—I don't know a thing. I allow myself to receive what I know.

I give up the Y factor, totally and completely. I don't need to possess what I know. I act and come from a place within of guidance and intuition, that is married with the present moment. I don't need to hold onto things so I won't forget them nor fear that I'll look like I'm a silly rabbit, or a floundering fool. Even more deeply, this means that I release all doubt about who I AM and about the nature of Allthatis. I do not need to know who I am.

I AM that I AM. I AM how I love to be. What I love to be, I AM.

This is deeper than the Third Circle. This release of the need to know releases *all* need to know. It means releasing all doubt.

Acting based on what you feel is giving up the need to choose based in what you think is right.

CaN #2—I am humble before God and I am free to Be as I AM.

All that I AM, all that I Love to Be, comes to Be through my Will as an extension of God's Will. I am nothing without God's Love. And I can choose as freely as I wish, for I am an extension of God.

This CaN really deals with the fact that I AM, therefore there is no need to try to be like God. I give up trying to be like God inanotsoniceway, of needing to be the only one, of trying to be Allthatis. I see that I am a part of God and there is no effort in that. I AM a many and a One. I AM the God of my Life. Knowing this, I find my humility, and need not try to be, nor deny, who I really Am.

Combined with CaN #1, this is the release from the Tree of Knowledge for Good and Bad.

CaN #3—I release the need to dwell on the idea of evil.

I do recognize energies exist that are not aligned with Love. I am not in Unbalanced Positive with this. However, I release the need to focus on the evil, for in doing so, I am seeing my power to not allow evil things to happen. I also see that I have choice, fully and completely, so I release the disempowering idea that I am being controlled or influenced by outside, negative forces. I also am aligned with the very deep truth that it is AllGood, and in simply loving, I am healing all that is negative. So why would I need to focus on evil?

CaN #4—I have FAITH in AllthatIs.

I have faith in the people I know and meet. I have faith in the Goodness of the Universe and all that is before me and all that can Be. I have faith that it is Good and will be Good. I give up all control and just allow the faith of who I Am and of Allthatis to embrace me.

Eighth Circle:

1) **There is nothing to worry about.** It is all unfolding as I love.

2) **There is nothing to hurry about.** There is time enough for everything. Balanced with: *You can do things as quickly and efficiently as you are able.*

3) **There is nothing to doubt.** I know what it feels like to doubt. As soon as I feel myself doubting, I clear it. I know what is in my Heart, so what is there to doubt?

4) **There is nothing to resist.** I allow myself to feel. As soon as I start to resist, I can resist a little more and then let go. Balanced with: *I overcome what does not serve the Love.*

5) **There is nothing I must try hard for.** I know what it feels like when I try too hard. As soon as I feel I am trying too hard, I can switch into allowishing. Balanced with: *I am dedicated to making things happen.*

6) **I give up all control.** I give up all control over others and myself. Balanced with: *I am in charge of my life.*

376

APPENDIX E:
BIBLIOGRAPHY

Abd-ru-shin, *Buddha—Life and Work of the Forerunner in India,* Grail Foundation Press, Gambier, Ohio, 1995

Bach, Richard. *Illusions: The Adventures of a Reluctant Messiah,* Dell Publishing, 1977.

Bailley, Phillip, M.D. *Homeopathic Psychology,* North Atlantic Books, 1995.

Besant, Annie., C. W. Leadbeater. *Occult Chemisty,* Health Research, 1907.

Bhagavad Gita, A New Translation, translated by Stephen Mitchell, Harmony Books, 2000.

Braden, Gregg. *Awakening to Zero Point, The Video,* Radio Bookstore Press, 1996.

Brennan, Barbara Ann. *Hands of Light: A Guide to Healing Through the Human Energy Field,* Bantam New Age Books, 1988.

Brennan, Barbara Ann. *Light Emerging: A Journey of Personal Healing,* Bantam New Age Books, 1993.

Castaneda, Carlos. *The Active Side of Infinity,* Harper Collins, 1998.

Castaneda, Carlos. *The Teachings of Don Juan: A Yaqui Way of Knowledge,* Washington Square Press, 1996.

Chopra, Dr. Deepak, M.D. *Seattle Center Talk,* May 18, 1991.

Dalai Lama, The. *The Dalai Lama's Book of Daily Meditations,* edited by Renuka Singh, Random House, Australia, 1998.

Danciger, Elizabeth. *Homeopathy: From Alchemy to Medicine,* Healing Arts Press, 1995.

Donne, John. *Poems of John Donne. vol I,* E. K. Chambers, ed. 51-52. London, Lawrence & Bullen, 1896.

Dossey, Larry, M.D. *Healing Words: The Power of Prayer and The Practice of Medicine*, Harper Collins, 1993.

Einstein, Albert: "What Life Means to Einstein: An Interview by George Sylvester Viereck," *The Saturday Evening Post*, October 26, 1929.

Gerber, Richard, M.D. *Vibrational Medicine: New Choices for Healing Ourselves*, Bear and Co., 1988.

Goleman, Daniel. *Emotional Intelligence: Why it can matter more than IQ*, Bantam Books, 1995.

Hamilton, Edward, M.D. *The Flora Homeopathica*, Edward, London, U.K., 1852. Reprinted by B. Jain Publishers, New Delhi, India, 1992.

Hurtak, J.J., with Desiree. *The Five Bodies*, Academy for Future Science, 1996.

Hurtak, J.J. *The Book of Knowledge: The Keys of Enoch*, The Academy for Future Science, 1987.

Jung, Carl G. *Memories, Dreams, Reflections*, edited by Aniela Jaffé, translated by Richard and Clara Winston, Vintage, New York, 1965.

Kazantzakis, Nikos. *The Saviors of God*, translated by Kimon Friar, Simon and Schuster, New York, 1960.

Keats, John. *Poetical Works of John Keats*, "Ode on Melancholy," London, Macmillan, 1884.

Kent, James Tyler. *Lectures on Homoeopathic Materia Medica*, Jain Publishing Company, New Delhi, 1980.

Lanctot, Guylaine, M.D. *The Medical Mafia: How to get out of it alive and take back our health and wealth*, Here's The Key, 1995.

Louise L. Hay and Friends. *Gratitude: A Way of Life*, Hay House, Inc., 1996.

Millman, Dan. *Way of the Peaceful Warrior: A Book that Changes Lives*, H.J. Kramer, Inc., 1984.

New World Translation of the Holy Scriptures, Watchtower Bible and Tract Society of New York, Inc. 1984.

Oates, David. *Reverse Speech Technology,* http://www.reversespeech.com/

Pierrakos, Eva and Judith Saly. *Creating Union: The Pathwork of Relationships,* Pathwork Press, 1993.

Reich, Wilhelm, M.D. *The Sexual Rights of Youth,* Wilhelm Reich Infant Trust Fund, 1983. Translated from German, Der Sexuelle Kampf der Jugend, 1932.*Rig Veda,* Tree of Life Publishing, 2001.

Schatz, Rabbi Moshe. *Sparks of the Hidden Light: Seeing the Unified Nature of Reality Through Kabbalah,* The Ateret Tiferet Institute, 1996.

Schiffe, Michel. *The Memory of Water: Homeopathy and the Battle of Ideas in the New Science,* Harper Collins, 1995.

Schlemmer, Phyllis V., transceiver. *The Only Planet of Choice: Essential Briefings from Deep Space,* 2nd Edition, Gateway Books, 1996.

Schucman, Helen. *A Course in Miracles,* Foundation for Inner Peace, 1996.

The Chumash: The Torah, Haftaros and Five Megillos With a Commentary Anthologized From the Rabbinic Writings, Stone Edition, by Rabbi Nosson Scherman, Mesorah Publications Inc., 1994.

The Essene Gospel of Peace, Translated by Edmond Bordeaux Szekely, International Biogenic Society, 1981.

Tsunetomo, Yamamoto. HAGAKURE: The Book of the Samurai, W.S.Wilson, translator. Kodansha Int'l Ltd., 1979

Tzu, Lao. *Tao Te Ching, The Witter Bynner Version,* Witter Bynner, 1944.

Tzu, Lao. *Tao Te Ching,* translation by Stephen Mitchell, Harper Perennial, 1988.

Walsch, Neale Donald. *Conversations with God: an uncommon dialogue, Book1,* Hampton Roads Publishing Company, 1996.

Walsch, Neale Donald. *Conversations with God: an uncommon dialogue, Book3,* Hampton Roads Publishing Company, 1997.

Williamson, Marianne. *A Return to Love: Reflections on the Principles in A course in Miracles,* HarperCollins, 1993.

Zaren, Ananda. *Core Elements of the Materia Medica of the Mind Volumes I and II,* Ulrich Burgdorf Homoeopathic Publishing House, Germany, 1994.